YOUR
SYMPTOMS
DIAGNOSED

YOUR SYMPTOMS DIAGNOSED

- *All symptoms listed alphabetically* -
- *Four-part arrangement for quick reference* -
- *Easy identification of likely conditions* -
- *Illustrations to aid location of symptoms* -
- *Suggested action and medical treatment* -

Dr Barrington Cooper and Dr Laurence Gerlis

HAMLYN

Editor: Neil Curtis
Designed and produced by Curtis Garratt Limited
The Old Vicarage, Horton cum Studley, Oxford OX9 1BT

First published in Great Britain in 1993
by Hamlyn, an imprint of Reed Consumer Books Limited
Michelin House, 81 Fulham Road, London SW3 6RB
and Auckland, Melbourne, Singapore and Toronto

A catalogue record for this book is available from the British Library

ISBN 0 600 57846 1 (paperback)
      0 600 58051 2 (hardback)

Printed in Great Britain

IMPORTANT ADVICE

As the introduction explains, *Your Symptoms Diagnosed* is
designed to help you quickly to reach informed conclusions
about any condition from which you may be suffering, the
causes leading up to it, whether or not medical help should
be sought and how quickly, what kind of self-medication can
be administered and for how long without seeking further
help. *Your Symptoms Diagnosed* is **not intended** to be a
substitute for the advice of a qualified medical practitioner,
and you should **always** consult a physician if any symptoms
from which you are suffering persist or worsen.

Every effort has been made to ensure that the information
contained in the book is as accurate, informed, and up-to-
date as possible at the time of going to press but medical and
pharmaceutical knowledge continues to progress, and every
patient has separate and unique needs which may ultimately
be resolved **only** by direct consultation with a physician.

The authors, editors, and publishers of this book cannot be
held liable for any errors or omissions, nor for any conse-
quences of using it.

Contents

The book and how to use it

Your Symptoms Diagnosed offers a completely new approach to self-diagnosis and assumes no prior medical or scientific knowledge. It enables the user quickly to reach informed conclusions about the condition from which he or she may be suffering, the causes leading up to it, whether or not medical help should be sought and how quickly, what kind of self-medication can be administered and for how long without seeking further help, the tests that might be carried out by a doctor or in hospital, the prescription medications that might be given, and any advice necessary to aid recovery after illness.

For ease of reference, *Your Symptoms Diagnosed* is divided into four parts. Part 1 is a straightforward list, in alphabetical order, of the symptoms from which someone is likely to suffer. Under each entry there is a further list, also in alphabetical order, of the conditions or illnesses of which the entry may be one symptom among several. These conditions are described by systems in Part 2 of the book and include: a brief description of the condition and the factors that are likely to have contributed to it; a more detailed description of the symptom; associated symptoms which may lead to a confirmation of the conditions; any tests that may be necessary, and any further action that should be taken before, during, and after the occurrence of the condition. Each entry is also given a symbol to provide an instant visual indication of its severity. Part 3 is a glossary of those medical and scientific terms which cannot be avoided in Part 2. Part 4 is an alphabetical listing of the conditions included in Part 2 and a comprehensive index to Part 2 of the book so that it is accessible in a number of ways.

Introduction

Your Symptoms Diagnosed completes a triad of health books with which we have sought to help to enable the individual to achieve increasing understanding, participation, and thus a sharing of control in medical situations. It is written for the general public, by which we mean the intelligent non-doctor who seeks to be appropriately informed about his or her health and that of the family directly and in relation to the changes that are taking place in our society. This book is designed to give the maximum amount of information for those who need it and seek it. Our experience is that people often want more information than was previously thought, and this book provides that information in a calm and unemotional way. Having said that, it must be realized that every cough is not lung cancer but it is up to the reader of this book to use the information provided in any way he or she wishes. We intend that *Your Symptoms Diagnosed* should answer the kinds of questions that our patients have asked us in the past. Very often, patients are aware of the worst possible outcome of any symptom and, if given the information, they can then put it into perspective. This seems to make more sense than hiding the basic truth.

Following directly upon its predecessors – *The Consumer's Guide to Prescription Medicines* and *The Consumer's Guide to Over the Counter Medicines* – this book expands the range of information available to you the reader. The three books together should be seen as a means of enablement to the individual in the unfamiliar world of health care; they should also enable patients to have well-informed discussions with friends, relatives, and advisers.

These books are not intended to be used as a 'home doctor' in the traditional sense nor to replace the advice of a physician but, on the contrary, to inform you more fully of the nature of your condition and the need for discriminating professional medical advice, and thus augment the shared value of such advice.

We have tried to cover a wide range of symptoms and relate those symptoms to possible causes. It is not absolutely comprehensive.

The wonders of the human body mean that almost any symptom can relate to almost any disease, and we apologize to those of you who cannot find your particular symptom and cannot relate it to the particular illness you have or think you have. All we can do is to outline where we believe the particular symptoms might lead and, of course, this is only a rough guide and is only our opinion. Opinions in medicine are as diverse as are opinions in art. *Your Symptoms Diagnosed* therefore represents a distilled version of some of our opinions. It does not guarantee total accuracy and reliability all the time. Of course, we cannot accept any responsibility for any consequence that may arise as a result of using this book. Every effort has been made to ensure accuracy but there may well be some errors and omissions. Nevertheless, we trust that this book will be a useful guide.

It is probably better to read this book when there is not a crisis at home or in the family. In other words, here is useful background reading to improve your knowledge about symptoms in general. Using anything in a crisis makes it much more liable to misinterpretation and misunderstanding. Perhaps this book, therefore, should be bedtime reading rather than part of a first-aid kit. Within the treatment of disorders listed, we outline investigations which may be carried out for the diagnosis of a condition. This is by no means an exhaustive list nor is it essential. It is not the idea that all the tests listed here must be carried out; these are merely a guide. Similarly, medications are listed which may be used to treat your condition. These are provided so that you might understand what is being done rather than to give you a list of things that must be done. Some detail is given on medications, whether prescription or over the counter, but readers are directed to our other books *A Consumer's Guide to Prescription Medicines* and *A Consumer's Guide to Over the Counter Medicines* which form part of this trilogy. Self-medication is no longer regarded as bad medicine. On the contrary, many patients are encouraged to self-diagnose and to self-medicate using over-the-counter medicines, some of which are very potent and available for treating a wide range of conditions. Of equal importance are the entries regarding further advice, because lifestyle changes are invaluable in the prevention and treatment of most conditions.

There are some situations we have deliberately left out of this book. The handbook is intended for adults, and we do not recommend its use for paediatric conditions, although it may apply in many cases. We have also left out congenital disorders. Many of the symptoms here may present as side-effects to medications and, where this is thought to be a possibility, we would advise you to consult the *Consumer's Guide to Prescription Medicines*, but we have not systematically included side-effects as causes of disease. It is intended that this book should concentrate on disease processes themselves rather than extraneous factors affecting the body and the disease process. We had always intended to write this trilogy. During the development phase we both had an opportunity to use the type of thinking that has gone into writing the entries for *Your Symptoms Diagnosed*. We can reassure the reader of *Your Symptoms Diagnosed* that our first-hand experience has indicated to us that this type of thinking is immensely valuable. Illness of all types creates a degree of sensitivity, indeed paranoia, where the overwhelming need is for more information more frequently.

Rapidly changing times have increased radically the range of health remedies available directly over the counter and from the alternative non-medical health care providers, and we believe this trend will continue. These books provide you with the information that you need to have available to you to help you find your way in this increasingly individually responsible health world.

We each practice medicine in our different but related roles in direct relationship with patients, and we are increasingly convinced that the intelligently informed individual is a more discriminating and co-operative patient and a more active partner in the health care process.

It is to this partnership that we dedicate this book.

Dr Barrington Cooper
Dr Laurence Gerlis
21 Devonshire Place
London W1
1993

The skeleton

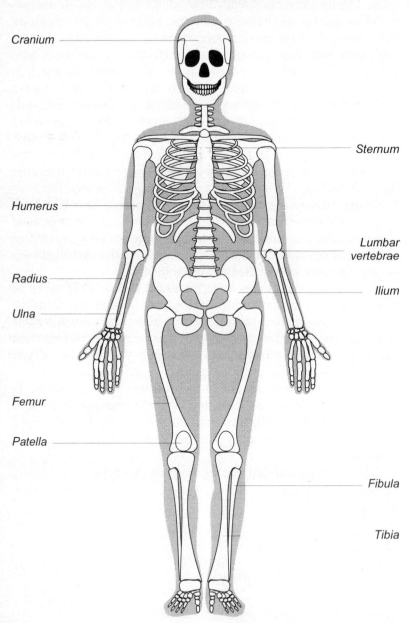

Cranium

Sternum

Humerus

Lumbar
vertebrae

Radius

Ilium

Ulna

Femur

Patella

Fibula

Tibia

The Organs

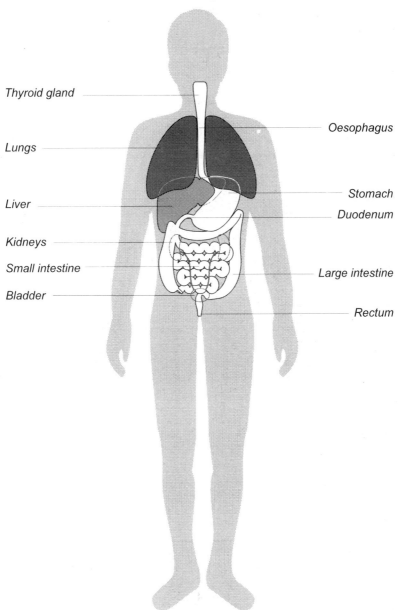

Thyroid gland

Oesophagus

Lungs

Liver

Stomach

Duodenum

Kidneys

Small intestine

Large intestine

Bladder

Rectum

The circulatory system

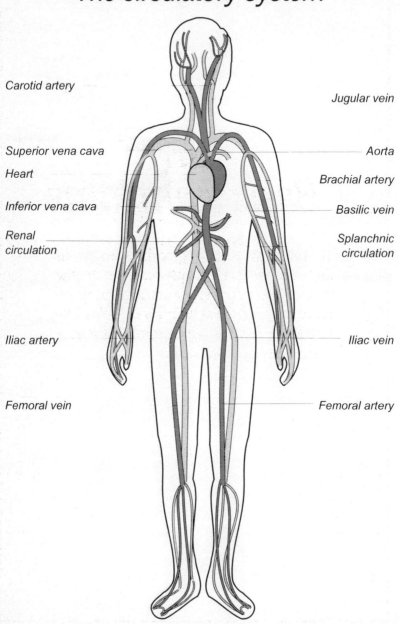

Carotid artery

Jugular vein

Superior vena cava

Aorta

Heart

Brachial artery

Inferior vena cava

Basilic vein

Renal circulation

Splanchnic circulation

Iliac artery

Iliac vein

Femoral vein

Femoral artery

Part I
Basic symptoms

To find any of the specific conditions included in this list, please refer to the index. Alternatively, you may simply refer to the chapter(s) mentioned – *See* The Digestive System, for example – for general reading on the topic.

Abdomen, pain in

Aortic aneurysm
Appendicitis
Bowel infections
Cystitis
Diseases of the ovary
Disorders of the pancreas
Duodenal ulcer
Endometriosis
Fibroids
Gall bladder disease or Cholecystitis
Gastric ulcer
Gastritis
Gastroenteritis
Hepatitis
Hiatus hernia
Inflammatory bowel disorders
Gall bladder disorder
Intestinal obstruction
Irritable bowel syndrome
Kidney stones and Kidney infections
Crohn's disease
Liver disorders
Malaria
Pancreas disorders
Pancreatitis
Pelvic infections
Peptic ulcer
Peritonitis
Pregnancy and its complications
Ulcerative colitis

See The Digestive System
Generalized Infections
Kidneys and Excretion
Reproductive System including Breasts.

Abdomen, rigidity of

Intestinal obstruction
Peptic ulcer
Peritonitis

See The Digestive System.

Abdomen, swelling

Ascites
Diseases of the ovary
Heart failure
Intestinal obstruction
Kidney disorders
Kidney failure
Liver disease
Obesity
Ovarian cysts
Pancreatitis
Peritonitis
Pregnancy and its complications

See The Digestive System
Heart and Circulation
Kidneys and Excretion
Reproductive System including Breasts.

Aches or Pains

Ankylosing spondylitis
Arthritis
Gout
DVT
Lumbago
M.E.
Sciatica

Slipped disc
Spondylitis
Tennis elbow

See Bones, Joints, and Muscles
Heart and Circulation

Allergy

Anaphylactic shock
Penicillin and drug allergy
Rhinitis
Urticaria
Wasp and bee stings

See Ear, Nose, and Throat Disorders
General Conditions
Lung Diseases
Skin Diseases

Amnesia

Addiction to alcohol
Alzheimer's disease
Anxiety
Brain tumour
CVA (Stroke)
Dementia
Depression
Drug and tranquillizer abuse
Pre-senile dementia
Senile dementia
Trauma/Head injury

See Addictions
Heart and Circulation
Nervous System

Psychological Disorders

Anxiety

Addiction to alcohol
Agitated depression
Anxiety states
Overactive thyroid
Phobias and obsessive compulsive disorders
Tranquillizer abuse

See Addictions
Endocrine Disorders
Psychological Disorders

Appetite, loss of

Anorexia nervosa
Depression
Duodenal ulcer
Heart failure
Hiatus hernia
Pancreatic cancer
Pancreatitis
Stomach cancer
Stomach ulcer (Gastric ulcer)

See The Digestive System
Heart and Circulation
Psychological Disorders

Balance, loss of

Acoustic neuroma
Labyrinthitis
Middle-ear infection (Otitis media)
Ménière's disease
Vestibulitis

See Ear, Nose, and Throat Disorders

Bleeding

Haemophilia
Leukaemia
Menorrhagia
See Blood Disorders
Reproductive System including Breasts

Bleeding from the back passage (Rectal bleeding)

Anal tear
Bowel cancer
Crohn's disease
Diverticulitis
Gastric or duodenal ulcer
Haemorrhoids
Inflamatory bowel disorders
Stomach cancer
Ulcerative colitis
See The Digestive System

Bleeding from the ear

Middle-ear infection (Otitis media)
Outer-ear infection (Otitis externa)
Trauma/Head injury
Wax

See Ear, Nose, and Throat Disorders
Nervous System

Bleeding from the mouth

Aphthous ulcers

Gingivitis
Gum disease
Salivary gland tumours

See Disorders of the Mouth

Bleeding from the nose

Addiction to illegal drugs (cocaine)
Epistaxis
Hypertension (High blood-pressure)
Rhinitis
Sinusitis
Trauma/Head injury

See Addictions
Ear, Nose, and Throat Disorders
Heart and Circulation
Nervous System

Bleeding in the sputum (Coughing up blood)

Bronchiectasis
Bronchitis
Lung cancer
Pleurisy
Pneumonia
Pulmonary embolus
Sinusitis
Tracheitis
Tuberculosis

See Lung Diseases

Bleeding in the urine

Bladder cancer

Cystitis
Endocarditis
Functional disorders of the bladder
Infections of the renal tract
Kidney cancer
Kidney failure
Kidney stones
Trauma

See Heart and Circulation
Kidneys and Excretion

Bleeding from the vagina

Antepartum haemorrhage
Cervical cancer
Diseases of the ovary
Diseases of the uterus and cervix
Ectopic pregnancy
Inter-menstrual bleeding
Menorrhagia
Menstruation
Pregnancy and its complications
Threatened miscarriage
Uterine prolapse
Vaginal diseases and infections
Vaginitis

See Reproductive System including Breasts

Blood in the semen

Diseases of the testes

See Reproductive System including Breasts

Blood, vomiting up (Haematemasis)

Hiatus hernia
Liver disorders
Oesophageal varices (Liver failure)
Oesophagitis
Peptic ulcer
Stomach cancer
Torn oesophagus

See The Digestive System

Bones, pain in

Serious bone disease including cancer and infection

See Bones, Joints, and Muscles

Bowel habits, persistent alteration in

Bowel cancer
Diverticulitis
Ulcerative colitis

See The Digestive System

Bowels, pain on opening

Anal tear
Anal fissure
Fistulae
Haemorrhoids

See The Digestive System

Breasts, pain or lumps in

Breast cancer

Breast cyst
Fibroids
Mastitis
Pregnancy
Premenstrual tension

See Reproductive System including Breasts

Breastbone, pressure on

Angina pectoris
See Heart and Circulation

Breathing, difficulty in

Anaphylactic shock
Anxiety
Asthma
Bronchitis, chronic
Deviated nasal septum
Emphysema
Heart attack
Kidney failure
Pleurisy
Pneumonia
Pneumothorax
Pulmonary embolism

See Ear, Nose, and Throat Disorders
Heart and Circulation
Kidneys and Excretion
Lung Diseases
Psychological Disorders

Breathlessness

Anaemia

Anxiety
Asthma
Bronchitis, chronic
Emphysema
Heart attack
Lung diseases
Pneumonia
Pneumonothorax
Sarcoid

See Blood Disorders
Heart and Circulation
Lung Diseases
Psychological Disorders.

Bruising

Haemophilia
Idiopathic thrombocytopenic purpura
Leukaemia
Lymphomas

See Blood Disorders

Chest pain

Abdominal disorders
Angina pectoris
Anxiety
Bornholm disease
Bronchitis
Gall bladder disorders
Heart attack
Indigestion
Lipid disorders
Pancreas disorders
Peptic ulcer

Pericarditis
Pleurisy
Pneumonia
Pneumothorax
Sarcoidosis
Spondylosis

See Bones, Joints, and Muscles
The Digestive System
Endocrine Disorders
Heart and Circulation
Lung Diseases
Psychological Disorders

Chest, phlegm on

Bronchitis, acute
Bronchitis, chronic
Emphysema
Pneumonia
Tracheitis
Sinusitis

See Lung Diseases

Collapse

Anaphylactic shock
Bowel perforation
Brain tumour
CVA
Grand mal epilepsy
Pancreatitis, acute

See The Digestive System
General Conditions
Heart and Circulation

Nervous System
See also Consciousness, loss of

Confusion

Addiction to alcohol
Addiction to illegal drugs
Alzheimer's disease
Anxiety
Dementia
Depression
Meningitis
Pre-senile dementia
Schizophrenia
Stroke (CVA)
Trauma/Head injury

See Addictions
Heart and Circulation
Nervous System
Psychological Disorders

Consciousness, loss of

Addiction to alcohol
Addiction to illegal drugs
Brain tumour
Circulatory collapse (Shock)
CVA
Diabetes
Encephalitis
Epilepsy
Heart attack
Hysteria
Ketoacidosis
Meningitis
Respiratory disorders

Schizophrenia
Septicaemia
Stroke
Trauma/Head injury

See Addictions
Endocrine Disorders
Generalized Infections
Heart and Circulation
Lung Diseases
Nervous System
Psychological Disorders

Constipation

Anorexia nervosa
Bowel cancer
Bowel obstruction
Depression
Diabetes
Intestinal obstruction
Laxative abuse
Peptic ulcer
Peritonitis
Thyroid, underactive (Myxoedema)

See The Digestive System
Endocrine Disorders
Nervous System
Psychological Disorders

Convulsions

Diabetes
Epilepsy
Hypoglycaemia
Meningitis

See Endocrine Disorders
Nervous System

Cough

Anxiety
Asthma
Bronchitis, chronic
Emphysema
Heart attack
Laryngitis
Pleurisy
Pneumonia
Respiratory infections, acute and chronic
Sinusitis
Tuberculosis

See Ear, Nose, and Throat Disorders
Heart and Circulation
Lung Diseases
Psychological Disorders

Cramp

Backache
Diabetes
Lumbar disc syndrome
Lumbago
Neuropathy
Polymyalgia
Slipped disc
See Bones, Joints, and Muscles
Endocrine Disorders
Nervous System

Daydreaming

Addiction to alcohol
Addiction to illegal drugs
Diabetes
Epilepsy; Petit mal

See Addictions
Endocrine Disorders
Nervous System
Psychological Disorders

Deafness

Acoustic neuroma
Brain tumour
Ear wax
Labyrithitis
Ménière's disease
Middle-ear infections (Otitis media)
Outer-ear infections (Otitis externa)
Perforated eardrum
Vestibulitis

See Ear, Nose, and Throat Disorders
Nervous System

Debility

Addiction to alcohol
Addiction to illegal drugs
AIDS
Anaemia
Anorexia nervosa
Cancer
Depression
Diabetes

Endocarditis
Epstein-Barr virus
Malaria
ME
Thyroid, underactive (Myxedema)

See Addictions
Blood Disorders
Bones, Joints, and Muscles
Endocrine Disorders
Generalized Infections
Heart and Circulation
Nervous System
Psychological Disorders

Depression

Addiction to alcohol
Addiction to illegal drugs
Malaria
ME
Multiple sclerosis
Premenstrual tension
Thyroid, underactive
Trauma/Head injury

See Addictions
Bones, Joints, and Muscles
Endocrine Disorders
Generalized Infections
Nervous System
Psychological Disorders
Reproductive System including Breasts

Diarrhoea

Bowel infections

Gastroenteritis
Gluten sensitivity (Coeliac disease)
Inflammatory bowel disorders
Intestinal infections
Irritable bowel syndrome
Crohn's disease
Peptic ulcer
Thyrotoxicosis
Ulcerative colitis

See The Digestive System
Endocrine Disorders

Dizziness

Acoustic neuroma
Labrynthitis
Middle-ear infection (Otitis media)
Ménière's disease
Vestibulitis

See Ear, Nose, and Throat Disorders
Nervous System

Ears, discharge from

Middle-ear infections (Otitis media)
Outer-ear infections (Otitis externa)
Wax

See Ear, Nose, and Throat Disorders

Ears, pain in

Dental problems
Ear wax
Glue ear

Middle ear infections (Otitis media)
Mumps
Perforated eardrum
Sinusitis
Throat infections
Tonsillitis

See Ear, Nose, and Throat Disorders
Diseases of the Mouth

Ears, ringing or other noises in

Ear wax
Labyrinthitis
Ménière's disease
Middle-ear infections (Otitis media)
Outer-ear infections (Otitis externa)
Tinnitus
Vestibulitis

See Ear, Nose, and Throat Disorders

Elation

Hypomania
Mania
Manic depressive disorders (Bipolar depression)
Multiple sclerosis

See Nervous System
Psychological Disorders

Eyes, dry

Conjunctivitis
Rheumatoid arthritis
Sjøgren's syndrome

See Bones, Joints, and Muscles
Disorders of the Eye

Eyes; flashes of light in

Detached retina
Glaucoma
Migraine

See Disorders of the Eye
Nervous System

Eyes, floaters

Iritis
Sarcoidosis
Uveitis

See Disorders of the Eye
Lung Diseases

Eyes, halos around objects

Glaucoma

See Disorders of the Eye

Eyes itching

Allergy (Blepharitis)
Conjunctivitis

See Disorders of the Eye

Eyes, loss of vision (sudden)

Detached retina
Glaucoma, acute

Haemorrhage
Retinal artery obstruction
Retinal vein obstruction
Uveitis, acute

See Disorders of the Eye

Eyes, pain in

Conjunctivitis
Detached retina
Eye disorders
Glaucoma
Haemorrhage
Iritis
Uveitis

See Disorders of the Eye

Eyes, red

Ankylosing spondylitis
Conjunctivitis
Glaucoma
Haemorrhage
Herpes infection (Dendritic ulcer)
Iritis
Measles
Uveitis

See Bones, Joints, and Muscles
Disorders of the Eye
Generalized Infections
Skin Disorders

Eyes, sensitive to light

Conjunctivitis
Glaucoma
Herpes infection (Dendritic ulcer)
Iritis
Uveitis

See Disorders of the Eye

Eyes, yellowness of

Disorders of the pancreas
Gall bladder disorders
Liver disorders

See The Digestive System

Eyes, watering

Allergy (Blepharitis)
Conjunctivitis
Herpes infection (Dendritic ulcer)
Migraine

See Disorders of the Eye
Nervous System

Facial pain

Migraine
Sinusitis
Toothache
Trigeminal neuralgia
See Diseases of the Mouth
Ear, Nose, and Throat Disorders
Nervous System

See also Headache.

Faintness or dizziness

Acoustic neuroma
Labrynthitis
Low blood-pressure
Hypoglycaemia
Middle-ear infection (Otitis media)
Ménière's disease
Vestibulitis

See Ear, Nose, and Throat Disorders
Endocrine Disorders
Heart and Circulation
Nervous System

Fear

Anxiety
Phobias and obsessive compulsive disorders

See Psychological Disorders

Fever

Cancer
Chicken pox
Dental abscess and caries
German measles
Hodgkin's disease
Malaria
Measles
Meningitis
Middle ear infection (Otitis media)
Osteomyelitis
Septicaemia

Shingles
Tuberculosis

See Blood Disorders
Bones, Joints, and Muscles
Diseases of the Mouth
Ear, Nose, and Throat Disorders
Generalized Infections
Lung Diseases
Skin Disorders

Flushing

Hypertension
Menopause
Phaeochromocytoma

See Endocrine Disorders
Heart and Circulation
Reproductive System including Breasts

Glands, swelling of

Chickenpox
Epstein-Barr virus
German Measles
Infectious mononucleosis
Lymphomas
Measles
Shingles

See Blood Disorders
Generalized Infections
Skin Disorders

Groin, pain or swelling in

Gall bladder disorders
Hernia
Irritable bowel syndrome
Osteoarthritis

See Bones, Joints, and Muscles
The Digestive System

Hair growth

Ovarian cysts

See Endocrine Disorders
Menopause
Reproductive System including Breasts
Skin Disorders

Hair loss

Alopecia
Myxoedema
Pituitary disorders
Postpartum hair loss
Psoriasis
Thyroid, underactive

See Endocrine Disorders
Generalized Infections
Skin Disorders

Hallucinations

Schizophrenia

See Generalized Infections

Nervous System
Psychological Disorders

Head, pain in

Brain tumour
Cervical spondylosis
Encephalitis
Hypertension (High blood pressure)
Meningitis
Middle-ear infection (Otitis media)
Migraine
Migrainous neuralgia
Temporal arteritis
Tooth infection
Trauma/Head injury
Trigeminal neuralgia

See Bones, Joints and Muscles
Disorders of the Eye
Ear, Nose, and Throat Disorders
Heart and Circulation
Nervous System
Diseases of the Mouth

Headache

Brain tumour
Cervical spondylosis
Encephalitis
Epstein-Barr virus
Hypertension (High blood pressure)
Malaria
Meningitis
Middle-ear infection (Otitis media)
Migraine
Migrainous neuralgia

Septicaemia
Temporal arteritis
Tooth infection
Trauma/Head injury
Trigeminal neuralgia

See Bones, Joints and Muscles
Disorders of the Eye
Ear, Nose; and Throat Disorders
Generalized Infections
Heart and Circulation
Nervous System
Diseases of the Mouth

Hearing, loss of

Acoustic neuroma
Brain tumour
Ménière's disease
Middle-ear infection (Otitis media)
Outer-ear infection (Otitis externa)
Perforated eardrum
Wax

See Ear, Nose, and Throat Disorders
Nervous System

Heart, palpitations in

Addiction to illegal drugs
Angina pectoris
Anxiety
Ectopic beats
Heart attack
Heart rhythm disturbances (arrhythmias)
Kidney failure

See Addictions
Heart and Circulation; Kidneys and Excretion
Psychological Disorders

Heartburn

Gastric ulcer
Hiatus hernia
Oesophagitis

See The Digestive System

Hoarseness

Swellings of the vocal cord (larynx)
Upper respiratory tract infections, acute

See Ear, Nose, and Throat Disorders

Impotence

Depression
Disorders of the pituitary gland

See Endocrine Disorders
Psychological Disorders

Incontinence

Functional disorders of the bladder
Prostate
Stress incontinence
Uterine prolapse

See Kidneys and Excretion
Reproductive System including Breasts

Indecisiveness

Depression

See Psychological Disorders

Indigestion

Hiatus hernia
Oesophagitis
Peptic ulcer
Stomach cancer

See The Digestive System

Insomnia

Anxiety
Depression
Thyroid, overactive

See Endocrine Disorders
Psychological Disorders

Intercourse, painful

Disorders of the cervix
Infertility; Prolapse
Vaginismus
Vaginitis

See Reproductive System including Breasts

Legs, aches or pains in

Cramps
Deep vein thrombosis
Intermittent claudication

Osteoarthritis
Peripheral artery disease
Rheumatoid arthritis
Varicose veins

See Bones, Joints, and Muscles
Heart and Circulation

Loins, pain in

Bladder cancer
Infections of the renal tract
Kidney cancer
Kidney stones

See Kidneys and Excretion

Memory, loss of

Addiction to alcohol
Alzheimer's disease
Dementia
Drug and tranquillizer abuse
Pre-senile dementia
Senile dementia
Trauma/Head injury

See Addictions
Nervous System
Psychological Disorders

Mood, rapid change of

Addiction to alcohol
Addiction to illegal drugs
Anxiety
Bi-polar depression

Depression
Menopause
Pre-senile dementia
Senile dementia

See Addictions
Psychological Disorders
Reproduction including Breasts

Mouth and tongue soreness

Epilepsy
Fungus infections
Iron and vitamin deficiency
Thrush

See Diseases of the Mouth
Nervous System

Mouth and tongue swelling

Epilepsy
Trauma/Head injury
Tumours of the mouth

See Diseases of the Mouth
Nervous System

Mouth, dry

Diabetes insipidus
Diabetes mellitus
Salivary glands

See Disorders of the Mouth
Ear, Nose, and Throat Disorders
Endocrine Disorders

Mouth, pain in

Dental abscess and caries

See Diseases of the Mouth

Muscle loss

AIDS

See Generalized Infections

Muscles, pain in

ME
Polymyalgia rheumatic

See Bones, Joints, and Muscles

Nail disorders

Calcium deficiency
Iron deficiency
Liver disease
Psoriasis
Trauma
Vitamin deficiency

See Blood Disorders
The Digestive System
Skin Disorders

Nausea

Addiction to alcohol
Appendicitis
Bowel obstruction

Brain haemorrhage
Brain tumour
Gall bladder disorders or cholecystitis
Gastritis
Gastroenteritis
Heart attack
Hepatitis
Hiatus hernia
Kidney disorders
Kidney failure
Ketoacidosis
Labrynthitis
Liver disease
Ménière's disease
Middle-ear infection (Otitis media)
Migraine
Pancreatitis
Peptic ulcer
Peritonitis
Pregnancy and its complications
Vestibulitis

See Addictions
The Digestive System
Ear, Nose, and Throat Disorders
Heart and Circulation
Kidneys and Excretion
Nervous System
Reproductive System including Breasts

Neck, stiff

Meningitis
osteoarthritis
Sports injuries

See Bones, Joints, and Muscles

Nervous System

Nose, bleeding from

Addiction to illegal drugs (cocaine)
Epistaxis
Hypertension (High blood-pressure)
Rhinitis
Sinusitis

See Addictions
Ear, Nose, and Throat Disorders
Heart and Circulation

Nose, blocked

Allergy
Coryza
Deviated nasal symptom
Rhinitis
Sinusitis

See Ear, Nose, and Throat Disorders

Nose, pain

Addiction to illegal drugs (cocaine)
Epistaxis
Hypertension (High blood-pressure)
Rhinitis
Sinusitis

See Addictions
Ear, Nose, and Throat Disorders
Heart and Circulation

Nose, running

Allergy
Coryza
Rhinitis
Sinusitis

See Ear, Nose, and Throat Disorders

Numbness or pins and needles

Carpal tunnel syndrome
Diabetes
Migraine
Multiple sclerosis
Neuropathy
Vitamin deficiency

See Blood Disorders
Bones, Joints, and Muscles
Endocrine Disorders
Nervous System

Pain in back

Ankylosing spondylitis
Rheumatoid arthritis
Lumbago
Osteoporosis
Peptic ulcer
Sciatica
Slipped disc
Spondylitis

See Bones, Joints, and Muscles
The Digestive System

Pain in hands

Carpal tunnel syndrome
Tennis elbow

See Bones, Joints, and Muscles
Nervous System

Pain in joints

Ankylosing spondylitis
Arthritis
Gout
Lumbago
Repetitive strain injury
Sciatica
Scleroderma
SLE
Slipped disc
Spondylitis

See Bones, Joints, and Muscles

Pain in legs

Arthritis
Deep vein thrombosis
Intermittent claudication
Malaria
Meniscus
Sports injuries
Varicose veins

See Bones, Joints, and Muscles
Generalized Infections
Heart and Circulation

Pain under right side of ribs

Gall bladder disorders

See The Digestive System

Pain/Swelling of salivary gland

Mumps
Tumour

See Ear, Nose, and Throat Disorders
Generalized Infections

Pain in testicles

Cancer of the testicle
Diseases of the testes
Epididymitis
Kidney diseases
Kidney stone
Orchitis
Polyarteritis nodosa
Tortion

See General Conditions
Kidneys and Excretion
Reproductive System including Breasts

Palpitations

Arrhythmia

See Heart and Circulation

Paralysis

Bell's palsy

Brain tumour
Multiple sclerosis
Motor neurone disease
Stroke (CVA)

See Heart and Circulation
Nervous System

Pelvis, pain in

Diseases of the uterus and cervix

See Reproductive System including Breasts

Penis, discharge from

Cystitis
Gonorrhoea
Non-specific urethritis
Venereal diseases

See Reproductive System including Breasts

Penis, sore on

Herpes
Syphilis
Thrush

See Reproductive System including Breasts

Period difficulties

Dysmenorrhea
Fibroids
Infertility
Menorrhagia

Ovarian cysts
See Endocrine Disorders
Reproductive System including Breasts

Period, excessive bleeding

Antepartum haemorrhage
Cervical cancer
Disorders of the cervix
Ectopic pregnancy;
Gynaecological disorders
Inter-menstrual bleeding
Menorrhagia
Menstruation
Pregnancy
Threatened miscarriage
Vaginitis

See Reproductive System including Breasts

Period, irregular

Disorders of the pituitary gland
Infertility.
See Endocrine Disorders
Reproductive System including Breasts

Pins and needles

Carpal tunnel syndrome
Diabetes; Multiple sclerosis
Neuropathy
Vitamin deficiency

See Blood Disorders
Endocrine Disorders
Nervous System

Rash

Acne
Athlete's foot
Cellulitis
Chickenpox
Dermatitis
Dhobi itch
Eczema
Fungus infections
German measles
Herpes
Impetigo
Measles
Meningitis
Psoriasis
Shingles
Skin infestations

See Generalized Infections
Nervous System
Skin Disorders

Rigidity

Meningitis
Parkinson's disease

See Nervous System

Scrotum, swelling in

Diseases of the testes

See Reproductive System including Breasts

Sensation, loss of

Brain tumour
Neuropathy
See Nervous System

Shivering chills

Coryza
Fever
Influenza
Septicaemia
See Ear, Nose, and Throat Disorders
Generalized Infections.

Skin infections

Cellulitis
Dhobi itch
Fungus infections
See Skin Disorders

Skin moles

Basal cell tumours
Haemangiomas
Malignant melanoma
Naevi
Warts

See Skin Disorders

Skin rash

Acne
Allergy
Athlete's foot

Cellulitis
Chickenpox
Dermatitis
Dhobi itch
Eczema
Fungus infections
German measles
Herpes
Impetigo
Measles
Psoriasis
Shingles
Skin infestations
SLE

See Generalized Infections
Skin Disorders

Skin warts

Haemangiomas
Lipid disorders
Malignant melanoma
Naevi
Warts

See Endocrine Disorders
Skin Disorders

Skin

dandruff
Blepharitis
Seborrhoeic dermatitis
Eczema
Psoriasis

See Disorders of the Eye
Skin Disorders

Skin, itching

Dermatitis
Eczema
Fungus infections
Kidney failure
Liver failure
Pruritis
Psoriasis
Skin infestations

See The Digestive System
Kidneys and Excretion
Skin Disorders

Skin, painful lesions

Basal cell carcinomas
Cellulitis
Dhobi itch
Fungus infections
Herpes
Ringworm
Squamous cell carcinoma

See Skin Disorders

Skin, stretch marks

Cushing's syndrome
Pregnancy

See Endocrine Disorders
Reproductive System including Breasts

Sleep, difficulties with

Anxiety
Depression
Thyroid, overactive (Thyrotoxicosis)

See Endocrine Disorders
Psychological Disorders

Sleep, excessive

Addiction to alcohol
Alzheimer's disease
Angina
Brain tumour
CVA (stroke)
Depression
Drug and tranquillizer abuse
Manic-depressive psychosis
Narcolepsy
Premenstrual tension
Pre-senile dementia
enile dementia
Thyroid
underactive (Myxoedema)
Trauma/Head injury

See Addictions
Endocrine Disorders
Generalized Infections
Heart and Circulation
Nervous System
Psychological Disorders
Reproductive System including Breasts

Slowed down

Addiction to alcohol
Addison's disease
Alzheimer's disease
Angina
Brain tumour
CVA (stroke)
Depression
Drug and tranquillizer abuse
Endocarditis
Head injury
Manic-depressive psychosis
M.E.
Pre-senile dementia
Senile dementia
Thyroid, underactive (Myxoedema)
Trauma/Head injury

See Addictions
Endocrine Disorders
Generalized Infections
Heart and Circulation
Nervous System
Psychological Disorders

Smell, loss of

Allergy
Brain tumour
Deviated nasal septum
Rhinitis
Sinusitis
Trauma/Head injury

See Ear, Nose, and Throat disorders
Nervous System

Smell, strange

Diabetes mellitus
Ketoacidosis
Mouth abscess
Sinusitis
Temporal lobe epilepsy

See Ear, Nose and Throat disorders
Endocrine disorders
Nervous System

Speech, difficulties with

Addiction to alcohol
Alzheimer's disease
Brain tumour
CVA (stroke)
Dementia
Drug and tranquillizer abuse
Motor-neurone disease
Parkinson's disease
Pre-senile dementia
Senile dementia
Tongue-tie
Trauma/Head injury

See Addictions
Disorders of the Mouth
Heart and Circulation
Nervous System
Psychological Disorders

Speeded up

Addiction to alcohol
Agitated depression

Cocaine
Drug and tranquillizer abuse
Ecstacy
Hypomania
Mania
Overactive thyroid

See Addictions
Endocrine Disorders
Psychological Disorders

Sweating

Hodgkin's disease
Lymphomas
Menopause
Thyrotoxicosis

See Blood Disorders
Endocrine Disorders
Generalized Infections
Reproductive System including Breasts

Swellings or lumps

Arthritis
Breast cancer
Breasts
Bursitis
Ganglion
Hernia
Hodgkin's disease
Lymphomas
Lipoma
Mumps
Sarcomas
Tennis elbow

Testicular cancer

See Blood Disorders
Bones, Joints, and Muscles
The Digestive System
Generalized Infections
Reproductive System including Breasts
Skin Disorders

Taste, loss of

Brain tumour
Sinusitis
Trauma/Head injury

See Ear, Nose, and Throat Disorders
Nervous System

Tension

Addiction to alcohol
Addiction to illegal drugs
Agitated depression
Anxiety states
Anxiety

See Addictions
Psychological Disorders

Thirst, excessive

Diabetes insipidus
Diabetes mellitus
Hypercalcaemia

See Endocrine Disorders

Throat, sore

Colds (Coryza)
Epstein-Barr Virus
Influenza
Tonsillitis
Upper respiratory infections
Viral diseases

See Ear, Nose, and Throat Disorders
Generalized Infections

Tiredness

see Debility

Toothache

Dental abcess
Dental caries

See Disorders of the Mouth
Ear, Nose, and Throat Disorders

Twitching and trembling

Benign tremor
Brain tumour
Epilepsy; Grand mal
Parkinson's disease
Petit mal
Stroke
Tourette's syndrome

See Nervous System

Unconsciousness

Addiction to alcohol
Addiction to illegal drugs
Brain tumour
Circulatory collapse (Shock)
CVA
Diabetes
Encephalitis
Heart attack
Hysteria
Ketoacidosis
Meningitis
Respiratory disorders
Schizophrenia
Stroke
Trauma/Head injury

See Addictions
Heart and Circulation
Lung Diseases
Nervous System
Psychological Disorders

Urination, difficulty with

Bladder cancer
Cystitis
Diabetes
Diseases of the prostate
Diseases of the testes
Functional disorders of the bladder
Kidney cancer
Multiple sclerosis
Stress incontinence
Uterine prolapse

See Kidneys and Excretion
Nervous System
Reproductive System including Breasts

Urination, frequency of

Diabetes mellitus
Hypercalcaemia
Kidney failure
Sarcoidosis

See Endocrine disorders
Kidneys and Excretion

Vagina, discharge from

Candida
Herpes
Pelvic infection
Thrush
Trichomona vaginitis
Venereal diseases

See Reproductive System including Breasts

See also Bleeding from vagina

Vagina, lump in

Syphilis
Bartholin cyst

See Reproductive System including Breasts

Vertigo

Acoustic neuroma

Labrynthitis
Ménière's disease
Middle-ear infection (Otitis media)
Vestibulitis

See Ear, Nose, and Throat disorders
Nervous System

Vision, blurring
Cataract
Conjunctivitis
Diabetes
Glaucoma
Iritis
Uveitis

See Disorders of the Eye

Vision, difficulties with

Brain haemorrhage
Brain tumour
Cataract
Conjunctivitis
Diabetes
Glaucoma
Iritis
Migraine
Multiple sclerosis
Retinal artery thrombosis
Retinal vein thrombosis
Uveitis

See Disorders of the Eye
Endocrine Disorders
Nervous System

Vision, double

Multiple sclerosis

See Disorders of the Eye
Nervous system

Vision, loss of

Brain tumour
Cataract
CVA (stroke)
Dendritic ulcer (herpes infections)
Diabetes
Diabetic retinopathy
Eye infections
Glaucoma
Hypertension (High blood pressure)
Hypertensive retinopathy
Multiple sclerosis
Retinal artery thrombosis
Retinal vein thrombosis

See Disorders of the Eye
Endocrine Disorders
Heart and Circulation
Nervous System

Voice, loss of

Laryngitis
Laryngeal cancer
Laryngeal warts
Singer's nodes
Sinusitis
Swellings of the vocal cords

See Ear, Nose, and Throat Disorders

Vomiting

Addiction to alcohol
Addiction to illegal drugs
Anorexia nervosa
Appendicitis
Bowel infections
Brain tumour
Bulimia
Epstein-Barr virus
Food poisoning
Gall bladder disorders (Cholecystitis)
Gastroenteritis
Heart attack
Hiatus hernia
Intestinal obstruction
Kidney failure
Liver failure
Migraine
Peptic ulcer
Peritonitis
Pulmonary embolus

See Addictions
The Digestive System
Generalized Infections
Heart and Circulation
Kidneys and Excretion
Nervous System
Psychological Disorders

See also Vertigo

Weakness

Addison's disease
AIDS
Anaemia
Coeliac disease
Coryza
Diabetes
Endocarditis
Hypokalemia
Influenza
Lymphomas
Malaria
ME
Migraine
Motor neurone disease
Myasthenia gravis
Polymyalgia rheumatica
Septicaemia

See Blood Disorders
Bones, Joints, and Muscles
The Digestive System
Endocrine Disorders
General Conditions
Generalized Infections
Heart and Circulation
Nervous System

Weight gain

Compulsive eating
Cushing's syndrome
Depression
Kidney failure
Obesity

Obsessive compulsive disorders
Underactive thyroid

See Endocrine Disorders
Kidneys and Excretions
Psychological Disorders

Weight loss

Addiction to alcohol
Addison's disease
Anorexia nervosa
Bulimia
Cancer (any organ)
Diabetes insipidus
Diabetes mellitus
HIV and AIDS
Inflammatory bowel disorders
Peptic ulcer
Thyroid, overactive
Tuberculosis

See Addictions
The Digestive System
Endocrine Disorders
General Conditions
Generalized Infections
Lung Diseases
Psychological Disorders

Wheezing

Asthma
Bronchitis

See Lung Diseases

Key to severity of condition

♥♥♥♥♥   immediately life threatening and potentially fatal

♥♥♥♥   potentially fatal

♥♥♥   very serious, may deteriorate to a fatal condition

♥♥   serious, and needs treatment

♥   minor

Part 2
Systems of the body and the conditions that affect them

Chapter 1

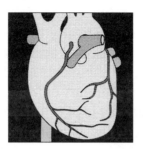

Heart and Circulation

Please refer to 'Important Advice' on page 4 at the beginning of this book; and remember, if you are in any doubt, consult a physician.

The function of the circulatory system is to move blood around the body. The heart works as a pump providing pressure to enable this circulation to take place. As with any plumbing system, failure can occur – failure or blockage of one of the pipes or blood vessels. The human heart is particularly vulnerable, and heart disease is the commonest cause of death in the Western world. The main cause of heart disease is hardening of the arteries, which impairs the blood supply to the heart muscle itself (coronary artery disease or atherosclerosis). This will show up as angina or heart attack. Abnormal heart rhythms (arrhythmias) and valve diseases will also affect

71

the heart. Excess pressure in the system will appear as hypertension (raised blood pressure) which will also cause leakage in any of the blood vessels. Most dramatically this can appear as a stroke or cerebrovascular accident (CVA). Clots within the system can cause blockage; the most dramatic is the pulmonary embolus where a blood clot travels from the legs to the lungs. Narrowing of the arteries to the legs may cause difficulty walking.

Apart from congenital abnormalities of the heart (i.e. heart defects that appear in the newborn child), most conditions are degenerative because of the effect of external factors, such as nicotine and unsuitable diets, on a heart that evolved to last for perhaps forty years. Early humans probably died of accidents and infections when the lifestyle was more dangerous and no appropriate treatment was available. The challenge of modern public health medicine, therefore, is to prevent heart disease by adapting to the new demands made upon the heart, i.e. to help it to last for 80 years or more despite highly refined diets and occasionally excessive external pressures.

Heart attack ♥♥♥♥♥

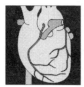 A heart attack is caused by a reduction in the blood flow to a part of the heart muscle and a subsequent clot in one of the coronary arteries. The factors which may precipitate a heart attack include: family history of heart disease; smoking; obesity; sedentary life style; high blood pressure; high cholesterol; high triglycerides.

Main symptom
Chest pain. The chest pain of a heart attack is typically central in the chest, severe, and vice-like or gripping. The pain may radiate to the left arm and jaw. Any chest pain can, however, indicate a heart attack.

Associated symptoms
Nausea, breathlessness, collapse, loss of consciousness, vomiting, loss of appetite, dizziness, death.

Action
Seek medical assistance immediately. While waiting for medical help, the patient should lie down. Clear patient's airway. Remove dentures. If trained first-aid assistance is available, carry out mouth-to-mouth resuscitation with cardiac massage. Patients should not be given alcoholic drinks or food. Avoid over-warming.

Tests
These include ECG (cardiograph), blood tests for heart enzymes, chest X-ray, blood tests for factors which may cause a heart attack, coronary angiography (X-ray of the coronary arteries using a dye); eventually exercise ECG test.

Emergency medications
The following medicines may be used by a qualified medical practitioner for the treatment of a heart attack: adrenalin, aspirin, bicarbonate drip, calcium chloride, diuretics, eminase, lignocaine, procainamide, streptokinase, TPA.

Other medications

The following medications may be given to a patient following a heart attack: anticoagulants, antihypertensives, anti-obesity drugs, aspirin, lipid-lowering agents.

Further advice

After recovery from a heart attack, you should lose weight, take up light regular exercise, stop smoking, eat a low-fat diet, and treat any other precipitating factors.

Angina pectoris

 Angina pectoris is a condition where pain in the heart is caused by an inadequate blood supply to the heart muscle. The condition is similar to, and may eventually lead to, a heart attack (*see* above). The factors that precipitate angina include: a family history of heart disease, smoking, obesity, a sedentary lifestyle, high blood pressure, high cholesterol, high triglycerides, cold weather.

Main symptom

Chest pain. Typically, the chest pain of angina pectoris is a central, gripping chest pain that may radiate to the left arm or jaw, and that may be worse on exercise, particularly in cold weather. The pain is relieved by rest. Any chest pain, however, that is worse on exercise and relieved by rest may be angina. Angina may sometimes come on at rest (atypical angina).

Associated symptoms

Nausea, breathlessness, collapse, dizziness, unconsciousness.

Action

Seek advice to investigate and treat angina. Pay particular attention to risk factors for heart disease and to treating these where possible.

Tests

Investigations for angina include: ECG, exercise ECG, chest X-ray, blood tests for precipitating factors, coronary angiography, thallium scanning of the heart, echocardiography.

Medications and treatment

Anti-anginal medications include ß-blockers and nitrates.

Further advice

After the treatment of the risk factors for heart disease, you may be investigated and considered for coronary artery bypass grafting (CABG) which replaces diseased arteries with fresh arteries or veins. You should lose weight, take light, regular exercise, stop smoking, and eat a low-fat diet. Angioplasty (balloon flattening of blockages) may also be used for treatment.

Hypertension ♥♥

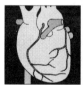

Hypertension or high blood pressure may be related to diseases in other parts of the body such as the kidney or adrenal glands. Hypertension may be an inherited disease, however, or have no known cause (essential hypertension). It is made worse by smoking, obesity, diabetes, high alcohol intake, and may lead to heart disease, stroke, kidney disease, or damage to the eyes.

Symptoms

Hypertension may be symptomless, but symptoms include those caused by stroke (*see* below) or heart disease. Headache may be a symptom of hypertension, as is nose bleeding or heavy bleeding elsewhere such as heavy menstrual bleeding.

Associated symptoms

These include those related to the eyes, kidneys, and

other organs which may be affected by hypertension.

Action
Hypertension should be treated by losing weight, stopping smoking, a low-salt diet, and treatment with antihypertensive drugs. If a cause for the hypertension may be identified and treated, investigations should be undertaken immediately.

Tests
These include: chest X-ray, ECG, kidney function tests, tests of the adrenal glands, routine blood tests.

Medications and treatment
Various types of drug lower blood pressure. These include diuretics, ACE inhibitors, and calcium antagonists.

Further advice
You should adopt a healthy lifestyle with light, regular exercise, no smoking, reduced alcohol intake, and weight loss.

Associated conditions
Low blood pressure (hypotension, *see also* shock) may also cause symptoms such as fatigue and headache. In some countries, heart drugs are given to increase blood pressure but this is not standard practice.

Heart failure

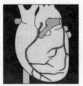 Heart failure is the failure of the heart to pump adequate blood through the body or through the lungs. It may be caused by diseases of the valves such as the mitral valve, aortic valve, or tricuspic valve. These valves function to prevent back-flow of blood within the heart. They may be damaged by rheumatic fever or other infections. Heart failure may also be

caused by high blood pressure or heart disease such as that described under angina or heart attack. Heart failure is a complication of having had a heart attack. Some conditions affect the heart muscle (cardiomyopathy) and these can lead to heart failure.

Main symptoms
Shortness of breath, swelling of ankles, fatigue, loss of appetite, poor exercise tolerance, swelling of the abdomen.

Action
Heart failure may be chronic or acute. Acute heart failure needs emergency treatment and patients should be treated in hospital.

Tests
Investigations for heart failure include chest X-ray, ECG, routine blood tests, kidney function tests, lung function tests, tests to identify cause of heart failure such as heart attack or high blood pressure.

Emergency medications
These include diuretics such as adrenalin, frusemide, inotropic drugs, noradrenalin.

Other medications
Medications for the long-term treatment of heart failure include Lanoxin, diuretics, other inotropic drugs, drugs to treat causes of heart failure, anti-arrhythmic drugs.

Further advice
Pay particular attention to fluid intake and output, general health, heart and kidney function. You should take light, regular exercise, stop smoking, reduce alcohol intake, and lose weight.

Cerebrovascular accident (stroke, CVA)

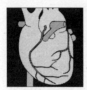 Strokes are due to brain damage caused by narrowing or blockage of an artery supplying the brain. The artery may be blocked by a clot (thrombus) which forms in the artery or by a travelling thrombus (embolus). Strokes may also be caused by brain haemorrhage related to high blood pressure or aneurysms (swellings of blood vessels) in the arteries in the brain.

Factors precipitating stroke include: heart disease, aneurysms, high blood pressure.

Symptoms

These are primarily nervous system symptoms related to the brain damage. They include collapse, unconsciousness, sudden death, paralysis of one half of the body, loss of speech, loss of sensation. Minor strokes (transient ischaemic attacks) may cause stroke symptoms that appear for a short time only. Small strokes may be relatively symptomless but may lead to progressive atherosclerotic dementia, i.e. a gradual loss of mental function.

Action

Transient ischaemic attacks or small strokes should be investigated and treated. Sudden stroke which appears as an emergency with collapse and paralysis needs to be treated as an emergency.

Tests

Investigations for stroke or suspected stroke include: chest X-ray, ECG, tests for causes of stroke, brain scan, MRI scan, arteriography of brain circulation, tests to identify possible site of embolus.

Medications and treatment

The treatment with drugs depends on the cause of the stroke. Thus, high blood pressure needs to be treated with antihypertensive drugs.

Clots or embolus need to be treated with blood-thinning drugs. Haemorrhage needs to be treated with measures to stop haemorrhage, including possible surgical treatment.

Further advice
Recovery from a stroke should include physiotherapy and speech therapy, and attention to any area of paralysis. Prevention of further strokes includes treatment of precipitating factors. Keep your blood pressure down, lose weight, stop smoking, and reduce alcohol intake.

Deep-vein thrombosis (DVT)

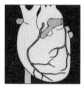 Deep-vein thrombosis is a condition where there is clotting of blood in one of the deeper veins, usually in the leg or pelvis. It is caused by prolonged bed rest, some diseases which increase the clotting of the blood, and some medications, such as the contraceptive pill, which increase clotting of the blood. Deep-vein thromboses are common after surgery, particularly surgery to the abdomen or pelvis, or gynaecological surgery.

Main symptoms
These include: pain and tenderness over the vein, swelling of the leg (oedema), difficulty and pain in walking. The thrombus in the leg may detach and cause a pulmonary embolus (*see* below). Deep-vein thrombosis may, therefore, lead to serious conditions including death.

Action
Deep-vein thrombosis needs to be diagnosed and treated quickly. Patients should rest with the leg elevated while medical assistance is sought.

Tests
These include: a venogram, and X-ray of the veins in the legs. In addition, routine investigations, such as chest X-ray, ECG, and blood tests, should be performed and a proper history taken to identify precipitating factors.

Medications and treatment
These include blood-thinning agents (anticoagulants) as well as general support such as elastic stockings which will support the leg. Prevention of deep-vein thrombosis is obtained in surgical patients by pre-operative administration of heparin by injection. Heparin, warfarin, and other anticoagulants may be used in treatment.

Further advice
If you have suffered from a deep-vein thrombosis, you should avoid medications, such as hormones, which may precipitate DVT. You should follow general advice about your health, such as losing weight, stopping smoking, taking light, regular exercise, and reducing alcohol intake.

Associated conditions
Superficial inflammation of the veins or phlebitis is similar but not as serious.

Pulmonary embolus

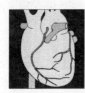
Pulmonary embolus is caused by a blood clot which travels to the lung and may block the lung or one of the blood vessels in the heart. Factors which may precipitate pulmonary embolus include deep-vein thrombosis (*see* above) and any blood-clotting disorder, previous or recent surgery, injury or damage to the veins in the leg or pelvis. Pulmonary embolus is a common complication of prolonged bed rest and hospitalization, particularly post-operative.

Main symptoms

These include onset of chest pain which may appear in a similar way to a heart attack. There is severe shortness of breath, and there may be collapse and sudden death. Pleuritic chest pain (that is, chest pain which is worse on taking a deep breath) may be a symptom of pulmonary embolus. Patients may cough up blood.

Action

Pulmonary embolus is a medical emergency. Patients should be rested and medical attention sought immediately. It is important to distinguish pulmonary embolus from a heart attack because different resuscitating methods will be required.

Tests

Investigations for suspected pulmonary embolus include: chest X-ray, lung perfusion scans (to test how much lung tissue is working), ECG, arteriography, blood tests for causes.

Medications and treatment

The treatment of pulmonary embolus includes urgent resuscitation and lung ventilation if required. Dissolving the clot and preventing further clots may require anticoagulant therapy which should be continued for several months. Prevention of pulmonary embolus is achieved by using heparin pre-operatively in surgical patients.

Associated conditions

Small multiple pulmonary emboli may appear without any symptoms. Eventually they may cause shortness of breath and possibly late presentation with full pulmonary embolus or pulmonary hypertension.

Peripheral arterial disease (intermittent claudication)

 Peripheral arterial disease is caused by a narrowing or blocking of the blood vessels in the lower limbs. This appears as intermittent claudication, a condition where there is pain in the legs on walking which is relieved by rest. It may also appear as sudden blockage of one of the arteries to the leg. Factors which precipitate peripheral arterial disease include smoking, obesity, high blood pressure and diabetes. Buerger's disease is a rare form of peripheral arterial disease, which is particularly sensitive to nicotine.

Symptoms

These include pain in the legs, particularly pain that is worse on walking and that is relieved by rest. Pain in the legs at night (rest pain) is also a symptom of this condition. Sudden blockage of an artery will result in a severely painful and white foot which needs emergency treatment. Progressive peripheral arterial disease may eventually lead to ulceration, infection, and gangrene.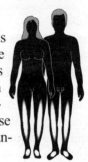

Action

Peripheral arterial disease needs investigation. Sudden onset of blockage of the main artery to the leg should be treated as an emergency. Patients should be rested and attempts made to warm the leg without overheating it.

Tests

Investigation of peripheral arterial disease include: arteriography to look at the state of the vessels, as well as general routine tests including chest X-ray, ECG, blood tests for clotting disorders or possible embolus. Doppler ultrasound methods can be used to assess blood flow in peripheral vessels.

Medications and treatment

Heparin or warfarin may be useful, and emergency surgical procedures may be necessary. In the longer term, several drugs are said to function as peripheral vasodilators to improve the blood supply. Examples: Hexopal, Opilon, Trental.

Further advice
Treatment of underlying conditions e.g. anaemia or diabetes is also part of the management of this condition. You should give up smoking, lose weight, take light, regular exercise, and reduce alcohol intake.

Associated conditions
Apart from Buerger's disease (*see* above), some people have poor circulation. This may be associated with conditions such as SLE or scleroderma (*see* below), but other people, particularly young women, have Raynaud's phenomenon where the small arteries in the hand are particularly sensitive to cold.

Pericarditis

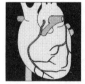 Pericarditis is inflammation of the pericardium or sac which surrounds the heart muscle. It is usually caused by a virus infection but sometimes occurs after bacterial infection, in association with endocarditis (*see* below), or after a heart attack. It may also be associated with conditions such as pleurisy.

Main symptom
Chest pain which may mimic the chest pain of a heart attack. Often this pain is related to posture, and, in this sense, the condition may be discriminated from a heart attack. The pain may radiate to the left arm and the jaw like the pain of a heart attack and may be associated with nausea, breathlessness, collapse, and fever.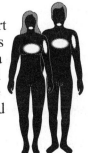

Action
Patients should be treated as if they have had a heart attack until the

definitive diagnosis of pericarditis has been made.

Tests
An ECG would show signs characteristic of pericarditis, and further investigations would include cardiac ultrasound, chest X-ray, blood tests.

Medications and treatment
These depend on the precipitating cause of pericarditis, and, if a bacterial infection has been found, antibiotics may be appropriate.

Further advice
If you have suffered an attack of pericarditis, you may be unfit and you should build up your exercise training gradually.

Endocarditis

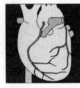 Endocarditis is a condition involving infection, usually by bacteria, of one of the valves inside the heart. This commonly affects the valves on the left side of the heart, particularly where these valves have been previously damaged by rheumatic fever. Valve disease can lead to heart failure and its associated symptoms. Endocarditis may arise after dental treatment in a person who has a damaged heart valve.

Symptoms
Minor debility, which progresses with gradual fatigue, anaemia, and weakness. Certain specific symptoms include painful nodules in the fingers and splinter haemorrhages under the nails. Traces of blood in the urine may also occur due to emboli affecting the kidney.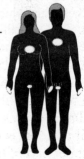

Action
The diagnosis needs to be made by an experienced clinician and treatment initiated.

Tests
These involve blood cultures, cardiac ultrasound, ECG, chest X-ray, kidney investigations, other routine blood tests. Swabs for infection, urine culture.

Medications and treatment
Usually the administration of an antibiotic such as penicillin. This needs to be continued for several weeks. Further treatment may be directed at correcting defects in the heart valve, including surgical treatment. Anticoagulants and other antithrombotic agents may be required.

Further advice
Patients should be advised to take preventative antibiotics before dental treatment.

Associated conditions
Endocarditis may be associated with myocarditis or pericarditis.

Heart rhythm disturbances (arrhythmias)

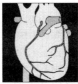Arrhythmias are caused by disturbances of the heart's electrical conducting system which can produce irregularities both detectable on ECG and of which the patient is aware. Serious arrhythmias can be fatal. There are various types of cardiac arrhythmias ranging from the simple ectopic beat through to atrial flutter, atrial fibrillation, and ventricular abnormalities, particularly ventricular fibrillation. Ventricular fibrillation is often the fatal end stage of a heart attack. The upper part of the heart is the atrium, while the lower part is the

ventricle. Both have muscles which may flutter (mild) or fibrillate (more severe).

Symptoms

The symptoms of arrhythmias depend on the type of rhythm disturbance. The symptoms may range from none at all to a feeling of a missed beat or an extra heartbeat, particularly after stress, fatigue, or high caffeine intake, irregular pulse rate. More severe arrhythmias may produce serious symptoms including collapse and death, the sensation of severe chest pain, breathlessness, or panic. The chest pain produced by arrhythmia may mimic the chest pain of angina or a heart attack and, indeed, may lead to either of these conditions. Some arrhythmias become worse when the patient is in certain situations or positions.

Action

An experienced first-aider may learn to massage the eyeballs or the neck to relieve the arrhythmia. Medical assistance should be sought urgently.

Tests

Tests include investigations for a heart attack and an urgent ECG, blood tests, chest X-ray, and investigation of the coronary circulation by coronary angiography.

Medications and treatment

The treatment of arrhythmias depends on the type of arrhythmia, but includes drugs such as lignocaine, calcium chloride, procainamide, bicarbonate. Milder arrhythmias can be treated with drugs such as Lanoxin, propanolol. Serious arrhythmias require DC shock with a defibrillating machine. A long-term pacemaker may be required.

Further advice

After recovery from arrhythmia, you should follow general advice as for other heart patients including weight loss, reducing nicotine and alcohol intake, and you should take light, regular exercise.

Shock ♥♥♥♥♥♥
(collapse, hypotension, anaphylactic shock)

Shock is caused by a sudden drop of blood pressure which may result from a severe allergy (anaphylactic shock), severe trauma as in a road traffic accident, loss of blood, or anything which precipitates a sudden decrease in blood pressure.

Main symptoms
Collapse, weakness, headache, inability to walk, inability to move limbs. Shock may result in death.

Action
Patients should be laid flat to improve the blood supply to the brain. Medical attention should be sought immediately. Patients should not be overwarmed with blankets because this will worsen shock. Obvious bleeding should be stopped where possible.

Tests
Investigations into the cause of shock should proceed immediately. These include ECG, chest X-ray, search for bleeding points, search for causes of allergy.

Medications and treatment
The main treatment for shock is to increase blood volume by giving plasma, blood, or fluids. Adrenalin, noradrenalin, isoprenaline, and other inotropic drugs will also bring up blood pressure.

Other medications
These can be used to treat the cause of shock, e.g. steroids, adrenalin, antihistamines for allergic shock, and specific treatments for heart attack if this is the cause.

Aortic aneurysm

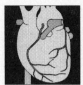

Aortic aneurysm is a swelling of the main artery leading to the heart. These aneurysms are most commonly found in the upper abdomen/lower chest area. The cause of aortic aneurysm is most commonly hardening of the arteries or arteriosclerosis. Occasionally aneurysms have been associated with previous syphilis infections, but these are rarely seen nowadays.

Main symptom
A swelling in the upper abdomen through which a pulse can clearly be felt. Occasionally, these aneurysms may dissect or rupture and this may appear as a medical emergency similar to a heart attack.

Action
If the patient is fit, aortic aneurysms will lend themselves to bypass surgery. The acute presentation of a ruptured or dissected aortic aneurysm should be treated as a medical emergency in the same way as a heart attack.

Tests
These involve routine tests such as abdomen and chest X-ray, ECG, coronary arteriography, and aortic angiogram.

Medications and treatment
Treatment of the acute condition includes treatment of shock with fluids, plasma, or blood, and treatment of associated conditions including kidney failure which can arise as a result of a dissecting aortic aneurysm.

Further advice
Because aortic aneurysms are related to hardening of the arteries, you should adopt similar changes to lifestyle as you would following a heart attack, i.e. you should lose weight, stop smoking, reduce alcohol intake, and take light, regular exercise.

Varicose veins ♥♥

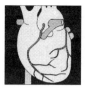 Varicose veins are caused by failure and incompetence of the veins in the legs which result in swelling of the veins and a collection of blood in those veins. Varicose veins may be precipitated by a family history, pregnancy, constipation, and a sedentary lifestyle.

Symptoms
Swelling of the veins in one or both legs which may sometimes be painful or bleed. Occasionally, varicose ulceration may be seen together with pigmentation on the inside of the ankle. Occasionally, varicose veins may bleed profusely.

Action
Bleeding varicose veins should be treated by local pressure. Avoid using a tourniquet because this may make the matter worse. Less urgent varicose vein treatment includes support stockings, injections, and surgery which is the main treatment for the condition.

Tests
Investigations include venograms and Doppler ultrasound.

Medications and treatment:
Paroven, for example, may relieve the pain from aching legs.

Further advice
After surgery, you should exercise regularly.

Associated conditions
Varicose veins are not usually associated with deep-vein thrombosis (*see* above) but there may be a superficial inflammation of the veins in the form of thrombophlebitis. Varicose veins in the scrotum can appear as a varicocoele.

Prescription Medicines

Acepril *see* Capoten

Adalat

An orange, liquid-filled capsule supplied at strengths of 5 mg, 10 mg and used as an anti-anginal treatment for angina, Raynaud's phenomenon.

Side effects: headache, flushes, fluid retention, dizziness, chest pain, rarely jaundice, gum swelling.
Caution: in patients with weak hearts, liver disease, or low blood pressure.
Not to be used for: children, pregnant women, nursing mothers, or patients suffering from severe low blood pressure.
Caution needed with: antihypertensives, cimetidine, quinidine.

Aldactide 50

A buff tablet supplied at a strength of 50 mg and used as a diuretic to treat congestive heart failure.

Side effects: breast enlargement, stomach upset, drowsiness, rash, sensitivity to light, blood changes.
Caution: in pregnant women, young patients, and in patients suffering from liver or kidney disease, gout, or diabetes. Your doctor may advise regular blood tests.
Not to be used for: nursing mothers or for patients suffering from severe kidney failure, progressive kidney failure, raised potassium levels.
Caution needed with: potassium supplements, lithium, digoxin, carbenoxolone, antihypertensives, ACE inhibitors.

Aldactone

A buff tablet or a white tablet according to strengths of 25 mg, 50 mg, 100 mg and used as a diuretic to treat congestive

heart failure, cirrhosis of the liver, fluid retention.

Side effects: breast enlargement, stomach upset, rash, drowsiness, headache, confusion.

Caution: in pregnant women or young patients, and in patients suffering from kidney or liver disease. Your doctor may advise regular blood tests.

Not to be used for: nursing mothers or for patients suffering from kidney failure or raised potassium levels.

Caution needed with: potassium supplements, carbenoxolone, digitalis, ACE inhibitors, antihypertensives.

Aldomet

A yellow tablet supplied at strengths of 125 mg, 250 mg, 500 mg and used as an antihypertensive to treat high blood pressure.

Side effects: sleepiness, headache, weakness, depression, slow heart rate, congestion of the nose, dry mouth, stomach upset, jaundice, blood changes.

Caution: in patients suffering from certain types of anaemia, history of liver disease, kidney disease, or patients undergoing anaesthesia. Your doctor may advise regular blood tests.

Not to be used for: patients suffering from liver disease, depression, phaeochromocytoma (a disease of the adrenal glands).

Caution needed with: tricyclics, MAOIs, other antihypertensives.

Aprinox

A white tablet supplied at strengths of 2.5 mg, 5 mg and used as a diuretic to treat fluid retention, high blood pressure.

Side effects: low potassium levels, rash, sensitivity to light, blood changes, gout, tiredness.

Caution: in pregnant women, nursing mothers, the elderly and for patients suffering from diabetes, severe kidney or liver disease, or gout.

Not to be used for: children or for patients suffering from urine

failure or severe or progressive kidney failure.
Caution needed with: lithium, digoxin, blood pressure-lowering drugs.

Arythmol

A white tablet supplied in strengths of 150 mg, 300 mg and used as an anti-arrhythmic drug to treat heart rhythm disturbances

Side effects: nausea, vomiting, dizziness, diarrhoea, constipation, headache, tiredness, skin rash, slow heart rate.
Caution: in the elderly, patients with pace makers, and in patients suffering from heart failure, liver and kidney disorders.
Not to be used for: children, pregnant women, or for patients suffering from uncontrolled heart failure, obstructive lung disease, electrolyte disturbances, some heart rhythm disturbances.
Caution needed with: other anti-arrhythmics, digoxin, warfarin, cimetidine, propanolol, metoprolol, rifampicin.

Atromid-S

A red capsule supplied at a strength of 500 mg and used as a lipid-lowering agent to treat elevated cholesterol.

Caution: in patients with low serum proteins. Your doctor may advise diet and other changes in lifestyle as well as regular blood tests.
Not to be used for: children, pregnant women, or for patients with a history of gall bladder problems or kidney or liver disease.
Caution needed with: anticoagulants, antidiabetic drugs, phenytoin.

Betaloc

A white, scored tablet supplied at strengths of 50 mg, 100 mg and used as a ß-blocker to treat angina, high blood pressure, and as additional treatment for overactive thyroid, migraine,

and heart rhythm defects.

Side effects: cold hands and feet, sleep disturbances, slow heart rate, tiredness, wheezing, heart failure, stomach upset, dry eyes, rash.

Caution: in pregnant women, nursing mothers, and in patients suffering from diabetes, kidney or liver disorders. May need to be withdrawn before surgery. Withdraw gradually. Your doctor may advise additional treatment with digoxin and diuretics.

Not to be used for: children or for patients suffering from heart block or failure, asthma.

Caution needed with: verapamil, antidiabetics, clonidine withdrawal, some anti-arrhythmic drugs and anaesthetics, some antihypertensives, ergotamine, cimetidine, sedatives, sympathomimetics, indomethacin.

Betim *see* **Blocadren**

Bezalip-Mono

A white tablet supplied at a strength of 400 mg and used as a lipid-lowering drug to treat high blood lipids.

Side effects: stomach upset, muscle aches, rash.

Caution: in patients with kidney disease. Your doctor may advise change in diet or lifestyle.

Not to be used for: children, pregnant women, nursing mothers, or for patients suffering from severe kidney or liver disease.

Caution needed with: anticoagulants, antidiabetics, MAOIs.

Blocadren

A blue, scored tablet supplied at a strength of 10 mg and used as a ß-blocker to treat angina, high blood pressure, migraine, and as a treatment following heart attack.

Side effects: cold hands and feet, sleep disturbances, slow heart rate, tiredness, wheezing, heart failure, stomach upset, dry eyes,

rash.
Caution: in pregnant women, nursing mothers, and in patients suffering from diabetes, kidney or liver disorders. May need to be withdrawn before surgery. Withdraw gradually. Your doctor may advise additional treatment with digoxin and diuretics.
Not to be used for: children, or for patients suffering from heart block or failure, asthma.
Caution needed with: verapamil, clonidine withdrawal, some anti-arrhythmic drugs and anaesthetics, some antihypertensives, ergotamine, antidiabetics, cimetidine, sedatives, sympathomimetics, indomethacin.

Britiazim

A white tablet supplied at a strength of 60 mg and used as a calcium antagonist to treat angina.

Side effects: slow heart rate, fluid retention, nausea, rash, headache.
Caution: your doctor may advise regular monitoring of heart rate, especially in elderly patients or in patients suffering from kidney or liver problems.
Not to be used for: children or for pregnant women, or in patients suffering from severe heart conduction defects.
Caution needed with: ß-blockers, digoxin.

Burinex

A white, scored tablet supplied at strengths of 1 mg, 5 mg and used as a diuretic to treat fluid retention associated with congestive heart failure, liver and kidney disease, including the nephrotic syndrome.

Side effects: low blood potassium, stomach discomfort, rash, cramps, blood changes, breast enlargement.
Caution: in pregnant women, nursing mothers, and in patients suffering from kidney or liver damage, diabetes, gout, enlarged prostate, or impaired urination. Your doctor may advise that potassium supplements may be needed.

Not to be used for: children or patients suffering from cirrhosis of the liver.
Caution needed with: lithium, digoxin, antihypertensives, some antibiotics.

Capoten

A mottled white, scored tablet, a mottled white, square tablet, or a mottled white, oval tablet according to strengths of 12.5 mg, 25 mg, 50 mg and used as an ace inhibitor in addition to diuretics and digoxin in the treatment of severe congestive heart failure, high blood pressure.

Side effects: rash, loss of taste, rarely a cough, blood changes, protein in the urine.
Caution: in patients suffering from kidney disease, auto-immune diseases, or patients undergoing anaesthesia, immune suppressant treatment, or who are taking leucopenic drugs. Your doctor may advise regular blood tests.
Not to be used for: pregnant women, nursing mothers, or for patients suffering from some heart valve diseases , kidney disease.
Caution needed with: potassium-sparing diuretics, potassium supplements, non-steroid anti-inflammatory drugs, vasodilators, clonidine, allopurinol, procainamide, probenecid, immunosuppressants.

Capozide

A white, scored tablet used as a diuretic/ACE inhibitor combination to treat high blood pressure.

Side effects: protein in the urine, low blood pressure, rash, loss of taste, blood changes, sensitivity to light, tiredness, rarely a cough.
Caution: in patients undergoing anaesthesia, immune suppressant treatment, or leucopenic drugs and those suffering from kidney disease, auto-immune diseases, diabetes, gout, liver disease.
Not to be used for: children, pregnant women, nursing mothers or for patients suffering from some heart valve diseases, kidney

disease.
Caution needed with: lithium, non-steroid anti-inflammatory drugs, allopurinol, procainamide, probenecid, immunosuppressants, vasodilators, clonidine, potassium-sparing diuretics, potassium supplements, antihypertensives.

Carace

A blue, oval tablet, a white, oval, scored tablet, a yellow, oval, scored tablet, or an orange, oval, scored tablet according to strengths of 2.5 mg, 5 mg, 10 mg, 20 mg and used as an ACE inhibitor to treat congestive heart failure in addition to diuretics and/or digoxin; high blood pressure.

Side effects: low blood pressure, kidney failure, swelling, rash, dizziness, headache, diarrhoea, cough, tiredness, palpitations, chest pains, weakness.
Caution: in nursing mothers and in patients suffering from kidney disease, severe congestive heart failure, or undergoing anaesthesia.
Not to be used for: children, pregnant women, or for patients suffering from some heart valve or lung diseases, or some types of fluid retention.
Caution needed with: potassium-sparing diuretics, potassium supplements, indomethacin, lithium, antihypertensives.

Cardene

A blue/white or blue/pale-blue capsule according to strengths of 20 mg, 30 mg and used as an anti-anginal, antihypertensive drug to treat chronic stable angina, high blood pressure.

Side effects: chest pain, dizziness, headache, swelling of lower limbs, flushing, feeling warm, palpitations and nausea.
Caution: in patients suffering from weak heart, congestive heart failure, or liver or kidney disease.
Not to be used for: children, pregnant women, nursing mothers, or for patients suffering from some heart valve diseases.

Caution needed with: digoxin, cimetidine.

Cedocard Retard

A yellow scored tablet or an orange scored tablet according to strengths of 20 mg, 40 mg and used as a nitrate treatment for angina.

Side effects: headache, flushes, dizziness.
Caution:
Not to be used for: children, or for patients suffering from severe low blood pressure, heart shock, severe anaemia, brain haemorrhage.
Caution needed with:

Cordarone X

A white, scored tablet supplied at strengths of 100 mg, 200 mg and used as an anti-arrhythmic drug to treat heart rhythm disturbances.

Side effects: corneal deposits, sensitivity to light, pulmonary alveolitis, nervous system, liver, heart, eye, and thyroid effects.
Caution: in pregnant women and in patients suffering from heart failure or allergy to iodine. Your doctor may advise thyroid, eyes, heart, and liver tests.
Not to be used for: nursing mothers or for patients suffering from cardiac shock, some types of heart block, thyroid disease.
Caution needed with: calcium antagonists, anticoagulants taken by mouth, ss-blockers, digoxin, anaesthetics, drugs to treat abnormal heart rhythm.

Cordilox

A yellow tablet supplied at strengths of 40 mg, 80 mg, 120 mg and used as a calcium antagonist to treat angina, high blood pressure, heart rhythm disturbances.

Side effects: constipation, flushes.
Caution: in patients suffering from some types of heart conduction block or failure, liver or kidney disease, slow heart rate, or low blood pressure.
Not to be used for: patients suffering from severe heart conduction block, very slow heart rates.
Caution needed with: ss-blockers, quinidine, digoxin.

Corgard

A pale-blue tablet supplied at strengths of 40 mg, 80 mg and used as a ß-blocker to treat heart rhythm disturbances, angina, high blood pressure, additional treatment in thyroid disease, migraine.

Side effects: cold hands and feet, sleep disturbances, slow heart rate, tiredness, wheezing, heart failure, stomach upset, dry eyes, rash.
Caution: in pregnant women, nursing mothers, and in patients suffering from diabetes, kidney or liver disorders, asthma. May need to be withdrawn before surgery. Withdraw gradually. Your doctor may advise additional treatment with diuretics or digoxin.
Not to be used for: children or for patients suffering from heart block or failure.
Caution needed with: verapamil, clonidine withdrawal, some anti-arrhythmic drugs and anaesthetics, reserpine, some antihypertensives, ergotamine, antidiabetics, cimetidine, sedatives, sympathomimetics, indomethacin.

Coversyl

A white tablet supplied at strengths of 2 mg, 4 mg and used as an ace inhibitor to treat high blood pressure, or as an additional treatment for congestive heart failure.

Side effects: rash, itching, flushing, severe allergy, low blood pressure, alteration of taste, nausea, stomach pain, tiredness, feeling of being unwell, headache, mild cough, blood changes,

protein in the urine.
Caution: in patients suffering from kidney disease, or undergoing surgery or anaesthesia.
Not to be used for: children, pregnant women, or nursing mothers.
Caution needed with: other antihypertensives, potassium supplements, some diuretics, lithium, antidepressants.

Deponit

Self-adhesive patches supplied in strengths of 5 mg, 10 mg and used as a nitrate preparation for the prevention of angina.

Side effects: headache, rash, dizziness.
Caution: reduce use of this treatment by replacing with oral nitrates.
Not to be used for: children.
Caution needed with:

Dirythmin SA

A white tablet supplied at a strength of 150 mg and used as an anti-arrhythmic drug to treat abnormal heart rhythm.

Side effects: anticholinergic effects.
Caution: in pregnant women, and in patients suffering from mild heart block, enlarged prostate, glaucoma, retention of urine, low potassium levels, heart failure, kidney or liver failure.
Not to be used for: children or for patients suffering from some types of heart block, heart muscle disease or shock.
Caution needed with: other similar drugs, ß-blockers, potassium-lowering drugs, anticholinergics.

Dyazide

A peach-coloured, scored tablet used as a diuretic to treat high blood pressure, fluid retention.

Side effects: nausea, diarrhoea, cramps, weakness, headache, dry mouth, rash, blood changes.
Caution: in pregnant women, nursing mothers, and in patients suffering from liver or kidney disease, diabetes, electrolyte changes, gout, pancreatitis.
Not to be used for: patients suffering from severe or progressive kidney failure, raised potassium levels, Addison's disease (a disease of the adrenal glands).
Caution needed with: potassium supplements, potassium-sparing diuretics, lithium, digoxin, antihypertensives, indomethacin, ACE inhibitors.

Elantan

A white, scored tablet supplied at strengths of 10 mg, 20 mg, 40 mg and used as a nitrate treatment for the prevention of angina, and in addition to other treatments for congestive heart failure.

Side effects: headache, flushes, dizziness.
Caution:
Not to be used for: children.
Caution needed with:

Frumil

An orange, scored tablet used as a potassium-sparing diuretic to treat fluid retention associated with heart failure, liver and kidney disease.

Side effects: feeling of being unwell, stomach upset, rash, blood changes.
Caution: in pregnant women, nursing mothers, and in patients suffering from liver or kidney disease, diabetes, electrolyte changes, enlarged prostate, gout, or impaired urination.
Not to be used for: children or for patients suffering from liver cirrhosis, progressive kidney failure, raised potassium levels.
Caution needed with: potassium supplements, potassium-sparing

diuretics, lithium, digoxin, some antibiotics (aminoglycosides, cephalosporins), antihypertensives, non-steroid anti-inflammatory drugs, ACE inhibitors.

Hexopal

A white, scored tablet supplied at a strength of 500 mg and used as a vasodilator to treat Raynaud's phenomenon (a condition caused by spasm of the blood vessels), intermittent claudication (difficulty walking caused by circulation disorders).

Side effects:
Caution: in pregnant women.
Not to be used for: children.
Caution needed with:

Hydergine

A white tablet supplied at strengths of 1.5 mg, 4.5 mg and used as a vasodilator as an additional treatment for elderly patients suffering from dementia.

Side effects: stomach upset, flushes, rash, blocked nose, cramps, headache, dizziness, low blood pressure when standing.
Caution: in patients suffering from slow heart rate.
Not to be used for: children
Caution needed with:

Hypovase

A white tablet, orange, scored tablet, or white, scored tablet according to strengths of 500 micrograms, 1 mg, 2 mg, 5 mg and used as a vasodilator to treat congestive heart failure, high blood pressure, Raynaud's phenomenon, additional treatment in urinary obstruction caused by prostate enlargement.

Side effects: loss of consciousness, dizziness, lassitude, dry mouth, blurred vision, rash.
Caution: in patients suffering from fainting when they urinate.
Not to be used for: children.
Caution needed with: antihypertensives.

Inderal LA

A lavender/pink capsule supplied at a strength of 160 mg and used as a ß-blocker to treat angina, high blood pressure, anxiety, migraine, and as an additional treatment for thyrotoxicosis.

Side effects: cold hands and feet, sleep disturbance, slow heart rate, tiredness, wheezing, heart failure, stomach upset, dry eyes, rash.
Caution: in pregnant women, nursing mothers, and in patients suffering from diabetes, kidney or liver disorders, asthma. May need to be withdrawn before surgery. Withdraw gradually. Your doctor may advise additional treatment with diuretics or digoxin. Potassium supplements may be needed.
Not to be used for: children or for patients suffering from heart block or failure.
Caution needed with: verapamil, clonidine withdrawal, some antihypertensives, anaesthetics, reserpine, cimetidine, sedatives, sympathomimetics, indomethacin, antidiabetics, ergotamine.

Innovace

A round white tablet, a white scored, or red or peach, triangular tablet according to strengths of 2.5 mg, 5 mg, 10 mg, 20 mg and used as an ace inhibitor to treat congestive heart failure, high blood pressure.

Side effects: low blood pressure, kidney failure, swelling, rash, headache, tiredness, dizziness, stomach upset, and rarely a cough.
Caution: fluid depletion may cause a marked drop in blood pressure. Dose of diuretic given may need to be reduced. Care in

patients suffering from some kidney diseases, severe heart failure, and in nursing mothers and patients being anaesthetized.
Not to be used for: children, pregnant women, or for patients suffering from some heart defects..
Caution needed with: other antihypertensives, lithium, potassium supplements, potassium-sparing diuretics.

ISMO

A white tablet or white, scored tablet according to strengths of 10 mg, 20 mg, 40 mg and used as a nitrate treatment for angina, and in addition to other treatment for congestive heart failure etc.

Side effects: headache, flushes, dizziness.
Caution:
Not to be used for: children.
Caution needed with:

Isoket Retard

A yellow, scored tablet or an orange, scored tablet according to strengths of 20 mg, 40 mg and used as a nitrate for the prevention of angina.

Side effects: headache, flushes, dizziness.
Caution:
Not to be used for: children or for patients suffering from uncompensated heart shock, severe low blood pressure, anaemia, brain haemorrhage.
Caution needed with:

Isordil

A white, scored tablet supplied at strengths of 10 mg, 30 mg and used as a nitrate for the prevention of angina, acute congestive heart failure.

Side effects: headache, flushes, dizziness, may make chest pain worse.
Caution: heart function should be checked in the case of heart failure.
Not to be used for: children.
Caution needed with:

Istin

White tablets supplied at strengths of 5 mg, 10 mg, and used to treat high blood pressure and poor blood supply to the heart (when associated with angina).

Side effects: headache, fluid retention, tiredness, nausea, flushing, dizziness.
Caution: in pregnant women, nursing mothers, and in patients suffering from liver disorder.
Not to be used for: children.
Caution needed with:

Kinidin Durules

A white tablet supplied at a strength of 250 mg and used as an anti-arrhythmic drug to treat abnormal heart rhythm.

Side effects: allergies, liver disease, quinine excess, heart muscle toxicity.
Caution: in patients with congestive heart failure, low blood pressure, rapid heart rate, low potassium levels.
Not to be used for: children, pregnant women, or for patients suffering from acute infection, myasthenia gravis (a muscle disorder), severe heart disease.
Caution needed with: digoxin, anticoagulants, antihypertensives, cimetidine.

Lanoxin

A white, scored tablet supplied at a strength of 0.25 mg used

as a heart muscle stimulant for digitalis treatment especially heart failure.

Side effects: stomach upset, visual changes, and heart rhythm changes.

Caution: the elderly and in patients suffering from heart block, potassium deficiency, lung disease, kidney and thyroid disorders.

Not to be used for: raised calcium levels, rapid heart rate, some heart muscle disorders.

Caution needed with: calcium injections and tablets, some diuretics, quinidine, lithium, antacids, antibiotics, other heart muscle stimulants.

Lasix

A white, scored tablet supplied at strengths of 20 mg, 40 mg and used as a diuretic to treat fluid retention, high blood pressure.

Side effects: stomach upset, rash, gout.

Caution: in pregnant women, nursing mothers, and in patients suffering from liver or kidney disease, gout, diabetes, enlarged prostate, impaired urination.

Not to be used for: patients suffering from liver cirrhosis.

Caution needed with: digoxin, lithium, aminoglycoside and cephalosporin antibiotics, antihypertensives, non-steroid anti-inflammatory drugs.

Lipostat

A pink, oblong tablet supplied at a strength of 10 mg, 20 mg, and used as a lipid-lowering agent to treat raised cholesterol.

Side effects: rash, muscle pain, headache, chest pain, nausea, vomiting, diarrhoea, tiredness.

Caution: in patients with a history of liver disease. Your doctor may advise regular tests during treatment.

Not to be used for: children, pregnant women, nursing mothers, or for patients suffering from liver disease.

Caution needed with: cholestyramine, colestipol.

Lopid

A white/maroon capsule and white oval tablet supplied at strengths of 300 mg, 600 mg and used as a lipid-lowering agent to treat raised lipid levels.

Side effects: stomach upset, rashes, impotence, headache, dizziness, painful extremities, muscle aches, blurred vision.
Caution: your doctor may advise a lipid check; blood count, and liver function should be checked before treatment; eyes, blood, and serum should be checked regularly.
Not to be used for: pregnant women, nursing mothers, alcoholics, or patients suffering from gallstones or liver disease.
Caution needed with: anticoagulants.

Lopresor

A pink, scored tablet or a pale-blue, scored tablet according to strengths of 50 mg, 100 mg and used as a ß-blocker to treat angina, for the prevention of heart muscle damage, high blood pressure, and as an additional treatment in thyrotoxicosis, migraine.

Side effects: cold hands and feet, sleep disturbance, slow heart rate, tiredness, wheezing, heart failure, stomach upset, dry eyes, rash.
Caution: in pregnant women, nursing mothers, and in patients suffering from diabetes, kidney or liver disorders, asthma. May need to be withdrawn before surgery. Withdraw gradually. Your doctor may advise additional treatment with diuretics or digoxin.
Not to be used for: children, or for patients suffering from heart block or failure.
Caution needed with: verapamil, clonidine withdrawal, some anti-arrhythmic drugs and anaesthetics, reserpine, some antihypertensives, ergotamine, cimetidine, sedatives, antidiabetics, sympathomimetics, indomethacin.

Lurselle

A white, scored tablet supplied at a strength of 250 mg and used as a lipid-lowering agent to treat elevated lipids.

Side effects: diarrhoea, stomach upset.
Caution: in patients suffering from heart disorders. Cease treatment 6 months before a planned pregnancy.
Not to be used for: children, pregnant women, or nursing mothers.
Caution needed with:

Maxepa

A clear, soft capsule used as a lipid-lowering agent to treat elevated lipids.

Side effects: nausea, belching
Caution: in patients suffering from bleeding disorders.
Not to be used for: children.
Caution needed with: anticoagulants

Mexitil

A red/purple capsule or a red capsule according to strengths of 50 mg, 200 mg and used as an anti-arrhythmic treatment for abnormal heart rhythm.

Side effects: stomach and brain disorders, low blood pressure.
Caution: in patients suffering from nerve conduction defects in the heart, low blood pressure, heart, liver, or kidney failure, Parkinson's disease.
Not to be used for: children.
Caution needed with:

Moduretic

A peach-coloured, diamond-shaped, scored tablet used as a potassium-sparing diuretic to treat high blood pressure,

congestive heart failure, liver cirrhosis with fluid retention.

Side effects: rash, sensitivity to light, blood changes, gout.
Caution: in patients suffering from diabetes, electrolyte changes, gout, kidney or liver damage
Not to be used for: children, pregnant women, nursing mothers, or for patients suffering from raised potassium levels, progressive or severe kidney failure.
Caution needed with: potassium supplements, potassium-sparing diuretics, digoxin, lithium, antihypertensives, ACE inhibitors.

Monit

A white, scored tablet supplied at a strength of 20 mg and used as a nitrate for the prevention of angina.

Side effects: headache, flushes, dizziness.
Caution:
Not to be used for: children.
Caution needed with:

Monocor

A pink tablet or a white tablet according to strengths of 5 mg, 10 mg and used as a ß-blocker to treat angina, high blood pressure.

Side effects: cold hands and feet, sleep disturbance, slow heart rate, tiredness, wheezing, heart failure, stomach upset, dry eyes, rash.
Caution: in pregnant women, nursing mothers, and in patients suffering from diabetes, kidney or liver disorders, asthma. May need to be withdrawn before surgery. Withdraw gradually. Your doctor may advise additional treatment with diuretics or digoxin.
Not to be used for: children or for patients suffering from heart block or failure..
Caution needed with: verapamil, clonidine withdrawal, some anti-arrhythmic drugs and anaesthetics, reserpine, some antihypertensives, ergotamine, cimetidine, sedatives,

antidiabetics, sympathomimetics, indomethacin.

Natrilix

A pink tablet supplied at a strength of 2.5 mg and used as a vasorelaxant to treat high blood pressure.

Side effects: low potassium level, nausea, headache.
Caution: in pregnant women and in patients suffering from severe kidney or liver disease.
Not to be used for: children, nursing mothers, or for patients suffering from severe liver failure or who have recently suffered a stroke.
Caution needed with: diuretics, anti-arrhythmics, digoxin, steroids, laxatives, lithium.

Navidrex

A white, scored tablet supplied at a strength of 0.5 mg and used as a diuretic to treat heart failure, fluid retention, high blood pressure.

Side effects: rash, sensitivity to light, blood changes, stomach upset, pancreatitis, headache, dizziness, tingling sensation, electrolyte and metabolic disturbances, lung and liver changes.
Caution: the elderly, and in patients suffering from diabetes, kidney or liver disease, gout, high blood lipid levels. Potassium supplements may be needed.
Not to be used for: pregnant women, nursing mothers, or for patients suffering from inability to produce urine or severe kidney failure, low sodium or potassium levels, Addison's disease, high calcium or uric acid levels.
Caution needed with: digoxin, lithium, antihypertensives, non-steroid anti-inflammatory drugs.

Nimotop

A white tablet supplied at a strength of 30 mg and used to

treat symptoms following stroke.

Side effects: low blood pressure, flushing, headache, changes in heart rate.
Caution: in pregnant women and in patients suffering from fluid retention or high blood pressure in the brain, kidney damage.
Not to be used for: children.
Caution needed with: ß-blockers, other similar drugs.

Nitrolingual

An aerosol used as a nitrate for the prevention and treatment of angina.

Side effects: headache, flushes, dizziness
Caution: do not inhale spray.
Not to be used for: children.
Caution needed with:

Olbetam

A red-brown/dark-pink capsule supplied at a strength of 250 mg and used as a lipid-lowering agent to treat elevated lipids.

Side effects: flushes, rash, redness, stomach upset, headache, general feeling of being unwell.
Caution:
Not to be used for: children, pregnant women, nursing mothers, or for patients suffering from stomach ulcer.
Caution needed with:

Opilon

A yellow tablet supplied at a strength of 40 mg and used as a vasodilator to treat Raynaud's syndrome.

Side effects: nausea, diarrhoea, vertigo, headache.
Caution: in patients suffering from diabetes, angina, recent heart attack.

Not to be used for: children, pregnant women, nursing mothers, or for patients who are sensitive to thymoxamine.
Caution needed with: tricyclic antidepressants, antihypertensives.

Paroven

A yellow capsule supplied at a strength of 250 mg and used as a vein constrictor to treat ankle swelling, varicose veins.

Side effects: stomach disturbances, flushes, headache.
Caution:
Not to be used for: children.
Caution needed with:

Praxilene

A pink capsule supplied at a strength of 100 mg and used as a blood vessel dilator to treat cerebral and peripheral vascular problems

Side effects: nausea, stomach pain.
Caution:
Not to be used for: children.
Caution needed with:

Questran

A powder in a sachet used as a lipid-lowering agent to treat elevated lipids, and to relieve some cases of diarrhoea and itching.

Side effects: constipation, vitamin K deficiency.
Caution: in pregnant women, nursing mothers, and patients on long-term treatment should take Vitamin A, D, K supplements.
Not to be used for: children under 6 years or for patients suffering from complete biliary blockage.
Caution needed with: digoxin, antibiotics, diuretics; allow 1 hour between treatment and any other drugs.

Ronicol
(Roche)

A white, scored tablet supplied at a strength of 25 mg and used as a vasodilator to treat poor circulation.

Side effects: flushes.
Caution: care in long-term treatment of diabetics.
Not to be used for: children.
Caution needed with:

Rythmodan

A yellow/green capsule or a white capsule according to strengths of 100 mg, 150 mg and used as an anti-arrhythmic treatment for abnormal heart rhythm

Side effects: anticholinergic effects, rarely jaundice, mood changes, low blood sugar.
Caution: in pregnant women, and in patients suffering from heart conduction block, heart,liver, and kidney failure, enlarged prostate, glaucoma, urine retention, low potassium levels.
Not to be used for: for patients suffering from severe heart conduction block, heart failure.
Caution needed with: ß-blockers, diuretics, anticholinergics, other anti-arrhythmics.

Sectral

A buff/white capsule or a buff/pink capsule according to strengths of 100 mg, 200 mg, or a white tablet supplied at a strength of 400 mg and used as a ß-blocker to treat angina, abnormal heart rhythm, or high blood pressure.

Side effects: cold hands and feet, sleep disturbance, slow heart rate, tiredness, wheezing, heart failure, stomach upset, dry eyes, rash.
Caution: in pregnant women, nursing mothers, and in patients suffering from diabetes, kidney or liver disorders, asthma. May

need to be withdrawn before surgery. Withdraw gradually. Your doctor may advise additional treatment with diuretics or digoxin. *Not to be used for:* children or for patients suffering from heart block or failure.

Caution needed with: verapamil, clonidine withdrawal, some anti-arrhythmic drugs and anaesthetics, reserpine, some antihypertensives, ergotamine, cimetidine, sedatives, antidiabetics, sympathomimetics, indomethacin.

Sorbid SA

A red/yellow capsule or a red/clear capsule according to strengths of 20 mg, 40 mg and used as a nitrate for the prevention of angina.

Side effects: flushes, headache, nausea.
Caution:
Not to be used for: children.
Caution needed with:

Staril

A white, diamond-shaped tablet supplied at strengths of 10 mg, 20 mg, and used as an ACE-inhibitor, to treat high blood pressure.

Side effects: dizziness, cough, stomach upset, palpitations, chest pain, rash, muscle/bone pain, tiredness, taste disturbance, severe allergy.
Caution: in patients suffering from liver or kidney damage, congestive heart failure, salt or body fluid depletion.
Not to be used for: children, pregnant women, nursing mothers.
Caution needed with: some diuretics, potassium supplements, non-steroid anti-inflammatory drugs, antacids, lithium, antihypertensives.

Suscard Buccal

A white tablet supplied at strengths of 1 mg, 2 mg, 3 mg, 5 mg and used as a nitrate to treat angina, acute heart failure, congestive heart failure.

Side effects: headache, flushes.
Caution:
Not to be used for: children.
Caution needed with:

Sustac

A pink, mottled tablet supplied at strengths of 2.6 mg, 6.4 mg, 10 mg and used as a nitrate for the prevention of angina.

Side effects: headache, flushes.
Caution:
Not to be used for: children.
Caution needed with:

Tambocor

A white, scored tablet supplied at strengths of 50 mg, 100 mg and used as an anti-arrhythmic treatment for abnormal heart rhythm.

Side effects: dizziness, disturbed vision, sensitivity to light, nausea, vomiting, liver disturbance, tingling, unsteadiness.
Caution: in pregnant women, patients fitted with pacemakers, and in patients suffering from kidney or liver problems, some heart muscle disorders. Your doctor may advise blood tests to check electrolytes and blood levels.
Not to be used for: children and for patients suffering from some heart disorders.
Caution needed with: digoxin and some other heart drugs.

Tenormin

An orange capsule supplied at a strength of 100 mg and used as a ß-blocker to treat angina, abnormal heart rhythm, high blood pressure.

Side effects: cold hands and feet, sleep disturbance, slow heart rate, tiredness, wheezing, heart failure, stomach upset, dry eyes, rash.

Caution: in pregnant women, nursing mothers, and in patients suffering from diabetes, kidney or liver disorders, asthma. May need to be withdrawn before surgery. Withdraw gradually. Your doctor may advise additional treatment with diuretics or digoxin.

Not to be used for: children or for patients suffering from heart block or failure.

Caution needed with: verapamil, clonidine withdrawal, some anti-arrhythmic drugs and anaesthetics, reserpine, some antihypertensives, ergotamine, cimetidine, sedatives, antidiabetics, sympathomimetics, indomethacin.

Tildiem Retard

A tablet supplied at strengths of 90 mg, 120 mg and used as a calcium antagonist to treat angina and high blood pressure.

Side effects: nausea, headache, rash, slow heart rate, ankle swelling, heart conduction block.

Caution: your doctor may advise that the heart rate be measured regularly especially in the elderly and in patients suffering from kidney or liver problems.

Not to be used for: children, pregnant women or for patients suffering from slow heart rate or heart block.

Caution needed with: ß-blockers, digoxin.

Tonocard

A yellow tablet supplied at a strength of 400 mg and used as an anti-arrhythmic drug to treat abnormal heart rhythms.

Side effects: tremor, dizziness, stomach upset, white cell changes, SLE (a multisystem disorder).
Caution: in the elderly and pregnant women, and in patients suffering from severe liver or kidney disease or uncompensated heart failure.
Not to be used for: children or patients suffering from heart conduction block.

Trandate

An orange tablet supplied at strengths of 50 mg, 100 mg, 200 mg, 400 mg and used as an alpha- and ß-blocker to treat angina with high blood pressure, high blood pressure of pregnancy.

Side effects: cold hands and feet, sleep disturbance, slow heart rate, tiredness, wheezing, heart failure, stomach upset, dry eyes, skin rash.
Caution: in pregnant women, nursing mothers, and in patients suffering from diabetes, kidney or liver disorders, asthma. May need to be withdrawn before surgery. Withdraw gradually. Your doctor may advise additional treatment with diuretics or digoxin.
Not to be used for: children or for patients suffering from heart block or failure.
Caution needed with: verapamil, clonidine withdrawal, some anti-arrhythmic drugs and anaesthetics, reserpine, some antihypertensives, ergotamine, cimetidine, sedatives, antidiabetics, sympathomimetics, indomethacin.

Transiderm-Nitro

Patches supplied at strengths of 5 mg, 10 mg and used as a nitrate for the prevention of angina and vein inflammation.

Side effects: headache, rash, dizziness.
Caution: in patients suffering from heart failure or who have recently had a heart attack. The treatment should be reduced gradually and replaced with decreasing doses of an oral nitrate.
Not to be used for: children, or for patients suffering from low

blood pressure, raised pressure in the brain, or heart muscle weakness.
Caution needed with:

Trasicor

A white tablet, a beige tablet, or an orange tablet according to strengths of 20 mg, 40 mg, 80 mg, 160 mg and used as a ß-blocker to treat angina, abnormal heart rhythm, high blood pressure, anxiety.

Side effects: cold hands and feet, sleep disturbance, slow heart rate, tiredness, wheezing, heart failure, stomach upset, dry eyes, skin rash.
Caution: in pregnant women, nursing mothers, and in patients suffering from diabetes, kidney or liver disorders, asthma. May need to be withdrawn before surgery. Withdraw gradually. Your doctor may advise additional treatment with diuretics or digoxin.
Not to be used for: patients suffering from heart block or failure.
Caution needed with: verapamil, clonidine withdrawal, some anti-arrhythmic drugs and anaesthetics, reserpine, some antihypertensives, ergotamine, cimetidine, sedatives, antidiabetics, sympathomimetics, indomethacin.

Trental

A pink, oblong tablet supplied at a strength of 400 mg and used as a blood cell altering drug to treat peripheral vascular problems.

Side effects: stomach disturbances, vertigo, flushes.
Caution: in patients suffering from low blood pressure, severe heart artery disease, kidney disease.
Not to be used for: children.
Caution needed with: antihypertensives.

Zestril

A white, pink, or red tablet according to strengths of 2.5 mg, 5 mg, 10 mg, 20 mg and used as an ace inhibitor to treat congestive heart failure in addition to diuretics and digoxin, high blood pressure.

Side effects: low blood pressure, kidney failure, rash, dizziness,diarrhoea, cough, tiredness, palpitations, chest pain, weakness, headache, nausea, severe allergy.
Caution: in nursing mothers and in patients suffering from kidney disease, congestive heart failure.
Not to be used for: children, pregnant women, or for patients suffering from some heart diseases or previous ellergy to ACE inhibitors.
Caution needed with: diuretics, potassium supplements, indomethacin, antihypertensives.

Zocor

A peach-coloured, oval tablet or a tan, oval tablet according to strengths of 10 mg, 20 mg and used as a lipid-lowering agent to treat raised cholesterol.

Side effects: headache, indigestion, diarrhoea, tiredness, rash, constipation, wind, nausea, muscle weakness.
Caution: in patients suffering from liver disease. Your doctor may advise liver and eye checks.
Not to be used for: pregnant women, nursing mothers, or for patients suffering from liver disease.
Caution needed with: digoxin, some anticoagulants, cyclosporin, gemifibrozil, nicotinic acid.

Over-the-counter Medicines

Cedocard Retard

A yellow scored tablet or an orange scored tablet according to strengths of 20 mg, 40 mg and used as a nitrate treatment for angina.

Side effects: headache, flushes, dizziness.
Caution:
Not to be used for: children, or for patients suffering from severe low blood pressure, heart shock, severe anaemia, brain haemorrhage..
Caution needed with:

Deponit

Self-adhesive patches supplied in strengths of 5 mg, 10 mg and used as a nitrate preparation for the prevention of angina.

Side effects: headache, rash, dizziness.
Caution: reduce use of this treatment by replacing with oral nitrates.
Not to be used for: children.
Caution needed with:

Elantan

A white, scored tablet supplied at strengths of 10 mg, 20 mg, 40 mg and used as a nitrate treatment for the prevention of angina, and in addition to other treatments for congestive heart failure.

Side effects: headache, flushes, dizziness.
Caution:
Not to be used for: children.
Caution needed with:

ISMO

A white tablet or white, scored tablet according to strengths of 10 mg, 20 mg, 40 mg and used as a nitrate treatment for angina, and in addition to other treatment for congestive heart failure etc.

Side effects: headache, flushes, dizziness.
Caution:
Not to be used for: children.
Caution needed with:

Isoket Retard

A yellow, scored tablet or an orange, scored tablet according to strengths of 20 mg, 40 mg and used as a nitrate for the prevention of angina.

Side effects: headache, flushes, dizziness.
Caution:
Not to be used for: children or for patients suffering from un-compensated heart shock, severe low blood pressure, anaemia, brain haemorrhage.
Caution needed with:

Isordil

A white, scored tablet supplied at strengths of 10 mg, 30 mg and used as a nitrate for the prevention of angina, acute congestive heart failure.

Side effects: headache, flushes, dizziness, may make chest pain worse.
Caution: heart function should be checked in the case of heart failure.
Not to be used for: children.
Caution needed with:

Nitrolingual

An aerosol used as a nitrate for the prevention and treatment of angina.

Side effects: headache, flushes, dizziness
Caution: do not inhale spray.
Not to be used for: children.
Caution needed with:

Sorbitrate

A yellow, oval, scored tablet or a blue, oval scored tablet according to strengths of 10 mg, 20 mg and used as a nitrate for the prevention of angina.

Side effects: flushes, headache, dizziness.
Caution:
Not to be used for: children.
Caution needed with:

Suscard Buccal

A white tablet supplied at strengths of 1 mg, 2 mg, 3 mg, 5 mg and used as a nitrate to treat angina, acute heart failure, congestive heart failure.

Side effects: headache, flushes.
Caution:
Not to be used for: children.
Caution needed with:

Sustac

A pink, mottled tablet supplied at strengths of 2.6 mg, 6.4 mg, 10 mg and used as a nitrate for the prevention of angina.

Side effects: headache, flushes.
Caution:
Not to be used for: children.

Caution needed with:

Transiderm-Nitro

Patches supplied at strengths of 5 mg, 10 mg and used as a nitrate for the prevention of angina and vein inflammation.

Side effects: headache, rash, dizziness.
Caution: in patients suffering from heart failure or who have recently had a heart attack. The treatment should be reduced gradually and replaced with decreasing doses of an oral nitrate.
Not to be used for: children, or for patients suffering from low blood pressure, raised pressure in the brain, or heart muscle weakness.
Caution needed with:

Vascardin

A white, scored tablet supplied at a strength of 10 mg, 30 mg and used as a nitrate treatment for angina, and as an additional treatment for congestive heart failure.

Side effects: headache, flushes.
Caution:
Not to be used for: children.
Caution needed with:

Chapter 2

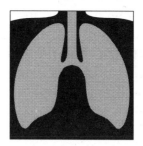

Lung Diseases

Please refer to 'Important Advice' on page 4 at the beginning of this book; and remember, if you are in any doubt, consult a physician.

The purpose of the respiratory system is to deliver oxygen from the atmosphere via the lungs into the circulation where it can then be passed to the tissues and function as a fuel for the activity of the organs of the body. The main lung disorders, such as asthma or bronchitis, emphysema or pneumonia, are caused because this system is open to attack from the outside air, notably from infection and pollutants. Self-pollution – cigarette smoking – and industrial pollution are the most common causes of lung disease, and increasing numbers of allergies are being seen that contribute to asthma.

Lung cancer is the most common cancer in

Western societies and is linked largely to cigarette smoking. The challenge for prevention and treatment of lung diseases in the twenty-first century is to deliver oxygen via the trachea, bronchi, and lungs, but limit the delivery of pollution. If this were achieved, lung disease would decrease dramatically.

Lung cancer
(carcinoma of the bronchus, squamous
cell carcinoma, adenocarcinoma, small cell
carcinoma, oatcell carcinoma)

Lung cancer, or carcinoma of the bronchus, is the commonest form of cancer. The vast majority of lung cancers occur in cigarette smokers, and passive smoking may be a factor in causing lung diseases. The appearance of mesothelioma (cancer of the lung lining) may occur 20-30 years after exposure to asbestos.

Main symptoms
Persistent cough, weight loss, coughing up blood, repeated chest infections, symptoms of secondary deposits particularly in the brain and bones. Some unusual presentations of lung cancer can occur with fluid retention and joint symptoms.

Action
Diagnosis should be made early. This condition may sometimes be picked up on routine chest X-ray. Examination of sputum for malignant cells can sometimes diagnose this condition.

Tests
Tests involve sputum cytology for malignant cells, chest X-ray, bronchoscopy with biopsy, bone scan, brain scan, routine blood tests.

Medications and treatment
Some lung cancers are amenable to surgery; others respond to chemotherapy and radiotherapy. Infections should be treated with appropriate antibiotics or antifungal medications.

Further advice
Lung cancer is best prevented by avoiding cigarette smoking. If you have suffered from lung cancer and been treated successfully, you should maintain a healthy lifestyle and not smoke.

Asthma

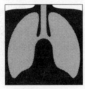 Asthma is a condition caused by spasm of the muscles in the bronchial tree (the tubes taking air from the mouth to the lungs) resulting in wheezing. Asthma may occur in adults or children and may be precipitated by allergic factors, cold, exercise, stress, or dust inhalation.

Symptoms
Typically coughing and wheezing, the cough often producing thick sputum.

Action
Severe asthma (status asthmaticus) is a medical emergency and help should be sought urgently. Less severe asthma may respond to humidification of the room, rest, and avoidance of precipitating factors.

Tests
Tests for asthma include lung function tests, particularly peak flow rate, chest X-ray, allergy tests.

Medications and treatment
Asthma treatments include bronchodilators and steroids. Anti-allergy treatments are also helpful.

Further advice
Where possible, you should avoid precipitating factors, and take

medications to prevent asthma attack rather than wait until it is well established.

Associated conditions
Asthma may be associated with hay fever and eczema and may run in allergic (atopic) families.

Acute lower respiratory infections ♥♥♥ (pleurisy, pneumonia, tracheitis, acute bronchitis)

These acute chest infections may be caused by bacteria, viruses, or fungi. They may be secondary to other respiratory infections (*see* ear, nose, and throat disorders).

Main symptoms
Cough with production of sputum, chest pain, fever, weakness, and associated debility with vomiting. Conditions such as pleurisy have a chest pain which is noticeably worse on taking a deep breath, and pleurisy may co-exist with pneumonia. The conditions may affect one lobe of the lung or all the lobes of both lungs (double pneumonia).

Action
Severe infections with severe fatigue and prostration require immediate medical treatment. General advice includes resting the patient in bed, avoiding smoking, humidifying the room, and maintaining a sensible room temperature — approximately 20 °C (68 °F). Patients should not be too warm.

Tests
Investigations for suspected pneumonia and other lower respiratory

infections include chest X-ray, blood tests including white cell count and sedimentation rate, culture of sputum for bacteria, and fungal swabs from the upper respiratory tract.

Medications and treatment
Antibiotics, including amoxycillin, ampicillin, cephalexin, Ciproxin, erythromycin, penicillin, Septrin, tetracycline, and trimethoprim, can be used for bacterial infections. Antifungal agents are used for fungal infections. Viral infections will not respond to such treatment and need general supportive care, including oxygen, humidifiers, and possibly bronchodilators.

Further advice
You may suffer from repeated lower respiratory tract infections. You should avoid smoking and contact with other irritants such as dust which may provoke chronic lower respiratory infections.

Chronic lower respiratory infections ♥♥ (including chronic bronchitis, emphysema, and bronchiectasis)

 Chronic lower respiratory infections may follow on from lung damage caused by repeated attacks of acute lower respiratory infections. They are more likely where there is poor hygiene and living conditions, cigarette smoking, poor nutrition, and a family history of such infections. Bronchiectasis is a condition where there are lung abscesses, and emphysema where there is breakdown of lung material. The most common is chronic bronchitis, and this is commonly caused by cigarette smoking.

Main symptoms
Chronic cough with overproduction of infected sputum. In addition,

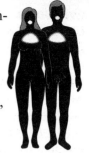

shortness of breath, repeated fevers, chest pain, general fatigue, and malaise are also symptoms.

Action
You should seek medical advice to treat the acute exacerbation of chronic bronchitis, bronchiectasis, and emphysema.

Tests
Tests for chronic lower respiratory infections include chest X-ray, sputum culture for bacteria and fungi, ECG, routine blood tests for white count and sedimentation rate.

Medications and treatment
You may need long-term oxygen therapy. In addition, you may require long-term antibiotic treatment, including amoxycillin, ampicillin, cephalexin, Ciproxin, erythromycin, penicillin, Septrin, tetracycline, and trimethoprim, with additional cover during acute exacerbations. Bronchodilators based on aminophylline or salbutamol may be helpful.

Further advice
You should stop smoking, take regular exercise, eat a healthy diet, and improve living conditions where possible to avoid dust, damp, and cold.

Pneumothorax

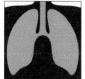 Pneumothorax is a condition in which air enters the space between the lung and the chest wall. Pneumothorax may be a spontaneous event arising from rupture of the lung or it may occur as a result of trauma. In the latter case, a dangerous type of pneumothorax may occur with increasing pressure and compression on the lung.

Symptoms

The classic symptom of pneumothorax is a sudden onset of severe chest pain and breathlessness. This can occur in otherwise fit and healthy individuals with no predisposing factors, although it may be exacerbated by changes in air pressure, such as during air travel or deep-sea diving. The patient may collapse through the shortness of breath and the pain. Pneumothorax caused by trauma will clearly also appear with symptoms of trauma itself, e.g. puncturing wound of the chest, gunshot wound, and so on.

Action

Immediate medical attention is required. Trained paramedics may wish to attempt to relieve the pressure caused by pneumothorax in an emergency situation by application of a needle which releases air from the chest and relieves lung compression.

Tests

Investigations for pneumothorax include chest X-ray, bronchoscopy, pleural biopsy.

Medications and treatment

The treatment of pneumothorax is surgical, but short-term oxygen and antibiotics may be required. Trauma needs to be attended to in its own right.

Further advice

If you are prone to recurrent spontaneous pneumothorax, you should avoid changes of barometric pressure or consider having preventative operations to obliterate the space between the lung and the chest wall.

Associated conditions

Haemothorax or haemopneumothorax is an additional complication of this condition where blood enters the space between the lung and the chest wall.

Tuberculosis ♥♥♥♥

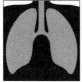 Tuberculosis is an infection by the tubercle bacillus and it usually causes diseases of the lungs although it may affect other parts of the body including the brain, the gut, and adrenal glands. It is associated with poor general nutrition and hygiene.

Symptoms
These include weight loss, fever, cough, production of sputum and blood.

Action
If it is suspected, tuberculosis must be fully investigated and treated under medical supervision.

Investigations
These include chest X-ray, sputum tests for tubercle bacilli, biopsy of suspected glands, stool tests for possible bacilli, blood tests particularly for changes in white cells and sedimentation rate. Investigations of tuberculous meningitis or cerebral tubercle would include lumbar puncture and brain scan.

Medications and treatment
There is a number of antituberculous drugs available, including Myambutol, Mynah, Rifadin, Rifater, Rifinah, Rimactane, Rimactazid, Zinamide, and streptomycin which is given by injection. Patients should be encouraged to rest, stop smoking, and, where possible, be isolated from susceptible contacts.

Further advice
If you are suffering from conditions that lower the immunity, such HIV infection or AIDS, you may also contract tuberculosis. You should be given appropriate supportive and immunological treatment. Tuberculosis can be prevented by a suitable programme of screening and vaccination as well as by pasteurization of milk and

improved social and housing conditions. Alcohol and diabetes may lower the immunity and predispose to tuberculosis. Occasionally tuberculous pleurisy, tuberculous laryngitis, or tuberculous infections of the gynaecological tract may occur.

Sarcoidosis

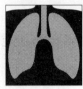 Sarcoidosis is a granulomatous disease whereby granulomata appear in various organs, including the lymph nodes, lungs, liver, spleen, eyes, bones. Granulomata are internal 'abscesses' sometimes of unknown cause. The cause of sarcoidosis not known.

Symptoms
There may be no symptoms with sarcoidosis but, occasionally, it appears with chest symptoms due to enlargement of lymph nodes in the chest. There may also be fever, arthritis, eye symptoms such as uveitis, skin rash, liver failure, enlargement of the spleen, or changes in the heart. Sarcoidosis may cause elevation of calcium in the blood or urine and so it may appear with thirst and frequency of urination or kidney stones.

Action
Sarcoidosis needs to be investigated and managed in a specialist centre.

Tests
These include chest X-ray, Kveim test, blood test measuring sedimentation rate, calcium levels, liver function, lung function tests, eye tests and examination, cardiac investigation.

Medications and treatment
The main drugs used for treatment of sarcoidosis are steroids.

Patients may not require any steroids but, occasionally, maintenance doses of Prednisolone of about 5 to 20 mg a day are required.

Further advice

If you are suffering from sarcoidosis, you may be vulnerable to infections, particularly if you are taking steroids. Therefore, you should try to maintain a good standard of general health and look out for any long-term side effects of the steroids.

Prescription Medicines

Alupent

An off-white, scored tablet supplied at a strength of 20 mg and used as an anti-asthma drug to treat bronchial spasm brought on by chronic bronchitis, asthma, emphysema.

Side effects: abnormal heart rhythm, tremor, nervous tension, headache, dilation of the veins, rapid heart rate.
Caution: in diabetics and patients suffering from high blood pressure.
Not to be used for: patients suffering from cardiac asthma, acute heart disease, overactive thyroid gland.
Caution needed with: MAOIs, tricyclics, sympathomimetics.

Atrovent

An inhaler used as an anticholinergic preparation to relieve blocked airways especially as a result of bronchitis.

Side effects: dry mouth, constipation, retention of urine.
Caution: in patients suffering from enlarged prostate, glaucoma.
Not to be used for:
Caution needed with:

Becotide

An aerosol supplied at a strength of 50 micrograms, 100 micrograms, 200 micrograms and used as a steroid to treat bronchial asthma.

Side effects: hoarseness, thrush.
Caution: in pregnant women, in patients transferring from steroids taken by mouth, or in patients suffering from tubercular lungs.
Not to be used for:
Caution needed with:

Berotec

An aerosol supplied at a strength of 0.1 mg and 0.2 mg and used as a bronchodilator to treat bronchial asthma, emphysema, bronchitis.

Side effects: headache, dilation of the blood vessels, nervous tension.
Caution: in pregnant women and in patients suffering from heart disease, angina, abnormal heart rhythms, high blood pressure, overactive thyroid gland.
Not to be used for:
Caution needed with: sympathomimetics.

Biophylline

A syrup used as a bronchodilator to treat bronchial spasm.

Side effects: rapid heart rate, stomach upset, headache, sleeplessness, nausea, abnormal rhythms.
Caution: in the elderly, pregnant women, nursing mothers, and in patients suffering from heart or liver disease, or peptic ulcer.
Not to be used for:
Caution needed with: cimetidine, erythromycin, ciprofloxacin, interferon, diuretics, steroids, some other bronchodilators.

Brelomax

A white, scored tablet supplied at a strength of 2 mg, and used as a bronchodilator to prevent and control bronchial spasm in conditions where airways are obstructed (such as asthma).

Side effects: low potassium levels, shaking, rapid or forceful heartbeat, mild headache, or nervous tension.
Caution: in patients suffering from diabetes, overactive thyroid, high blood pressure, epilepsy or heart/circulation disorder.
Not to be used for: children under 10 years, or for patients suffering from kidney or liver failure, other liver disorders.
Caution needed with: steroids, theophylline.

Bricanyl

A white, scored tablet supplied at a strength of 5 mg and used as a bronchodilator to treat bronchial spasm brought on by asthma, bronchitis, or emphysema.

Side effects: shaking of the hands, dilation of the blood vessels, tension, headache.
Caution: in pregnant women and in diabetics, or in patients suffering from high blood pressure, abnormal heart rhythms, heart muscle disorders, overactive thyroid gland, angina.
Not to be used for:
Caution needed with: sympathomimetics.

Bronchodil

An aerosol supplied at a strength of 0.5 mg and used as a bronchodilator to treat bronchial asthma, bronchitis, emphysema.

Side effects: shaking of hands, nervous tension, headache, dilation of the blood vessels.
Caution: in pregnant women and in patients suffering from heart muscle disorders, angina, high blood pressure, abnormal heart

rhythms, overactive thyroid gland.
Not to be used for: children under 6 years.
Caution needed with: sympathomimetics.

CAM

A syrup used as a bronchodilator to treat bronchial spasm.

Side effects: nervousness, sleeplessness, restlessness, dry mouth, cold hands and feet, abnormal heart rhythms.
Caution: in patients suffering from diabetes.
Not to be used for: infants under 3 months or for patients suffering from heart disease,high blood pressure, overactive thyroid gland.
Caution needed with: MAOIs

Choledyl

A pink tablet or a yellow tablet according to strengths 100 mg, 200 mg and used as a bronchodilator to treat bronchial spasm brought on by chronic bronchitis or asthma.

Side effects: rapid heart rate, sleeplessness, nausea, change in heart rhythms, stomach upset.
Caution: in pregnant women, nursing mothers, and in patients suffering from heart or liver disease or peptic ulcer. Diabetics should avoid syrup.
Not to be used for: children under 3 years.
Caution needed with: cimetidine, erythromycin, ciprofloxacin, interferon, steroids, diuretics, some other bronchodilators.

Duovent

An aerosol used as a bronchodilator to treat blocked airways.

Side effects: headache, dry mouth, dilation of the blood vessels.
Caution: in patients suffering from glaucoma, enlarged prostate, high blood pressure,overactive thyroid gland, heart muscle

disease, angina, abnormal heart rhythms.
Not to be used for: children under 6 years.
Caution needed with: sympathomimetics.

Exirel

An olive green/turquoise-blue capsule or a beige/turquoise-blue capsule according to strengths of 10 mg, 15 mg and used as a bronchodilator to treat bronchial spasm brought on by bronchial asthma, bronchitis, emphysema.

Side effects: shaking of the hands, nervous tension, headache, dilation of the blood vessels.
Caution: in pregnant women and in patients suffering from high blood pressure, abnormal heart rhythms, angina, heart muscle disease, overactive thyroid.
Not to be used for: children.
Caution needed with: sympathomimetics.

Franol

A white tablet used as a bronchodilator to treat blocked airway brought on by chronic bronchitis or bronchial asthma.

Side effects: nausea, stomach upset, headache, sleeplessness, rapid or abnormal heart rate, anxiety, tremor.
Caution: in the elderly, nursing mothers, and in patients suffering from kidney, heart or liver disease, stomach ulcer, agitation, overactive thyroid, glaucoma, enlarged prostate, adrenal tumour.
Not to be used for: children, pregnant women, or for patients suffering from coronary heart disease, high blood pressure, some blood disorders.
Caution needed with: cimetidine, erythromycin, ciprofloxacin, MAOIs, tricyclics, sympathomimetics, interferon, the contraceptive pill.

Intal

A yellow/clear spincap (delivery capsule) supplied at a strength of 20 mg and used as an anti-asthmatic drug for the prevention of bronchial asthma.

Side effects: passing cough, irritated throat, rarely bronchial spasm.
Caution:
Not to be used for:
Caution needed with:

Intal Compound

An orange/clear spincap (delivery capsule) used as an anti-asthmatic drug for the prevention of bronchial asthma.

Side effects: passing cough, irritated throat, headache, abnormal heart rhythms, rapid heart rate, dilation of the blood vessels, rarely bronchial spasm.
Caution: in patients suffering from diabetes, high blood pressure.
Not to be used for: patients suffering from heart disease, overactive thyroid, cardiac asthma.
Not to be used with: MAOIs, sympathomimetics, tricyclics.

Lasma

A white, elongated, scored tablet supplied at a strength of 300 mg and used as a bronchodilator to treat brochial spasm brought on by asthma, bronchitis, emphysema.

Side effects: rapid heart rate, nausea, stomach upset, headache, abnormal heart rhythms.
Caution: in pregnant women, nursing mothers, and in patients suffering from heart or liver disease, or stomach ulcer.
Not to be used for: children.
Caution needed with: cimetidine, erythromycin, ciprofloxacin, interferon, steroids, diuretics, other bronchodilators.

Medihaler-EPI

An aerosol supplied at a strength of 0.28 mg and used as a sympathomimetic additional treatment for sensitivity to drugs or stings due to previous exposure.

Side effects: nervousness, shaking hands, dry mouth, stomach pain.
Caution: in patients suffering from diabetes.
Not to be used for: patients suffering from heart disease, high blood pressure, overactive thyroid, abnormal heart rhythm.
Caution needed with: MAOIs, tricyclics, other sympathomimetics.

Medihaler-Iso

An aerosol supplied at a strength of 0.08 mg and used as a ß-agonist to treat bronchial asthma, chronic bronchitis.

Side effects: rapid or abnormal heart rate, dry mouth, nervousness.
Caution: in pregnant women, and in patients suffering from diabetes, high blood pressure.
Not to be used for: patients suffering from heart disease, overactive thyroid.
Caution needed with: MAOIs, sympathomimetics, tricyclics.

Myambutol

A yellow tablet or a grey tablet according to strengths of 100 mg, 400 mg and used as an anti-tubercular, additional treatment and preventive drug for tuberculosis.

Side effects: visual changes, eye inflammation.
Caution: in nursing mothers and in patients suffering from kidney disease. Eyes should be checked regularly.
Not to be used for: patients suffering from inflamation of the optic nerve.
Caution needed with:

Mynah

A yellow tablet or orange tablet according to different strengths and used as an anti-tuberculous drug combination for the prevention and treatment of tuberculosis.

Side effects: visual changes, eye inflammation, hepatitis, sleeplessness, restlessness, rheumatic disorders.
Caution: in nursing mothers, in patients with a history of epilepsy, or patients suffering kidney or liver disease, chronic alcoholism. Eyes should be tested regularly.
Not to be used for: children or or patients suffering from inflammation of the optic nerve.
Caution needed with: alcohol.

Oxivent

An aerosol supplied at a strength of 100 micrograms per dose, and used as an anticholinergic treatment for asthma and other diseases associated with breathing obstruction.

Side effects: irritation, nausea, dry mouth, anticholinergic effects.
Caution: in patients suffering from glaucoma, enlarged prostate, wheezing, or coughing. Avoid the eyes.
Not to be used for: children, pregnant women, nursing mothers, or for patients sensitive to atropine or ipratropium bromide.
Caution needed with:

Phyllocontin Continus

A pale-yellow tablet supplied at a strength of 225 mg and used as a bronchodilator to treat left ventricular or congestive heart failure, bronchial spasm associated with asthma, chronic bronchitis, emphysema.

Side effects: nausea, stomach upset, headache, brain stimulation.
Caution: in pregnant women, nursing mothers, and in patients suffering from other forms of heart disease, liver disease, stomach ulcer.

Not to be used for:
Caution needed with: cimetidine, erythromycin, ciprofloxacin, interferon, steroids, diuretics, some other bronchodilators.

Pulmadil

An aerosol supplied at a strength of 0.2 mg and used as a bronchodilator to treat bronchial spasm brought on by chronic bronchitis, bronchial asthma.

Side effects: headache, dilation of the blood vessels.
Caution: in pregnant women and in patients suffering from abnormal heart rhythms, high blood pressure, overactive thyroid, heart muscle disorders, angina.
Not to be used for:
Caution needed with: sympathomimetics.

Pulmicort

An aerosol supplied at a strength of 200 micrograms and used as a steroid to treat bronchial asthma.

Side effects: hoarseness, thrush of the mouth and throat.
Caution: in pregnant women, in patients suffering from tuberculosis of the lungs, and in those transferring from steroids taken by mouth.
Not to be used for:
Caution needed with:

Rifadin

A red/blue capsule or a red capsule according to strengths of 150 mg, 300 mg and used as an antibiotic in the additional treatment for tuberculosis, and other infections. Used to prevent meningitis in susceptible patients

Side effects: symptoms similar to influenza, rash, stomach and liver disturbances, orange-coloured urine and faeces.

Caution: in the elderly, pregnant women, nursing mothers, underfed or very young infants, and in patients suffering from liver disease.
Not to be used for: patients suffering from jaundice.
Caution needed with: anticoagulants, digoxin, antidiabetics, contraceptive pill, steroids, cyclosporin, dapsone, phenytoin, quinidine, some analgesics.

Rifater

A pink/beige tablet used as an antibiotic combination to treat tuberculosis of the lungs.

Side effects: flu-like symptoms, skin reactions, stomach and liver disturbances, change in urine colour, insomnia, muscle twitch, mental disturbance.
Caution: in the elderly, pregnant women, nursing mothers and in patients suffering from liver disease, gout, or coughing blood.
Not to be used for: patients suffering from jaundice.
Caution needed with: anticoagulants, digoxin, quinidine, steroids, the contraceptive pill, dapsone, analgesics, antidiabetics taken by mouth, cyclosporin, phenytoin, some painkillers.

Rifinah

A pink tablet or an orange, oval-shaped tablet according to strength and used as an antibiotic combination to treat tuberculosis.

Side effects: sleeplessness, muscle twitching, flu-like symptoms, skin reactions, stomach and liver disturbances, orange urine and faeces.
Caution: in pregnant women, nursing mothers, the elderly, and patients suffering from liver disease, or with a history of epilepsy.
Not to be used for: children or for patients suffering from jaundice.
Caution needed with: anticoagulants, digoxin, steroids, the

contraceptive pill, antidiabetics, cyclosporin, dapsone, phenytoin, quinidine, some painkillers.

Rimactane

A red capsule or a brown/red capsule according to strengths of 150 mg, 300 mg and used as an antibiotic in the additional treatment for tuberculosis and other similar infections. Used to prevent meningitis in susceptible patients.

Side effects: flu-like symptoms, skin reactions, stomach and liver disturbances, orange urine and faeces.
Caution: in the elderly, pregnant women, nursing mothers, or in very young undernourished patients, and in patients suffering from liver disease, porphyria (a rare blood disorder).
Not to be used for: patients suffering from jaundice.
Caution needed with: anticoagulants, contraceptive pill, steroids, digoxin, antidiabetics, cyclosporin, dapsone, phenytoin, quinidine, indigestion remedies, anticholinergics, some painkillers.

Serevent

An aerosol supplied at a strength of 25 micrograms per dose, and used as a bronchodilator to treat asthma and chronic bronchitis,

Side effects: low potassium levels, breathing difficulty, headache, tremor, palpitations.
Caution: in pregnant women and nursing mothers.
Not to be used for: children, or for emergency use.
Caution needed with: ss-blockers.

Tilade

An aerosol supplied at a strength of 2 mg and used as a bronchial anti-inflammatory drug to treat blocked airway, bronchial asthma, asthmatic bronchitis, asthma.

Side effects: headache, nausea.
Caution: in pregnant women.
Not to be used for: children.
Caution needed with:

Ventide

An aerosol supplied at a strength of 100 micrograms and used as a bronchodilator and steroid to treat asthma.

Side effects: hand shaking, nervous tension, headache, hoarseness, thrush, dilation of the blood vessels.
Caution: in pregnant women, and in patients suffering from overactive thyroid gland, heart muscle disease, abnormal heart rhythms, angina, high blood pressure, tuberculosis of the lungs, or in those transferring from steroids taken by mouth.
Not to be used for:
Caution needed with: sympathomimetics.

Ventolin

A pink tablet supplied at strengths of 2 mg, 4 mg and used as a bronchodilator to treat bronchial spasm brought on by bronchial asthma, chronic bronchitis, emphysema. Also used to stop premature labour.

Side effects: rapid heart rate, anxiety, rise in blood sugar level, shaking of the hands, nervous tension, dilation of the blood vessels, headache.
Caution: in patients suffering from thyrotoxicosis, diabetes, or cardiovascular disease. Heart rate of mother and foetus should be monitored carefully when used for treatment of premature labour.
Not to be used for: children under 2 years, or for patients suffering from antepartum haemorrhage, toxaemia of pregnancy, cord compression, threatened abortion, or conditions where prolonging the pregnancy may be dangerous.
Caution needed with: ß-blockers, other bronchodilators, sympathomimetics.

Zaditen

A white, scored tablet supplied at a strength of 1 mg and used as an antihistamine preparation for the prevention of bronchial asthma, and the treatment of allergic rhinitis, conjunctivitis.

Side effects: drowsiness, reduced reactions, dizziness, dry mouth, excitement, weight gain.
Caution:
Not to be used for: children under 2 years, pregnant women, nursing mothers.
Caution needed with: alcohol,sedatives, antidiabetics taken by mouth, other antihistamines.

Zinamide

A white, scored tablet supplied at a strength of 500 mg and used as an anti-tubercular drug in the additional treatment for tuberculosis.

Side effects: hepatitis.
Caution: in patients with a history of gout or diabetes. Your doctor may advise that liver function and blood should be checked regularly.
Not to be used for: children or for patients suffering from liver disease.
Caution needed with:

Antibiotics

Amoxil

A maroon/gold capsule supplied at a strength of 250 mg, 500 mg and used as a broad-spectrum penicillin to treat respiratory, ear, nose, and throat, urinary, venereal, and soft tissue infections. Also for dental abscess, and to prevent infection of

the heart during dental procedures

Side effects: stomach upset, allergy.
Caution: in patients suffering from glandular fever.
Not to be used for: patients suffering from penicillin allergy.
Caution needed with:

Ciproxin

Tablets supplied at strengths of 250 mg, 500 mg, and used as an antibiotic to treat infections of the ear, nose, throat, urinary system, respiratory system, skin, soft tissues, bone, joints, stomach, and gonorrhoea (a venereal disease), and major infections.

Side effects: stomach and intestinal disturbances, dizziness, headache, tiredness, confusion, convulsions, rash, pain in the joints, changes in blood, liver, or kidneys, blurred vision, rapid heart rate.
Caution: in patients suffering from severe kidney disease or with a history of convulsions. Plenty of liquid should be drunk.
Not to be used for: children, growing youngsters unless absolutely necessary, and pregnant women or nursing mothers.
Caution needed with: theophylline, antacids, alcohol, anticoagulants, non-steroid anti-inflammatory drugs, cyclosporin.

Erythrocin

A white, oblong tablet supplied at strengths of 250 mg, 500 mg and used as an antibiotic to treat infections, including acne.

Side effects: stomach disturbances, allergies.
Caution: in patients suffering from liver disease.
Not to be used for: children.
Caution needed with: theophylline, anticoagulants taken by mouth, carbamazepine, digoxin, terfenadine, astemizole.

Flagyl

An off-white tablet or an off-white, capsule-shaped tablet according to strengths of 200 mg, 400 mg and used as an antibacterial treatment for trichomoniasis, non-specific vaginitis, other infections, dysentery, abscess of the liver, ulcerative gingivitis (gum disease).

Side effects: stomach upset, furred tongue, unpleasant taste, allergy, rash, swelling, brain disturbances, dark-coloured urine, nerve changes, seizures, white cell changes.
Caution: in patients with brain disorder caused by liver disease. Short-term high-dose treatment should not be used for pregnant women or nursing mothers.
Not to be used for:
Caution needed with: alcohol, phenobarbitone, anticoagulants taken by mouth.

Floxapen

A black/caramel-coloured capsule supplied at strengths of 250 mg, 500 mg and used as a penicillin treatment for skin, soft tissue, ear, nose, and throat, and other infections.

Side effects: allergy, stomach disturbances.
Caution:
Not to be used for: patients suffering from penicillin allergy.
Caution needed with:

Keflex

A dark green/white capsule or dark green/light green capsule supplied at strengths of 250 mg, 500 mg and used as a cephalosporin antibiotic to treat respiratory, soft tissue, urine, and skin infections.

Side effects: allergic reactions, stomach disturbances.
Caution: in patients suffering from kidney disease or who are very sensitive to penicillin.

Not to be used for:
Caution needed with: loop diuretics.

Monotrim

A white, scored tablet supplied at strengths of 100 mg, 200 mg and used as an antibiotic to treat infections, urine infections.

Side effects: stomach disturbances, skin reactions.
Caution: in the elderly and in patients suffering from kidney disease from folate deficiency (vitamin deficiency). Your doctor may advise regular blood tests.
Not to be used for: infants under 6 weeks, pregnant women, or for patients suffering from severe kidney disease where regular blood tests cannot be made.
Caution needed with:

Negram

A pale-brown tablet supplied at a strength of 500 mg and used as an antiseptic to treat urinary and stomach infections.

Side effects: stomach upset, disturbed vision, rash, blood changes, seizures, sensitivity to light.
Caution: in pregnant women, nursing mothers and in patients suffering from liver or kidney disease. Keep out of the sunlight.
Not to be used for: infants under 3 months or for patients with a history of convulsions, porphyria (a rare blood disorder).
Caution needed with: anticoagulants, probenecid, antibacterials.

Penbritin

A black/red capsule supplied at strengths of 250 mg, 500 mg and used as a penicillin to treat respiratory, ear, nose, and throat infections, gonorrhoea, soft tissue infections, urinary infections.

Side effects: allergy, stomach disturbances.
Caution: in patients suffering from glandular fever.
Not to be used for: patients suffering from penicillin allergy.
Caution needed with:

Septrin

A white tablet or an orange, dispersible tablet used as an antibiotic to treat respiratory, stomach, and skin infections.

Side effects: nausea, vomiting, tongue inflammation, rash, blood changes, folate (vitamin) deficiency, rarely skin changes.
Caution: in the elderly, nursing mothers, and in patients suffering from kidney disease. Your doctor may advise that patients undergoing prolonged treatment should have regular blood tests.
Not to be used for: pregnant women, new-born infants, or for patients suffering from severe kidney or liver disease, or blood changes.
Caution needed with: folate inhibitors, anticoagulants, anticonvulsants, antidiabetics.

Tetracycline Tablets

An orange tablet supplied at a strength of 250 mg and used as an antibiotic treatment for infections.

Side effects: stomach disturbances, allergy, additional infections.
Caution: in patients suffering from liver or kidney disease.
Not to be used for: children, nursing mothers, or women during the latter half of pregnancy.
Caution needed with: milk, antacids, mineral supplements, the contraceptive pill.

Vibramycin

A green capsule supplied at a strength of 100 mg and used as a tetracycline treatment for pneumonia, respiratory, stom-

ach, soft tissue, eye, and urinary infections.

Side effects: stomach disturbances, allergy, additional infections, oesophagitis, allergy, raised blood pressure in the brain.
Caution: in patients suffering from liver disease.
Not to be used for: children, nursing mothers, women in the last half of pregnancy, or even for pregnant women at all unless no other treatment is possible.
Caution needed with: antacids, mineral supplements, barbiturates, carbamazepine, phenytoin.

Zinnat

A white tablet supplied at strengths of 125 mg, 250 mg and used as a cephalosporin antibiotic to treat respiratory, ear, nose, and throat, skin, soft tissue, and urinary infections.

Side effects: stomach disturbances, allergy, colitis, blood changes, thrush, change in liver chemistry, headache, interference with some blood tests.
Caution: in pregnant women, nursing mothers, and in patients who are sensitive to penicillin.
Not to be used for:
Caution needed with:

Over-the-counter Medicines

Biophylline

A syrup used as a bronchodilator to treat bronchial spasm.

Side effects: rapid heart rate, stomach upset, headache, sleeplessness, nausea, abnormal rhythms.
Caution: in the elderly, pregnant women, nursing mothers, and in patients suffering from heart or liver disease or peptic ulcer.
Not to be used for:
Caution needed with: cimetidine, erythromycin, ciprofloxacin, interferon.

Brovon

A solution used as a bronchodilator to treat bronchial spasm brought on by chronic bronchitis, bronchial asthma, emphysema.

Side effects: nervousness, tremor, dry mouth, abnormal heart rhythms.
Caution: in patients suffering from diabetes.
Not to be used for: children or for patients suffering from heart disease, high blood pressure, overactive thyroid gland.
Caution needed with: sympathomimetics.

Cam

A syrup used as a bronchodilator to treat bronchial spasm.

Side effects: nervousness, sleeplessness, restlessness, dry mouth, cold hands and feet, abnormal heart rhythms.
Caution: in patients suffering from diabetes.
Not to be used for: patients suffering from heart disease, high blood pressure, overactive thyroid gland.
Caution needed with: MAOIs.

Choledyl

A pink tablet or a yellow tablet according to strengths of 100 mg, 200 mg and used as a bronchodilator to treat bronchial spasm brought on by chronic bronchitis or asthma.

Side effects: rapid heart rate, stomach upset, sleeplessness, nausea, change in heart rhythms.
Caution: in pregnant women, nursing mothers, and in patients suffering from heart or liver disease or peptic ulcer. Diabetics should avoid syrup.
Not to be used for: children under 3 years.
Caution needed with: cimetidine, erythromycin, ciprofloxacin, interferon.

Rynacrom Spray

A spray used as an anti-allergy treatment for allergic rhinitis.

Side effects: temporary itching nose, rarely bronchial spasm.
Caution:
Not to be used for:
Caution needed with:

Theodrox

A white tablet used as a bronchodilator to treat bronchial spasm brought on by asthma, chronic bronchitis.

Side effects: rapid heart rate, stomach upset, headache, sleeplessness, abnormal heart rhythms.
Caution: in the elderly, pregnant women, nursing mothers, and in patients suffering from heart or liver disease or peptic ulcer.
Not to be used for: children.
Caution needed with: cimetidine, erythromycin, ciprofloxacin, interferon.

Visclair

A yellow tablet supplied at a strength of 100 mg and used as a mucus softener to treat bronchitis, phlegm.

Side effects: stomach upset.
Caution:
Not to be used for: children under 5 years.
Caution needed with:

Chapter 3

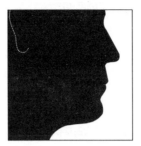

Ear, Nose, and Throat Disorders

Please refer to 'Important Advice' on page 4 at the beginning of this book; and remember, if you are in any doubt, consult a physician.

The nose and throat effectively form the upper respiratory tract, and their purpose and function are linked to those of the respiratory system described in Chapter 2. Like the respiratory system, they are prone to infections and tumours, and, like most of the illnesses in this category, disorders of the nose and throat are caused by pollution and infection.

The ear is anatomically related to the nose and throat but has evolved to provide hearing and balance capabilities to the human body. Its association with the throat leaves it prone to repeated infections. The hearing mechanism uses the ear-drum plus delicate bones in the middle ear to relay sounds to the inner ear which shares its activity with the balance mechanism. Thus, ear conditions may be associated with balance disorders. The greatest challenges presented by ear, nose, and throat disorders are the effective prevention, detection, and treatment of infections.

Acute upper respiratory tract infections ♥ *(including rhinitis, coryza, influenza, laryngitis, tonsillitis, sinusitis, scarlet fever)*

 These upper respiratory tract infections are very common causes of minor illness. Most of them are caused by viruses (especially coryza and influenza) and some are caused by a bacterial infection (particularly sinusitis and tonsillitis). They may often co-exist or, indeed, one of these infections may lead on to one of the others. It is appropriate, therefore, to consider them together because treating one will treat all.

Main symptoms
Sore throat, blocked and runny nose, nasal discharge, hoarseness, cough, fever, shivering, shaking, aches and pains, malaise.

Action
Many of these conditions will respond to self-medication for a few days at least, and a number of preparations are listed at the end of this chapter for self-treatment of these conditions. Symptoms which persist for more than seven days may require medical treatment, however.

Tests
Minor infections which do not respond to self-medication may require medical attention. Tests where necessary would include sinus X-ray, chest X-ray, analysis of sputum or discharge for bacteria.

Medications and treatment
Bacterial infections are treated with antibiotics including amoxycillin, ampicillin, cephalexin, Ciproxin, erythromycin, Flagyl, penicillin, Septrin, tetracycline, and trimethoprim. Viral infections will respond to supportive treatment. Paracetamol and aspirin are useful to control fever and aches and pains in the limbs, and you should drink

155

plenty of non-alcoholic fluids.

Further advice
Bed rest in the acute stage of an upper respiratory infection is useful. You should not get too warm even though you may feel shivery.

Associated conditions
Allergic rhinitis may appear like an acute rhinitis (nose infection), but it is caused by allergy. It will respond to antihistamine treatment, and patients should avoid allergic precipitating factors (*see* asthma).

Vestibulitis and labyrinthitis ♥

These conditions are caused by infection or inflammation of the balance mechanism of the inner ear (labyrinth). The infection is often a viral infection, but attacks of labyrinthitis or vestibulitis may occur without obvious infective cause.

Main symptoms
Vertigo, dizziness, and nausea, which may be associated with deafness and buzzing in the ears (*see* Ménière's disease).

Action
Acute attacks may respond simply to bedrest. A viral infection should be treated in the same way as acute upper respiratory tract infections such as sinusitis. Severe symptoms or symptoms that persist for more than seven days require medical attention.

Tests
If medical attention is required, labyrinthine function tests may be performed as well as hearing tests and brain scan.

Medications and treatment
Drugs such as Serc, Stemetil, or Stugeron may be useful for controlling the severe symptoms of labyrinthitis or vestibulitis.

Further advice
If you are prone to recurrent attacks, you should avoid smoking and drinking alcohol, and any other factors, such as air travel, which may bring on the attacks.

Associated conditions
See tinnitus, Ménière's disease.

Otitis media (middle-ear infection) ♥

Otitis media is an infection of the middle ear which occurs in adults and children. It is usually a bacterial infection.

Main symptoms
Severe pain in the middle ear, deafness particularly in response to changes in air pressure (i.e. while flying), fever, and other symptoms of an infection.

Action
Middle-ear infections usually need treatment, but often they resolve spontaneously when the eardrum ruptures to release the infection. This occurs by the slight tearing of the eardrum, and a sudden decrease in pain. You should seek medical advice, however, to check the integrity of the ear and to prescribe appropriate medications.

Tests
Routine testing is not normally carried out for middle-ear infection. Chronic ear infections with mastoiditis may require more intensive

investigation, however, including brain scan.

Medications and treatment
Antibiotics, including amoxycillin, ampicillin, cephalexin, Ciproxin, erythromycin, Flagyl, penicillin, Septrin, tetracycline, and trimethoprim, are best used for middle-ear infections and are usually given by mouth. Antibiotic eardrops are not suitable for this condition.

Further advice
You should avoid air travel during and after middle-ear infection. Avoid swimming, particularly diving deep into swimming pools where bacteria may lurk.

Associated conditions
Otitis externa (external-ear infection) is a similar condition affecting the outer ear. It may respond to antibiotic drops.

Ear wax ♥

Ear wax is a benign condition where the external ear is blocked by production of wax glands in the outer ear.

Main symptoms
Deafness on the affected side, occasionally with pain when the wax presses on the eardrum.

Action
It is not usually possible to remove ear wax using cotton buds and it is best not to poke cotton buds into the ear at all. Self-medication with the appropriate drops may be helpful, but syringing by a medical practitioner or nurse is often curative.

Tests
Routine testing is not appropriate.

Medications and treatment
Ear drops, such as Cerumol or Earex, may dissolve wax without the need for syringing.

Further advice
If you are suffering from ear wax, you should avoid swimming or air travel.

Associated conditions
Otitis externa may give rise to similar symptoms but it requires treatment with antibiotics.

Swellings of the vocal cords (larynx)   ♥♥♥

Swellings of the vocal cords can be malignant (carcinoma of the larynx) or benign, (particularly laryngeal warts and singers' nodules). All are more common in smokers, and singers' nodules are common among public speakers and in people who use their voices for professional purposes. Some people have multiple laryngeal papillomata (warts on the larynx) which may be viral in origin.

Main symptoms
Hoarseness and loss of voice. Some singers find that they are unable to reach notes that are usually achievable.

Action
You should be referred to an ear, nose, and throat specialist if one of these symptoms persists for longer than would be expected from just a simple upper respiratory infection such as laryngitis. Laryngitis would normally re-

solve after one to two weeks.

Tests
Direct laryngoscopy, i.e. examination of the vocal cords, should be carried out by an experienced ear, nose, and throat specialist.

Medications and treatment
After biopsy of the lesion, surgical removal or laser treatment may be appropriate. Some patients with multiple papillomata respond to interferon therapy.

Further advice
You should rest your voice, stop smoking, and reduce alcohol intake.

Associated conditions
Other conditions, such as laryngeal pouches or laryngitis, may give rise to similar symptoms.

Ménière's disease (and tinnitus)

Ménière's disease is a condition whereby the patient suffers from vertigo or dizziness, deafness, and buzzing in the ear (tinnitus). The cause of Ménière's disease is unknown, but it may be related to changes in lymph pressure in the inner ear.

Main symptoms
Tinnitus, deafness, and dizziness or vertigo. These symptoms may occur without warning several times a day and then with remissions for several days or weeks before recurring again without provocation.

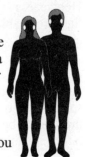

Action
If you have a severe attack of Ménière's disease, you

should lie down. If the attacks recur, you should seek medical advice.

Tests
Vestibular function tests and brain scan should be carried out to exclude acoustic neuroma, a rare tumour of the eighth cranial nerve which may mimic Ménière's disease.

Medications and treatment
Attacks of Ménière's disease respond to drugs such as Stemetil. Other drugs, such as Serc, may be useful in the long term.

Further advice
You should avoid swimming, diving, and air travel where possible. Cigarette smoking may make the condition worse.

Associated conditions
You may suffer from recurrent attacks of tinnitus without full-blown Ménière's disease. Tinnitus is a distressing symptom which may have no underlying cause and may disappear eventually.

Epistaxis (nose bleed)

Nose bleeding is a common symptom which usually resolves spontaneously but may sometimes need investigating for underlying causes.

Symptoms
Profuse bleeding from one, or occasionally both, nostrils. It may often occur spontaneously without warning, but typically occurs at moments of high stress and anxiety.

Action
Apply pressure to the appropriate side of the nose, and

161

sit up leaning slightly forward. Putting your head between your knees is not helpful because this will increase the pressure in the nose. You should not lie flat because this will encourage blood to gather in the back of the throat. Persistent heavy epistaxis requires medical attention.

Tests
Nose bleeds may be a symptom of high blood pressure or tumours. Therefore, a brain scan may be required. Investigation of high blood pressure may also be required.

Medications and treatment
The treatment of nose bleeding is essentially surgical, whereby cautery is applied to the bleeding point to arrest bleeding.

Further advice
If you suffer from recurrent nose bleeds, you should avoid persistent nose picking!

Deviated nasal septum

Deviated nasal septum is a condition in which the cartilage in the centre of the nose is twisted. This may occur as a result of injury or trauma, but it may also happen spontaneously.

Main symptom
Difficulty in breathing, particularly at night and especially when lying on one side. Symptoms of sinusitis may also occur.

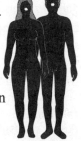

Action
Self-medication may be appropriate, but this condition often needs surgical intervention.

Tests

Examination of the nose is usually enough to make a diagnosis of this condition.

Medications and treatment

Nasal decongestants and antihistamines may improve the symptoms of this condition, but essentially an operation, called a submucous resection, is carried out to correct the twist in the nasal septum.

Further advice

Stop smoking to prevent this and similar conditions from recurring.

Swellings of the salivary gland, particularly the parotid gland ♥♥

 The parotid gland is a large salivary gland on each side of the jaw. There is a number of causes of swelling of the parotid gland including chronic infection, benign tumour, malignant tumour, and mumps (acute parotitis).

Symptoms

Swelling of the gland or glands and pain. Mumps and chronic parotitis may be associated with fever. The gland is often exquisitely painful.

Action

Seek medical advice to make the diagnosis.

Tests

Chronic infections of the parotid gland or suspected tumours may be investigated by arteriography or a sialogram.

Medications and treatment

Mumps and parotitis should be treated with painkillers and antibiotics, including amoxycillin, ampicillin, cephalexin, Ciproxin, erythromycin, Flagyl, penicillin, Septrin, tetracycline, and trimethoprim, where necessary. Benign or malignant tumours of the parotid gland require surgical intervention.

Further advice

Chronic parotitis may be associated with a high alcohol and nicotine intake, so you should drink less alcohol and stop smoking.

Associated conditions

Stone in the salivary duct may also cause swelling of the salivary gland and this needs to be investigated surgically. Mumps may be associated with other conditions such as swelling of the testicles (orchitis), inflammation of the pancreas gland (pancreatitis), and inflammation of the eyes (uveitis).

Prescription Medicines

Cerumol

Drops used as a wax softener to remove wax from the ears.

Side effects:
Caution:
Not to be used for: inflammation of the outer ear, dermatitis, eczema, perforated ear drum.
Caution needed with:

Flagyl

An off-white tablet or an off-white, capsule-shaped tablet according to strengths of 200 mg, 400 mg and used as an antibacterial treatment for trichomoniasis, non-specific

vaginitis, other infections, dysentery, abscess of the liver, ulcerative gingivitis (gum disease).

Side effects: stomach upset, furred tongue, unpleasant taste, allergy, rash, swelling, brain disturbances, dark-coloured urine, nerve changes, seizures, white cell changes.
Caution: in patients with brain disorder caused by liver disease. Short-term high-dose treatment should not be used for pregnant women or nursing mothers.
Not to be used for:
Caution needed with: alcohol, phenobarbitone, anticoagulants taken by mouth.

Serc

A white tablet supplied at a strength of 8 mg, 16 mg and used as a histamine-type drug to treat vertigo, tinnitus, and hearing loss caused by Ménière's disease.

Side effects: stomach upset.
Caution: in patients suffering from bronchial asthma, stomach ulcer.
Not to be used for: children or patients suffering from phaeochromocytoma (a disease of the adrenal glands).
Caution needed with:

Stemetil

A cream tablet or a cream, scored tablet according to strengths of 5 mg, 25 mg and used as a anti-sickness medication for minor mental and emotional problems, schizophrenia and other mental disorders, vertigo caused by Ménière's disease, severe nausea, vomiting.

Side effects: brain disturbances, anticholinergic effects, ECG and hormone changes, allergies, reduced judgement and abilities, rarely extrapyramidal effects, jaundice, blood disorder.
Caution: in the elderly, nursing mothers, and in patients suffering

from cardiovascular disease, undiagnosed or prolonged vomiting.
Not to be used for: patients in an unconscious state, pregnant
women, or patients suffering from bone marrow depression, liver
or kidney disease, Parkinson's disease.
Caution needed with: sedatives, alcohol, analgesics,
antihypertensives, antidepressants, anticholinergics,
anticonvulsants, antidiabetics.

Stugeron

**A white, scored tablet supplied at a strength of 15 mg and
used as an antihistamine treatment for vestibular disorders,
travel sickness.**

Side effects: drowsiness, reduced reactions, rarely skin eruptions.
Caution: in pregnant women, nursing mothers, and in patients
suffering from liver or kidney disease, glaucoma, epilepsy, or
enlarged prostate.
Not to be used for: children under 5 years.
Caution needed with: alcohol, sedatives, some antidepressants
(MAOIs), anticholinergics.

Antibiotics

Amoxil

**A maroon/gold capsule supplied at a strength of 250 mg, 500
mg and used as a broad-spectrum penicillin to treat respiratory, ear, nose, and throat, urinary, venereal, and soft tissue
infections. Also for dental abscess, and to prevent infection of
the heart during dental procedures**

Side effects: stomach upset, allergy.
Caution: in patients suffering from glandular fever.
Not to be used for: patients suffering from penicillin allergy.
Caution needed with:

Ciproxin

Tablets supplied at strengths of 250 mg, 500 mg, and used as an antibiotic to treat infections of the ear, nose, throat, urinary system, respiratory system, skin, soft tissues, bone, joints, stomach, and gonorrhoea (a venereal disease), and major infections.

Side effects: stomach and intestinal disturbances, dizziness, headache, tiredness, confusion, convulsions, rash, pain in the joints, changes in blood, liver, or kidneys, blurred vision, rapid heart rate.

Caution: in patients suffering from severe kidney disease or with a history of convulsions. Plenty of liquid should be drunk.

Not to be used for: children, growing youngsters unless absolutely necessary, and pregnant women or nursing mothers.

Caution needed with: theophylline, antacids, alcohol, anticoagulants, non-steroid anti-inflammatory drugs, cyclosporin.

Erythrocin

A white, oblong tablet supplied at strengths of 250 mg, 500 mg and used as an antibiotic to treat infections, including acne.

Side effects: stomach disturbances, allergies.
Caution: in patients suffering from liver disease.
Not to be used for: children.
Caution needed with: theophylline, anticoagulants taken by mouth, carbamazepine, digoxin, terfenadine, astemizole.

Flagyl

An off-white tablet or an off-white, capsule-shaped tablet according to strengths of 200 mg, 400 mg and used as an antibacterial treatment for trichomoniasis, non-specific vaginitis, other infections, dysentery, abscess of the liver, ulcerative gingivitis (gum disease).

Side effects: stomach upset, furred tongue, unpleasant taste, allergy, rash, swelling, brain disturbances, dark-coloured urine, nerve changes, seizures, white cell changes.
Caution: in patients with brain disorder caused by liver disease. Short-term high-dose treatment should not be used for pregnant women or nursing mothers.
Not to be used for:
Caution needed with: alcohol, phenobarbitone, anticoagulants taken by mouth.

Floxapen

A black/caramel-coloured capsule supplied at strengths of 250 mg, 500 mg and used as a penicillin treatment for skin, soft tissue, ear, nose, and throat, and other infections.

Side effects: allergy, stomach disturbances.
Caution:
Not to be used for: patients suffering from penicillin allergy.
Caution needed with:

Keflex

A dark green/white capsule or dark green/light green capsule supplied at strengths of 250 mg, 500 mg and used as a cephalosporin antibiotic to treat respiratory, soft tissue, urine, and skin infections.

Side effects: allergic reactions, stomach disturbances.
Caution: in patients suffering from kidney disease or who are very sensitive to penicillin.
Not to be used for:
Caution needed with: loop diuretics.

Monotrim

A white, scored tablet supplied at strengths of 100 mg, 200

mg and used as an antibiotic to treat infections, urine infections.

Side effects: stomach disturbances, skin reactions.
Caution: in the elderly and in patients suffering from kidney disease from folate deficiency (vitamin deficiency). Your doctor may advise regular blood tests.
Not to be used for: infants under 6 weeks, pregnant women, or for patients suffering from severe kidney disease where regular blood tests cannot be made.
Caution needed with:

Negram

A pale-brown tablet supplied at a strength of 500 mg and used as an antiseptic to treat urinary and stomach infections.

Side effects: stomach upset, disturbed vision, rash, blood changes, seizures, sensitivity to light.
Caution: in pregnant women, nursing mothers and in patients suffering from liver or kidney disease. Keep out of the sunlight.
Not to be used for: infants under 3 months or for patients with a history of convulsions, porphyria (a rare blood disorder).
Caution needed with: anticoagulants, probenecid, antibacterials.

Penbritin

A black/red capsule supplied at strengths of 250 mg, 500 mg and used as a penicillin to treat respiratory, ear, nose, and throat infections, gonorrhoea, soft tissue infections, urinary infections.

Side effects: allergy, stomach disturbances.
Caution: in patients suffering from glandular fever.
Not to be used for: patients suffering from penicillin allergy.
Caution needed with:

Septrin

A white tablet or an orange, dispersible tablet used as an antibiotic to treat respiratory, stomach, and skin infections.

Side effects: nausea, vomiting, tongue inflammation, rash, blood changes, folate (vitamin) deficiency, rarely skin changes.
Caution: in the elderly, nursing mothers, and in patients suffering from kidney disease. Your doctor may advise that patients undergoing prolonged treatment should have regular blood tests.
Not to be used for: pregnant women, new-born infants, or for patients suffering from severe kidney or liver disease, or blood changes.
Caution needed with: folate inhibitors, anticoagulants, anticonvulsants, antidiabetics.

Tetracycline Tablets

An orange tablet supplied at a strength of 250 mg and used as an antibiotic treatment for infections.

Side effects: stomach disturbances, allergy, additional infections.
Caution: in patients suffering from liver or kidney disease.
Not to be used for: children, nursing mothers, or women during the latter half of pregnancy.
Caution needed with: milk, antacids, mineral supplements, the contraceptive pill.

Vibramycin

A green capsule supplied at a strength of 100 mg and used as a tetracycline treatment for pneumonia, respiratory, stomach, soft tissue, eye, and urinary infections.

Side effects: stomach disturbances, allergy, additional infections, oesophagitis, allergy, raised blood pressure in the brain.
Caution: in patients suffering from liver disease.
Not to be used for: children, nursing mothers, women in the last half of pregnancy, or even for pregnant women at all unless no

other treatment is possible.
Caution needed with: antacids, mineral supplements, barbiturates, carbamazepine, phenytoin.

Zinnat

A white tablet supplied at strengths of 125 mg, 250 mg and used as a cephalosporin antibiotic to treat respiratory, ear, nose, and throat, skin, soft tissue, and urinary infections.

Side effects: stomach disturbances, allergy, colitis, blood changes, thrush, change in liver chemistry, headache, interference with some blood tests.
Caution: in pregnant women, nursing mothers, and in patients who are sensitive to penicillin.
Not to be used for:
Caution needed with:

Over-the-counter Medicines

Actidil

A white, scored tablet supplied at a strength of 2.5 mg and used as an antihistamine to treat allergies.

Side effects: drowsiness, reduced reactions, rarely skin eruptions.
Caution: in patients suffering from liver or kidney disease.
Not to be used for:
Caution needed with: alcohol, sedatives, some antidepressants (MAOIs).

Actifed Compound

A linctus used as an antihistamine to treat cough, congestion.

Side effects: drowsiness, reduced reactions.
Caution: in patients suffering from liver or kidney disease.

Not to be used for: children under 2 years
Caution needed with: alcohol, sedatives, some antidepressants
(MAOIs).

Afrazine

A spray or nasal drops used as a sympathomimetic treatment for blocked nose.

Side effects: itching nose, headache, sleeplessness, rapid heart rate.
Caution: in patients suffering from overactive thyroid gland, diabetes, coronary disease. Do not use for extended periods.
Not to be used for:
Caution needed with: MAOIs.

Avomine

A white, scored tablet supplied at a strength of 25 mg and used as an antihistamine treatment for travel sickness, nausea, vomiting, vertigo.

Side effects: drowsiness, reduced reactions, rarely skin eruptions.
Caution: in patients suffering from liver or kidney disease.
Not to be used for: children under 5 years.
Caution needed with: alcohol, sedatives, some antidepressants
(MAOIs).

Beecham's Powders

Beecham's Powders contain aspirin and caffeine; powder capsules have paracetamol, caffeine, and phenylephrine. Beecham's Hot Lemon is paracetamol with ascorbic acid (vitamin C). The main caution is to observe total daily dose of asprin or paracetamol.

Benylin Day and Night

Benylin Day and Night contains paracetamol and is a useful tablet preparation for treating the common cold.

Side effects: drowsiness, reduced reactions.
Caution: in patients suffering from liver or kidney disease.

Benylin Expectorant

A syrup used as an antihistamine, expectorant, and sputum softener to treat cough, bronchial congestion.

Side effects:
Caution:
Not to be used for: children under 1 year.
Caution needed with:

Coldrex

Coldrex contains paracetamol, caffeine, phenylephrine and ascorbic acid. Mildly stimulant and pain relieving — caffeine may cause tremors.

Contac 400

Contac 400 contains phenylpropanolamine as a sympathomimetic and chlorpheniramine as an antihistamine.

Side effects: drowsiness, reduced reactions.

Copholco

A linctus used as an opiate, expectorant to treat laryngitis, inflammation of the windpipe.

Side effects: constipation.
Caution: in patients suffering from asthma.

Not to be used for: children under 5 years, or for patients suffering from liver disease.
Caution needed with: MAOIs.

Copholcoids

A black pastille used as an opiate, expectorant to treat dry cough.

Side effects: constipation.
Caution: in patients suffering from asthma.
Not to be used for: children under 5 years or for patients suffering from liver disease
Caution needed with: MAOIs.

Daneral SA

An orange tablet supplied at a strength of 75 mg and used as an antihistamine to treat allergies.

Side effects: drowsiness, reduced reactions.
Caution: in nursing mothers.
Not to be used for:
Caution needed with: sedatives, MAOIs, alcohol.

Davenol

A linctus used as an antihistamine, sympathomimetic, and opiate preparation to treat cough.

Side effects: constipation, drowsiness, reduced reactions, anxiety, hands shaking, irregular or rapid heart rate, dry mouth, excitement, rarely skin eruptions.
Caution: in patients suffering from asthma, kidney disease, diabetes.
Not to be used for: children under 5 years or for patients suffering from liver disease, heart or thyroid disorders.
Caution needed with: MAOIs, alcohol, sedatives, tricyclics.

Day Nurse

Day Nurse contains paracetamol, ascorbic acid, phenylpropanolamine, dextromethorphan, and alcohol. It is available in tablet and liquid form. Night Nurse omits the stimulant sympathomimetic. Side effects are similar to those of Actifed.

Dimotane Expectorant

A liquid used as an antihistamine, expectorant, and sympathomimetic treatment for cough.

Side effects: anxiety, hands shaking, rapid or abnormal heart rate, dry mouth, brain stimulation.
Caution: in patients suffering from diabetes.
Not to be used for: children under 2 years or for patients suffering from cardiovascular problems, overactive thyroid gland.
Caution needed with: MAOIs, tricyclics, alcohol, sedatives, anticholinergics.

Dimotane Plus

A liquid used as an antihistamine and sympathomimetic treatment for allergic rhinitis.

Side effects: drowsiness, reduced reactions, rarely stimulant effects.
Caution: in nursing mothers and in patients suffering from bronchial asthma.
Not to be used for: patients suffering from glaucoma, comatose states, brain damage, epilepsy, retention of urine, cardiovascular problems, overactive thyroid gland.
Caution needed with: MAOIs, tricyclics, alcohol, sedatives, anticholinergics.

Dimotapp LA

A brown tablet used as an antihistamine and sympathomimetic treatment for catarrh, allergic rhinitis, sinusitis.

Side effects: drowsiness, reduced reactions, rarely stimulant effects.
Caution: in nursing mothers and in patients suffering from bronchial asthma.
Not to be used for: patients suffering from glaucoma, comatose states, brain damage, epilepsy, retention of urine, cardiovascular problems, overactive thyroid gland.
Caution needed with: MAOIs, tricyclics, alcohol, sedatives, anticholinergics.

Dramamine

A white, scored tablet supplied at a strength of 50 mg and used as an antihistamine treatment for vertigo, nausea, vomiting, travel sickness.

Side effects: drowsiness, reduced reactions, rarely skin eruptions.
Caution: in patients suffering from liver or kidney disease.
Not to be used for:
Caution needed with: alcohol, sedatives, some antidepressants (MAOIs).

Eskornade Spansule

A grey/clear capsule used as an antihistamine and sympathomimetic to treat congestion, running nose, and phlegm brought on by common cold, rhinitis, flu, sinusitis.

Side effects: drowsiness.
Caution: in patients suffering from diabetes.
Not to be used for: patients suffering from cardiovascular problems, overactive thyroid gland.
Caution needed with: MAOIs, tricyclics, alcohol.

Expulin

A linctus used as an antihistamine, opiate, and sympathomimetic treatment for cough and congestion.

Side effects: constipation, drowsiness, reduced reactions, anxiety, hands shaking, irregular or rapid heart rate, dry mouth, excitement, rarely skin eruptions.
Caution: in patients suffering from asthma, kidney disease, diabetes.
Not to be used for: children under 5 years, or for patients suffering from liver disease, heart or thyroid disorders.
Caution needed with: MAOIs, alcohol, sedatives, tricyclics.

Expurhin

A linctus used as an antihistamine and sympathomimetic treatment for congestion, phlegm, and running nose in children.

Side effects: drowsiness, reduced reactions, anxiety, hands shaking, irregular or rapid heart rate, dry mouth, excitement, rarely skin eruptions.
Caution: in patients suffering from liver or kidney disease, diabetes.
Not to be used for: infants under 3 months, or for patients suffering from heart or thyroid disorders.
Caution needed with: alcohol, sedatives, some antidepressants (MAOIs), tricyclics.

Fenostil Retard

A white tablet supplied at a strength of 2.5 mg and used as an antihistamine treatment for rhinitis, urticaria, hay fever, other allergies.

Side effects: drowsiness, reduced reactions.
Caution: in nursing mothers.
Not to be used for: children.

Caution needed with: alcohol, sedatives, MAOIs.

Galcodine

A linctus supplied at a strength of 15 mg and used as an opiate to treat dry cough.

Side effects: constipation.
Caution: in patients suffering from asthma.
Not to be used for: infants under 1 year, or for patients suffering from liver disease.
Caution needed with: MAOIs.

Galenphol

A liquid supplied at a strength of 5 mg and used as an opiate to treat dry cough.

Side effects: constipation.
Caution: in patients suffering from asthma.
Not to be used for: infants under 1 year, or for patients suffering from liver disease.
Caution needed with: MAOIs.

Galpseud

A white tablet supplied at a strength of 60 mg and used as an sympathomimetic to treat congestion of the nose, sinuses, and upper respiratory tract.

Side effects: anxiety, hands shaking, irregular or rapid heart rate, dry mouth, excitement.
Caution: in patients suffering from diabetes.
Not to be used for: children under 2 years, or for patients suffering from heart or thyroid disorders.
Caution needed with: MAOIs, tricyclics.

Guanor

A liquid used as an expectorant, antihistamine, mucus softener to treat cough, bronchial congestion.

Side effects: drowsiness, reduced reactions, rarely skin eruptions.
Caution: in patients suffering from liver or kidney disease.
Not to be used for: infants under 1 year.
Caution needed with: alcohol, sedatives, some antidepressants (MAOIs).

Haymine

A yellow tablet used as an antihistamine and sympathomimetic treatment for allergies.

Side effects: drowsiness, reduced reactions, dizziness.
Caution:
Not to be used for: children, or for patients suffering from overactive thyroid gland, high blood pressure, coronary thrombosis.
Caution needed with: alcohol, sedatives, MAOIs.

Hayphryn

A spray used as a sympathomimetic, antihistamine treatment for blocked nose resulting from allergy.

Side effects:
Caution: in patients suffering from overactive thyroid gland, cardiovascular disease; do not use for periods longer than 7 days.
Not to be used for: children under 7 years
Caution needed with: MAOIs.

Histalix

A syrup used as an antihistamine, expectorant, and sputum softener to treat bronchial and nasal congestion.

Side effects: drowsiness, reduced reactions, rarely skin eruptions.
Caution: in patients suffering from liver or kidney disease.
Not to be used for:
Caution needed with: alcohol, sedatives, MAOIs.

Histryl Spansule

A pink/clear capsule supplied at a strength of 5 mg and used as an antihistamine to treat rhinitis, severe allergic conditions, insect bites and stings, allergies to food or other drugs.

Side effects: drowsiness, reduced reactions, dry mouth, blurred vision, dizziness.
Caution: in nursing mothers.
Not to be used for: children.
Caution needed with: alcohol, sedatives, MAOIs.

Lemsip

Lemsip contains paracetamol, caffeine, and phenylephrine. Mildly stimulant and pain relieving — caffeine may cause tremors.

Lergoban

An off-white tablet supplied at a strength of 5 mg and used as an antihistamine to treat allergies.

Side effects: drowsiness, reduced reactions, dizziness, headache, flushing, anorexia, dry mouth.
Caution: in nursing mothers.
Not to be used for: children.
Caution needed with: alcohol, sedatives, MAOIs.

Lotussin

A linctus used as an antihistamine, antussive treatment for cough.

Side effects: drowsiness, reduced reactions, constipation, rarely skin eruptions.
Caution: in patients suffering from kidney disease, asthma.
Not to be used for: infants under 1 year, or for patients suffering from liver disease.
Caution needed with: alcohol, sedatives, some antidepressants (MAOIs).

Neophryn

A spray or nasal drops used as a sympathomimetic treatment for blocked nose.

Side effects:
Caution: in patients suffering from cardiovascular disease or overactive thyroid. Do not use for longer than 7 days.
Not to be used for: children under 7 years
Caution needed with: MAOIs.

Noradran

A syrup used as an antussive to treat bronchitis, bronchial asthma.

Side effects: sedation, dry mouth, nervousness, restlessness, hands shaking, abnormal heart rhythm, stomach upset.
Caution: in patients suffering from heart or liver disease, diabetes.
Not to be used for: children under 5 years, or for patients suffering from high blood pressure, overactive thyroid, coronary disease, cardiac asthma
Caution needed with: MAOIs, sympathomimetics, tricyclics, alcohol, cimetidine, erythomycin, interferon, ciprofloxaxin.

Optimine

A white, scored tablet supplied at a strength of 1 mg and used as an antihistamine and serotonin antagonist (hormone blocker) to treat bites and stings, itch, allergic rhinitis, urticaria.

Side effects: drowsiness, reduced reactions, greater appetite, anorexia, nausea, headache, anticholinergic effects.
Caution:
Not to be used for: infants under 1 year or for patients suffering from prostate enlargement, retention of urine, glaucoma, peptic ulcer causing blockage.
Caution needed with: sedatives, MAOIs, alcohol.

Otrivine-Antistin

A spray or drops used as a sympathomimetic, antihistamine treatment for hay fever, allergic rhinitis.

Side effects: itching nose, headache, sleeplessness, rapid heart rate.
Caution: Do not use for extended periods.
Not to be used for: children.
Caution needed with: MAOIs.

Pavacol-D

A mixture containing opiate and demulcents used to treat cough.

Side effects: constipation.
Caution: in patients suffering from asthma.
Not to be used for: infants under 1 year, or for patients suffering from liver disease.
Caution needed with: MAOIs.

Periactin

A white, scored tablet supplied at a strength of 4 mg and used as an antihistamine , serotonin antagonists (hormone blocker) to improve appetite and to treat allergies, itchy skin conditions.

Side effects: anticholinergic effects, reduced reactions, drowsiness, excitement.

Caution: in pregnant women, and in patients suffering from bronchial asthma, raised eye pressure, overactive thyroid, cardiovascular disease, high blood pressure.

Not to be used for: newborn infants, nursing mothers, the elderly, or patients suffering from glaucoma, enlarged prostate, bladder obstruction, retention of urine, stomach blockage, peptic ulcer, or debilitation.

Caution needed with: alcohol, sedatives, MAOIs.

Phenergan

A blue tablet supplied at a strength of 10 mg, 25 mg and used as an antihistamine to treat allergies.

Side effects: drowsiness, reduced reactions, dizziness, disorientation, sensitivity to light, convulsions on high doses, extrapyramidal reactions (shaking and rigidity).

Caution:

Not to be used for: infants under 1 year

Caution needed with: alcohol, sedatives, MAOIs.

Phensedyl

A linctus used as an antihistamine, opiate, sympathomimetic treatment for cough.

Side effects: constipation, drowsiness, reduced reactions, anxiety, hands shaking, irregular or rapid heart rate, dry mouth, excitement, rarely skin eruptions.

Caution: in patients suffering from asthma, kidney disease,

diabetes.
Not to be used for: children under 2 years, or for patients suffering from liver disease, heart or thyroid disorders.
Caution needed with: MAOIs, alcohol, sedatives, tricyclics.

Pholcomed-D

A linctus used as an opiate and bronchial relaxant to treat dry, irritating cough.

Side effects: constipation.
Caution: in patients suffering from asthma.
Not to be used for: children under 1 year, or for patients suffering from liver disease.
Caution needed with: MAOIs.

Pholtex

A liquid used as an opiate and antihistamine treatment for dry cough.

Side effects: constipation.
Caution: in patients suffering from asthma.
Not to be used for: children under 5 years, or for patients suffering from liver disease.
Caution needed with: MAOIs.

Piriton

A cream-coloured tablet supplied at a strength of 4 mg and used as an antihistamine treatment for allergies.

Side effects: drowsiness, reduced reactions, dizziness, excitation.
Caution: in nursing mothers.
Not to be used for:
Caution needed with: MAOIs, sedatives, alcohol.

Polleneze

Polleneze contains astemozole and is a useful antihistamine for hay fever.

Side effects: drowsiness, reduced reactions, dizziness, excitation.
Caution: in nursing mothers.

Pro-Actidil

A white tablet supplied at a strength of 10 mg and used as an antihistamine treatment for allergies.

Side effects: drowsiness, reduced reactions, rarely skin eruptions.
Caution: in nursing mothers, and in patients suffering from liver or kidney disease.
Not to be used for: children.
Caution needed with: MAOIs, sedatives, alcohol.

Stugeron

A white, scored tablet supplied at a strength of 15 mg and used as an antihistamine treatment for vestibular disorders, travel sickness.

Side effects: drowsiness, reduced reactions, rarely skin eruptions.
Caution: in patients suffering from liver or kidney disease.
Not to be used for: children under 5 years.
Caution needed with: MAOIs, sedatives, alcohol.

Sudafed

A red tablet supplied at a strength of 60 mg and used as a sympathomimetic treatment to relieve congestion of the nose, sinuses, and upper respiratory tract.

Side effects: anxiety, tremor, rapid or abnormal heart rate, dry mouth, brain stimulation.
Caution: in patients suffering from diabetes.

Not to be used for: patients suffering from cardiovascular disorders, overactive thyroid.
Caution needed with: MAOIs, tricyclics.

Sudafed Plus

A white, scored tablet used as an antihistamine, sympathomimetic treatment for allergic rhinitis.

Side effects: drowsiness, rash, disturbed sleep, rarely hallucinations.
Caution: in patients suffering from raised eye pressure, enlarged prostate.
Not to be used for: infants under 2 years, or for patients suffering from severe high blood pressure, coronary artery disease, overactive thyroid.
Caution needed with: MAOIs, sympathomimetics, furazolidone alcohol.

Tavegil

A white, scored tablet supplied at a strength of 1 mg and used as an antihistamine treatment for allergic rhinitis, dermatoses, urticaria, allergy to other drugs.

Side effects: drowsiness, reduced reactions, rarely dizziness, dry mouth, palpitations, gastro-intestinal disturbances.
Caution:
Not to be used for:
Caution needed with: MAOIs, sedatives, alcohol.

Tercoda

A syrup used as an opiate, expectorant, antussive, sputum softener to treat bronchitis.

Side effects: constipation.
Caution: in patients suffering from asthma.

Not to be used for: children, or for patients suffering from liver disease.
Caution needed with: MAOIs.

Terpoin

An elixir used as an opiate treatment for dry cough.

Side effects: constipation.
Caution: in patients suffering from asthma.
Not to be used for: children under 5 years, or for patients suffering from liver disease.
Caution needed with: MAOIs.

Thephorin

A white tablet supplied at a strength of 25 mg and used as an antihistamine to treat allergies.

Side effects: dry mouth, stomach upset, rarely drowsiness.
Caution:
Not to be used for: children.
Caution needed with: MAOIs, sedatives, alcohol, anticholinergics.

Triludan

A white, scored tablet supplied at a strength of 60 mg and used as an antihistamine treatment for allergies including hay fever and rhinitis.

Side effects: rash, sweating, headache, mild stomach disturbances.
Caution:
Not to be used for: children under 6 years.
Caution needed with:

Uniflu & Gregovite C

A red, oblong tablet and a yellow tablet used as an analgesic, opiate, antussive, xanthine, antihistamine treatment for cold and flu symptoms.

Side effects: constipation, drowsiness, reduced reactions, anxiety, hands shaking, irregular or rapid heart rate, dry mouth, excitement, rarely skin eruptions.
Caution: in patients suffering from asthma, kidney disease, diabetes.
Not to be used for: children, or for patients suffering from liver disease, heart or thyroid disorders.
Caution needed with: MAOIs, sedatives, alcohol, tricyclics.

Vick

Vicks preparations contain basic ingredients similar to Day Nurse. In addition, there is an expectorant which contains guaiphenesin and citrate, and a Medinite preparation which has ephedrine, doxylamine, and alcohol. Vicks Sinex spray contains oxymetalozine, menthol, camphor and eucalyptol. Vicks throat spray and vapour rub are also available. The side effects of these preparations depend upon the main ingredients but they should be treated similarly to Actifed.

Chapter 4

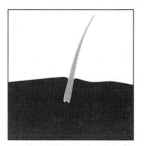

Skin Disorders

Please refer to 'Important Advice' on page 4 at the beginning of this book; and remember, if you are in any doubt, consult a physician.

Our skin separates us from the outside world. It must be maintained in good condition and re-newed, and must also be a self-lubricating and self-servicing system. This need for constant renewal can lead to some conditions where there is an imbalance between replacing skin and re-moving damaged skin. Thus, conditions, such as psoriasis, eczema, and dermatitis, can be caused by overgrowth of skin in association with other factors such as allergy to external agents. To some extent, therefore, many skin diseases are related to our environment. The most dangerous of all, skin cancer, is directly related to overexposure to ultraviolet light, that is, sunlight.

Many internal conditions, such as viruses, may appear as a skin rash, but this is valuable as a signalling process rather than suggesting any real defect in the skin. The skin is also prone to infections. Appendages to the skin, such as hair follicles and pores, are also prone to infections and illness. Hair loss and abnormal hair growth are often caused by a medical disorder.

Therefore, we must try to prevent and treat skin diseases in the context that the skin itself needs protection against a variety of external assaults.

Although they may be alarming, very few skin conditions are, in fact, contagious. Impetigo is contagious, however, and the rash that accompanies chicken pox or measles indicate a contagious condition.

Skin tumours, warts, and swellings

 Any swelling or tumour of the skin can be alarming. In this category we include skin tumours, such as malignant melanoma, basal cell carcinoma, squamous cell carcinoma, haemangiomas, lipomas, warts, and naevi. Of these, only malignant melanoma is particularly serious although, occasionally, lipomas may turn out to be liposarcomas which are malignant.

Many skin conditions, including melanoma and basal cell carcinoma, are made worse by exposure to sunlight and therefore occur in fair-skinned people living in tropical areas. Many warts are caused by viruses but, in general terms, the remainder of the skin lesions in this category have no known cause.

Main symptoms
A lump or bump in the skin which may bleed or ulcerate. Particularly serious signs to look for are the failure of a cut to heal, bleeding of a skin lesion, itching, change in size, shape, or colour, and the presence of associated or satellite lesions. These may indicate malignancy. Lipomas are usually painless lumps; warts have a crusty appearance; haemangiomas are collections of blood while naevi are often like large moles.

Action
You should seek medical attention if the lump or ulcer changes in any way. (*See* above).

Tests
The main test of any skin lesion is a biopsy. An incision is carried out and the fragments are examined under a microscope.

Medications and treatment
Most of these conditions require surgical excision. Occasionally

warts may respond to local wart remedies. Malignant conditions may need chemotherapy and/or radiotherapy.

Further advice
In general, you should avoid overexposure to sunlight and wear sunblocks.

Skin rash associated with fever ♥

 Skin rash associated with fever is most commonly caused by a virus infection. Notably these include measles, German measles, chickenpox, and shingles. In all cases the rash is generally contagious on the body or torso.

Main symptoms
Rash and fever. The rash of measles is slightly redder than the rather pink rash of German measles. Chickenpox consists of small fluid-filled blisters whereas shingles, which is caused by the same virus as chickenpox, affects one side of the body only and in one limited area. There is often considerable pain associated with shingles. Chickenpox may affect the lungs; German measles can cause glandular swelling, particularly at the back of the neck; while measles can cause reddening of the eyes and infection of the brain (encephalitis).

Action
Most of these virus infections are self-limiting, and, apart from medical attention to make the diagnosis, will respond to bedrest.

Tests
Occasionally blood tests may be required to confirm the diagnosis. Chest X-ray or lumbar puncture may be considered if complications occur.

Medications and treatment

Shingles responds to Zovirax and, recently, doctors have started to use Zovirax for chickenpox. Measles and German measles do not respond to current antiviral therapy. German measles is severely damaging to the unborn child, and so pregnant women should avoid contact with German measles. Shingles pain may continue for a very long time but it can be alleviated by painkillers. Encephalitis is a rare but late complication of measles. Glandular fever treated with ampicillin may result in a rash, and scarlet fever may cause a rash with fever. (*See* acute upper respiratory tract infections.)

Skin infections

 Bacteria, fungi, and viruses can cause skin infections. Bacterial infections usually give rise to acne, cellulitis, or impetigo. Fungus infections are quite common in the form of ringworm, athlete's foot, dhobi itch, and simple fungal plaques. The most common viral infections of the skin are herpes simplex, or cold sore, as well as herpes zoster or shingles. Occasionally, bacterial infections may cause a granuloma or swelling. All these conditions are contagious.

Main symptoms

Spots and a possible itchy rash. Dhobi itch affects the groin and athlete's foot affects the spaces between the toes. Acne is most common on the face, chest, and back whereas impetigo can often affect the face. Cellulitis is a spreading skin infection which can occur anywhere. Cold sores are usually found on the upper lip and are made worse at times of stress or menstruation.

Action

Self-medication with a local cleansing agent may resolve a bacterial infection and over-the-counter antifungal preparations can also be used. Cold sores often disappear spontaneously but may require prescription medication.

Tests
In difficult cases, scrapings may be taken for microscopic examination.

Medications and treatment
Antibiotics, particularly tetracycline and clindamycin, are useful for skin infections such as acne. Erythromycin is useful for treating acne as well as cellulitis and impetigo. Antifungal agents, such as Canesten, are useful for fungal infections, and Zovirax Cream valuable in the treatment of cold sores.

Further advice
Pay particular attention to hygiene, including washing clothes regularly, and avoid poor diet high in chocolate.

Associated conditions
Acne rosacea is a condition similar to acne which also responds to tetracycline therapy. It is not thought to be due to a bacterial infection and its cause is unknown.

Dermatitis and eczema

 Eczema and dermatitis are related conditions where there is itching and scaling of the skin with thickening. The condition is made worse if you scratch the affected area. Dermatitis may be an allergic phenomenon, e.g. contact dermatitis, where allergy to factors, such as soap powder, may bring it on. Eczema may also have an allergic component but, fundamentally, it is a disease associated with an allergic or atopic family, i.e. patients with eczema may suffer from or have relatives with asthma or hay fever.

Symptoms
Itchy or scaly rash which may bleed on contact. The rash may be found in the folds of skin such as behind the knees and in the elbows, and in areas where there is contact with chemicals, such as on the hands.

Action
Avoiding contact by wearing rubber gloves or using barrier creams may often be helpful. Simple remedies may resolve the conditions but severe conditions may require medical intervention.

Tests
The main test for this condition is biopsy of the skin or patch tests to check for skin allergies.

Medications and treatment
Eczema and dermatitis often respond to mild steroids such as Eumovate and hydrocortisone, or stronger steroids such as Betnovate or Dermovate. Strong steroids should be used with extreme caution.

Further advice
Anxiety and stress may provoke these conditions, so you should try to control these as part of your general disease management.

Associated conditions
Seborrhoeic dermatitis, which is similar to dermatitis, may affect the scalp. Blepharitis is an eczema condition affecting the eyes.

Psoriasis

Psoriasis is a skin disorder distinct from, but in many ways similar to, eczema. Its cause is not known. Psoriasis is not contagious.

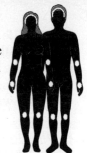

Main symptoms
An itchy, scaly rash, predominantly on the outside of the elbows, knees, in the hair, and on the hands. It is associated with changes to the hair and nails. Psoriasis can appear on any part of the body and may be quite extensive. The rash is quite red in appearance and may have a violet hue.

Action
Simple remedies may help psoriasis, and self-medication may be appropriate.

Tests
The main tests for psoriasis are skin biopsy in which a microscopic examination of the skin will confirm a diagnosis.

Medications and treatment
Self-medication with coal tar may be appropriate but prescription drugs, such as Dovonex, may be needed for the more severe cases. Cytotoxic drugs may also be useful. Ultraviolet A light is often used in association with psoriasis treatments. Steroids may result in some improvement.

Further advice
Stress and exposure to sunlight may worsen psoriasis. Diet may also affect the condition.

Associated conditions
Psoriasis may cause changes to nails as well as hair loss.

Hair loss (alopecia)

Alopecia may be partial or complete. There are many causes of alopecia but, in some cases, the origin may not be known. Pregnancy (hair loss after pregnancy is known as post-partum hair loss), iron or vitamin deficiency, underactive thyroid gland, psoriasis, dermatitis, skin infestation such as lice or scabies, and chemotherapy may all cause hair loss.

Symptoms
Partial or complete hair loss. The hair loss may well be in clumps. There may be associated precipitating factors, such as psoriasis, or symptoms of underactive thyroid gland.

Action
Slight loss of hair, such as might occur after pregnancy, can be ignored because the condition will resolve itself. Severe alopecia needs medical attention.

Tests
Blood tests, such as thyroid function tests, for precipitating causes are appropriate. Skin biopsy may be necessary.

Medications and treatment
Minoxodil lotion has been used to treat alopecia. Thyroid replacement or iron and vitamin replacement should be used to treat precipitating causes.

Further advice
Trying to improve general health, reducing stress, and improving diet may stop alopecia worsening.

Associated conditions
Male pattern baldness may occur early and may result in almost complete alopecia. Minoxodil lotion may be helpful in some cases. Some conditions appear with excessive hair growth; particularly, these are hormonal conditions, such as polycystic ovaries or tumours, that produce excess male hormone. A full hormone investigation is required in such cases.

Pruritis (itch) and skin allergy (including urticaria)

 Pruritis or itch may be a symptom of other conditions (*see* eczema, dermatitis, psoriasis, skin swellings) but it may be a condition in its own right without any known underlying cause, or associated with generalized allergy. Severe allergy may result in urticaria, a condition where there is generalized swelling of skin and underlying tissues. Very commonly, drugs may cause allergies, skin rashes, and skin eruptions. These may be itchy.

Main symptom
Itching.

Actions
If possible, do not scratch, and seek medical advice.

Tests
Allergy tests and skin biopsies are very important.

Medications and treatment
Antihistamines and steroid creams, including Betnovate, Calmurid, Clarityn, Epogam, Eumovate, Eurax, Hismanal, Phenergan, Piriton, Sudafed, Triludan, Zaditen, and Zirtek, may provide symptomatic improvement in cases of pruritis, but a full investigation is necessary if symptoms persist for more than a few days.

Further advice
Hot showers may make symptoms worse and, generally, sunlight is bad for itchy skin. Take extra care about medications, such as penicillin, where allergy is suspected.

Skin infestations (lice and scabies)

 These conditions are caused by skin infestation with small insects. They occur in areas of poor hygiene or when people live in very close communities such as in boarding schools.

Main symptoms
An itchy rash, and small eggs or insects can often be seen on the skin.

Action
Improve general hygiene, including washing sheets and blankets, but persistent infestation requires medical attention.

Tests
Skin biopsies are often used; examination of insects and eggs under the microscope will fix the diagnosis.

Medications and treatment
Ascabiol, Clinicide, Lyclear, Quellada.

Further advice
Attention to general hygiene, avoiding overcrowding, and regularly washing hair and linen should prevent this condition.

Associated conditions
Pubic lice are a venereally contracted condition where insects may be seen on the pubic hair.

Diseases of the nails

 The main conditions affecting the nails are infection (paronychia) and ingrowing toenail. The nails may also be altered by conditions such as psoriasis or calcium and vitamin deficiency. Iron deficiency may cause changes in nail shape. Trauma to the hands often causes nail disfigurement. Fungus infections may affect the nails.

Main symptoms
Obvious change in the shape, texture, and colour of the nail or an infection next to the nail as in ingrowing toenail or paronychia.

Action
These conditions may respond to self-medication, but, if they persist, you should seek medical attention.

Tests
Biopsy culture of nail scrapings may be required, and investigation of underlying causes (e.g. anaemia or psoriasis) may resolve the cause of nail problems.

Medications and treatment
Nail disorders, such as ingrowing toenail, are usually treated surgically but they may respond to local use of antiseptics and antibiotics. Paronychia should also respond to antibiotics, and fungus infections will respond to local nail paints, such as Trosyl, or antifungal tablets, such as Grisovin. The underlying causes of nail disorders (e.g. anaemia) should receive the appropriate treatment for that condition.

Further advice
Good general health and hygiene will maintain healthy strong nails.

Prescription Medicines

Adcortyl

A cream used as a steroid treatment for dermatitis, psoriasis, external ear infections, sunburn, insect bites and stings.

Side effects: fluid retention, suppression of adrenal glands, thinning of the skin may occur.
Caution: use for short periods of time only.
Not to be used for: patients suffering from acne or any other skin infections caused by tuberculosis, ringworm, viruses, or fungi, or continuously especially in pregnant women.
Caution needed with:

Alphaderm

A cream used as a steroid and wetting agent to treat eczema, dermatitis.

Side effects: fluid retention, suppression of adrenal glands. Thinning of the skin may occur.
Caution: use for short periods of time only.
Not to be used for: patients suffering from acne or any other skin infections caused by tuberculosis, ringworm, viruses, or fungi, or continuously especially in pregnant women.
Caution needed with:

Alphosyl

A cream used as an anti-psoriatic to treat psoriasis.

Side effects: irritation, sensitivity to light.
Caution:
Not to be used for: patients suffering from acute psoriasis.
Caution needed with:

Alphosyl HC

A cream used as an anti-psoriatic and steroid treatment for psoriasis.

Side effects: thinning of the skin, fluid retention, suppression of adrenal glands.
Caution: in pregnant women, and in patients on extended treatment – withdraw gradually.
Not to be used for: children under 5 years, or for patients suffering from acne or other skin infections unless otherwise directed, or continuously especially in pregnancy.
Caution needed with:

Ascabiol

An emulsion used as an insect-destroying drug to treat scabies, pediculosis.

Side effects: irritation.
Caution: keep out of the eyes.
Not to be used for:
Caution needed with:

Calmurid HC

A cream used as a steroid, wetting agent and skin softener to treat dry hyperkeratotic eczema and other skin disorders.

Side effects: fluid retention, suppression of adrenal glands, thinning of the skin may occur.
Caution: use for short periods of time only.
Not to be used for: patients suffering from acne or any other skin infections caused by tuberculosis, ringworm, viruses, or fungi, or continuously especially in pregnant women.
Caution needed with:

Canesten

A solution used as an antifungal treatment for fungal inflammation and infection of the outer ear, skin, and nails.

Side effects: local irritation, allergy.
Caution:
Not to be used for:
Caution needed with:

Clarityn

A white, oval, scored tablet supplied at a strength of 10 mg and used as an antihistamine treatment for allergic rhinitis and other allergies.

Side effects: tiredness, headache, nausea.
Caution:
Not to be used for: children under 2 years, pregnant women, or nursing mothers.
Caution needed with:

Clinicide

A liquid used as a pediculicide to treat lice of the head and pubic areas.

Side effects:
Caution: keep out of the eyes.
Not to be used for:
Caution needed with:

Dermovate

A cream used as a steroid treatment for psoriasis, eczema, other skin disorders where there is inflammation

Side effects: fluid retention, suppression of adrenal glands, thinning of the skin may occur.

Caution: adults check after 4 weeks; children check after 1 week; use for short periods of time only.
Not to be used for: patients suffering from acne or any other skin infections caused by tuberculosis, ringworm, viruses, or fungi, or continuously especially in pregnant women.
Caution needed with:

Diprosalic

An ointment used as a steroid and skin softener to treat hard skin and dry skin disorders.

Side effects: fluid retention, suppression of adrenal glands, thinning of the skin may occur.
Caution: use for short periods of time only.
Not to be used for: patients suffering from acne or any other skin infections caused by tuberculosis, ringworm, viruses, or fungi, or continuously especially in pregnant women.
Caution needed with:

Dovonex

An ointment used to treat mild to moderate psoriasis.

Side effects: irritation, dermatitis.
Caution: in pregnant women and nursing mothers. Avoid the face.
Not to be used for: children, or for patients suffering from disorders of calcium metabolism.
Caution needed with:

Epogam

An oil-filled capsule supplied at a strength of 40 mg and used to relieve the symptoms of eczema.

Side effects: nausea, headache.
Caution: in patients suffering from epilepsy.

Not to be used for: children under 1 year.
Caution needed with:

Eumovate Cream

A cream used as a steroid treatment for mild eczema and other skin disorders.

Side effects: fluid retention, suppression of adrenal glands, thinning of the skin may occur.
Caution: use for short periods of time only.
Not to be used for: patients suffering from acne or any other skin infections caused by tuberculosis, ringworm, viruses, or fungi, or continuously especially in pregnant women.
Caution needed with:

Eurax

A lotion used as a scabicide to treat scabies and itchy skin conditions.

Side effects:
Caution: keep out of the eyes, and avoid areas of broken skin.
Not to be used for: patients suffering from acute exudative dermatitis.
Caution needed with:

Gregoderm

An ointment used as a steroid, antibacterial treatment for psoriasis, itch of the anal and genital area, and other skin disorders where there is also inflammation and infection.

Side effects: fluid retention, suppression of the adrenal glands, thinning of the skin may occur.
Caution: use for short periods of time only.
Not to be used for: continuously especially for pregnant women, or for patients suffering from acne or any other tubercular, fun-

gal, viral, or ringworm infections.
Caution needed with:

Grisovin

A white tablet supplied at strengths of 125 mg, 500 mg and used as an antifungal treatment for infections of the nails, skin, and scalp.

Side effects: drowsiness, gastric upset, headache, allergies, sensitivity to light, rarely precipitation of SLE (a rare collagen disease).
Caution: in pregnant women and in patients on prolonged treatment.
Not to be used for: patients suffering from porphyria (a rare blood disease), liver disease, SLE (a rare collagen disease).
Caution needed with: barbiturates, coumarin anticoagulants, alcohol, the contraceptive pill.

Haelan

A cream used as a steroid treatment for skin disorders.

Side effects: fluid retention, suppression of the adrenal glands, thinning of the skin may occur.
Caution: use for short periods of time only.
Not to be used for: continuously especially for pregnant women, or for patients suffering from acne, or any other tubercular, viral, fungal, or ringworm skin infections.
Caution needed with:

Halciderm

A cream used as a steroid treatment for acute skin disorders.

Side effects: fluid retention, suppression of the adrenal glands, thinning of the skin may occur.
Caution: do not dilute the cream. Use for short periods of time

only.

Not to be used for: continuously especially for pregnant women, or for patients suffering from other tubercular, fungal, viral, or ringworm infections.

Caution needed with:

Hismanal

A white, scored tablet supplied at a strength of 10 mg and used as an antihistamine treatment for hay fever, allergic rhinitis, skin allergies.

Side effects: rarely drowsiness or gain in weight, heart rhythm disturbance.

Caution: women of child-bearing age should take steps to avoid conception during and for some weeks after the treatment.

Not to be used for: children under 6 years, pregnant women.

Caution needed with: ketoconazole, erythromycin, itraconazole.

Hydrocortistab Tablets

A white, scored tablet supplied at a strength of 20 mg and used as a steroid for replacement treatment in adrenocortical deficiency, inflammation in allergies, and rheumatic and collagen diseases.

Side effects: high blood sugar, thin bones, mood changes, ulcers, high blood pressure, fluid retention, potassium loss, muscle weakness.

Caution: in pregnant women, in patients who have had recent bowel surgery, or who are suffering from inflamed veins, psychiatric disorders, virus infections, some cancers, some kidney diseases, thinning of the bones, ulcers, tuberculosis, other infections, high blood pressure, glaucoma, epilepsy, diabetes, underactive thyroid, liver disease, stress. Withdraw gradually.

Not to be used for:

Caution needed with: phenytoin, phenobarbitone, ephedrine, rifampicin, diuretics, anticholinesterases, digoxin, antidiabetic agents, anticoagulants, non-steroid anti-inflammatory drugs.

Locoid-C

A cream/ointment used as an antibacterial and steroid to treat eczema, psoriasis, and other skin conditions which are also infected with bacteria or fungi.

Side effects: fluid retention, suppression of adrenal glands, thinning of the skin may occur.
Caution: use for short periods of time only.
Not to be used for: continuous use, especially on pregnant women, or for patients suffering from acne or any other tubercular or viral infection of the skin.
Caution needed with:

Lyclear

A conditioning lotion applied to the head to treat head lice.

Side effects:
Caution: in children under 2 years, pregnant women, and nursing mothers. Avoid eyes.
Not to be used for: infants under 6 months.
Caution needed with:

Metosyn

A cream used as a steroid treatment for allergic and other skin conditions where there is also inflammation.

Side effects: fluid retention, suppression of adrenal glands, thinning of the skin may occur.
Caution: use for short periods of time only.
Not to be used for: patients suffering from acne or any other skin infections caused by tuberculosis, ringworm, viruses, or fungi, or continuously especially in pregnant women.
Caution needed with:

Modrasone

A cream used as a steroid treatment for skin disorders.

Side effects: fluid retention, suppression of adrenal glands, thinning of the skin may occur.
Caution: use for short periods of time only.
Not to be used for: patients suffering from acne or any other skin infections caused by tuberculosis, ringworm, viruses, or fungi, or continuously especially in pregnant women.
Caution needed with:

Nerisone

A cream used as a steroid treatment for skin disorders.

Side effects: fluid retention, suppression of adrenal glands, thinning of the skin may occur.
Caution: do not use for longer than 3 weeks for children under 4 years; do not use for prolonged periods for other patients.
Not to be used for: patients suffering from acne or any other skin infections caused by tuberculosis, ringworm, viruses, or fungi, or continuously especially in pregnant women.
Caution needed with:

Phenergan

A blue tablet supplied at strengths of 10 mg, 25 mg and used as an antihistamine treatment for allergies, nausea, vomiting, and for sedation (if recommended by a doctor).

Side effects: drowsiness, reduced reactions, dizziness, disorientation, sensitivity to light, anticholinergic effects, extrapyramidal reactions (shaking and rigidity).
Caution:
Not to be used for: infants under 1 year.
Caution needed with: sedatives, MAOIs, alcohol.

Piriton

A cream-coloured tablet supplied at a strength of 4 mg and used as an antihistamine treatment for allergies.

Side effects: drowsiness, reduced reactions, dizziness, excitation.
Caution: in pregnant women and nursing mothers.
Not to be used for:
Caution needed with: sedatives, MAOIs, alcohol.

Propaderm

A cream used as a steroid treatment for skin disorders.

Side effects: fluid retention, suppression of adrenal glands, thinning of the skin may occur.
Caution: use for short periods of time only.
Not to be used for: patients suffering from acne or any other skin infections caused by tuberculosis, ringworm, viruses, or fungi, or continuously especially in pregnant women.
Caution needed with:

Quellada

A lotion used as a scabicide to treat scabies.

Side effects:
Caution: keep out of the eyes.
Not to be used for: infants under 1 month.
Caution needed with:

Quinocort

A cream used as a steroid, antifungal, antibacterial treatment for skin disorders where there is also infection.

Side effects: fluid retention, suppression of adrenal glands, thinning of the skin may occur.
Caution: use for short periods of time only.

Not to be used for: patients suffering from acne or any other skin infections caused by tuberculosis, ringworm, viruses, or fungi, or continuously especially in pregnant women.
Caution needed with:

Regaine

A liquid used as a hair restorer to treat hair loss in men and women.

Side effects: dermatitis.
Caution: in patients suffering from low blood pressure, and on broken skin.
Not to be used for: children.
Caution needed with:

Synalar

An ointment used as a steroid treatment for skin disorders.

Side effects: fluid retention, suppression of adrenal glands, thinning of the skin may occur.
Caution: use for short periods of time only.
Not to be used for: patients suffering from acne or any other skin infections caused by tuberculosis, ringworm, viruses, or fungi, or continuously especially in pregnant women.
Caution needed with:

Topilar

A cream used as a steroid treatment for skin disorders, psoriasis.

Side effects: fluid retention, suppression of adrenal glands, thinning of the skin may occur.
Caution: use for short periods of time only.
Not to be used for: patients suffering from acne or any other skin infections caused by tuberculosis, ringworm, viruses, or fungi, or

continuously especially in pregnant women.
Caution needed with:

Triludan

A white, scored tablet supplied at a strength of 60 mg and used as an antihistamine treatment for allergies including hay fever and rhinitis.

Side effects: rash, sweating, headache, mild stomach disturbances, rapid heart beat.
Caution: in patients suffering from liver disease or some heart irregularities.
Not to be used for: children under 3 years.
Caution needed with: ketoconazole, erythromycin, itraconazole.

Trosyl

A solution used as an antifungal treatment for infections of the nails.

Side effects: mild irritation.
Caution:
Not to be used for: pregnant women.
Caution needed with:

Zaditen

A white, scored tablet supplied at a strength of 1 mg and used as an antihistamine preparation for the prevention of bronchial asthma, and the treatment of allergic rhinitis, conjunctivitis.

Side effects: drowsiness, reduced reactions, dizziness, dry mouth, excitement, weight gain.
Caution:
Not to be used for: children under 2 years, pregnant women, nursing mothers.

Caution needed with: alcohol,sedatives, antidiabetics taken by mouth, other antihistamines.

Zirtek

A white, oblong, scored tablet supplied at a strength of 10 mg and used as an antihistamine treatment for rhinitis, allergy.

Side effects: drowsiness, dizziness, headache, agitation, stomach disturbances, dry mouth.
Caution: in pregnant women and in patients suffering from kidney disease.
Not to be used for: children, nursing mothers.
Caution needed with: sedatives, alcohol.

Zovirax

A blue, shield-shaped tablet supplied at strengths of 200 mg, 400 mg, 800 mg and used as an antiviral treatment for genital herpes, other skin herpes, shingles.

Side effects: irritation (local use).
Caution: in patients suffering from kidney damage; drink plenty of fluids.
Not to be used for:
Caution needed with: probenecid.

Over-the-counter Medicines

Anaflex Cream

A cream used as an antibacterial and antifungal treatment for skin infections.

Acetoxyl

A gel used as an antibacterial and skin softener to treat acne.

Side effects: irritation, peeling.
Caution: keep out of the eyes, nose, and mouth; children should use the weaker gel.
Not to be used for:
Caution needed with:

Acnegel

A gel used as an antibacterial and skin softener to treat acne.

Side effects: irritation, peeling.
Caution: keep out of the eyes, nose, and mouth.
Not to be used for:
Caution needed with:

Acnidazil

A cream used as an antibacterial and skin softener to treat acne.

Side effects: irritation, peeling.
Caution: keep out of the eyes, nose, and mouth.
Not to be used for:
Caution needed with:

Acriflex

Acriflex is a cream containing chlorhexidine gluconate as a disinfectant. It may be useful to soothe burns and to prevent secondary infection.

Alphosyl

A cream used as an anti-psoriatic to treat psoriasis.

Side effects: irritation, sensitivity to light.
Caution:
Not to be used for: patients suffering from acute psoriasis.
Caution needed with:

Anthisan

Anthisan is a topical antihistamine cream containing mepyramine maleate 2 %. It is used for the treatment of allergic skin reactions and allergies.

Aquasept

A solution used as a disinfectant for skin and body cleansing and disinfecting.

Side effects:
Caution: keep out of the eyes.
Not to be used for:
Caution needed with:

Bacticlens

A solution in a sachet used as a disinfectant to clean the skin, wounds, or broken skin.

Side effects: throw away any remaining solution straight away after use.
Caution:
Not to be used for:
Caution needed with:

Balneum with Tar

A bath oil used as an emolient and antipsoriatic to treat eczema, itchy or thickening skin disorders, psoriasis.

Side effects:
Caution:
Not to be used for: children under 2 years or for patients suffering from wet or weeping skin problems or where the skin is badly broken.
Caution needed with:

Baltar

A liquid used as an antipsoriatic treatment for psoriasis, dandruff, eczema, dermatoses of the scalp.

Side effects:
Caution: keep out of the eyes.
Not to be used for: children under 2 years or for patients suffering from wet or weeping dermatoses or where the skin is badly broken.
Caution needed with:

Benoxyl 5

A cream used as an antibacterial and skin softener to treat acne.

Side effects: irritation, peeling.
Caution: keep out of the eyes, nose, and mouth.
Not to be used for:
Caution needed with:

Benzagel

A white gel used as an antibacterial and skin softener to treat acne.

Side effects: irritation, peeling.
Caution: keep out of the eyes, nose, and mouth.
Not to be used for:
Caution needed with:

Betadine Ointment

An ointment used as an antiseptic to treat ulcers.

Side effects: rarely irritation.
Caution: in patients sensitive to iodine.
Not to be used for:
Caution needed with:

Betadine Scalp and Skin Cleanser

A solution used as an antiseptic and detergent to treat acne, seborrhoeic scalp and skin disorders.

Side effects: rarely irritation or sensitivity.
Caution:
Not to be used for:
Caution needed with:

Betadine Spray

A spray used as an antiseptic to treat infected cuts, wounds, and burns.

Side effects:
Caution: keep out of the eyes.
Not to be used for: patients suffering from non-toxic colloid goitre
Caution needed with:

Brasivol

A paste used as an abrasive to treat acne.

Side effects:
Caution:
Not to be used for: patients suffering from visible superficial arteries or veins on the skin.
Caution needed with:

Caladryl

Caladryl is a preparation of calamine lotion containing an antihistamine and camphor.

Calamine lotion

Calamine lotion is a zinc-containing pink solution which is especially useful in chicken pox to reduce itch. It can also be used in other irritating skin conditions. Other preparations of calamine include Caladryl.

Callusolve

A paint used as a skin softener to treat warts.

Side effects:
Caution: apply only to warts and avoid healthy skin.
Not to be used for: treating warts on the face or anal and genital areas
Caution needed with:

Canesten

A solution used as an antifungal treatment for fungal inflammation and infection of the outer ear, skin, and nails.

Side effects: local irritation.
Caution:
Not to be used for:
Caution needed with:

Capitol

A gel used as an antibacterial treatment for dandruff and other similar scalp disorders.

Side effects:

Caution: in patients sensitive to iodine.
Not to be used for:
Caution needed with:

Carbo-Dome

A cream used as an antipsoriatic treatment for psoriasis.

Side effects: irritation, sensitivity to light.
Caution:
Not to be used for: patients suffering from acute psoriasis.
Caution needed with:

Ceanel Concentrate

A liquid used as an antibacterial, antifungal treatment for psoriasis, seborrhoeic inflammation of the scalp.

Side effects:
Caution: keep out of the eyes.
Not to be used for:
Caution needed with:

Cetavlex

A cream used as an antiseptic to treat minor cuts and wounds, nappy rash.

Side effects: irritation, peeling.
Caution:
Not to be used for:
Caution needed with:

Cetavlon PC

A liquid used as a disinfectant to treat dandruff.

Side effects: .

Caution: keep out of the eyes.
Not to be used for:
Caution needed with:

Cetriclens

A solution in a sachet used as a disinfectant for cleansing broken skin and dirty wounds.

Side effects:
Caution: throw away any unused solution straight away after use
Not to be used for:
Caution needed with:

Chlorasol

A solution in a sachet used as a disinfectant for cleaning and removing dead skin from ulcers.

Side effects: irritation.
Caution: keep away from the eyes and clothes; throw away any remaining solution immediately.
Not to be used for: internal use.
Caution needed with:

Chymoral Forte

An orange tablet supplied at a strength of 100, 000 units and used as an enzyme to treat acute inflammatory swelling.

Side effects: stomach disturbance.
Caution: in patients sensitive to iodine.
Not to be used for:
Caution needed with:

Clearasil

Clearasil is available as a cream, gel, and soap. It contains

triclosan and sulphur to clean and disinfect the skin, and is used in the treatment of acne.

Clinitar Cream

A cream used as an antipsoriatic treatment for psoriasis, eczema.

Side effects: sensitivity to light.
Caution:
Not to be used for: patients suffering from pustular psoriasis
Caution needed with:

Conotrane

A cream used as an antiseptic for protecting the skin from water, nappy rash, bed sores.

Cradocap

A shampoo used as an antiseptic treatment for cradle cap, scurf cap.

Cuplex

A gel used as a skin softener to treat warts, corns, and callouses.

Side effects:
Caution: do not apply to healthy skin.
Not to be used for: warts on the anal or genital areas
Caution needed with:

CX Powder

A powder used as a disinfectant to clean and disinfect the skin and prevent infection.

Daktarin Cream

A cream used as an antifungal treatment for infections of the skin and nails.

Debrisan

A powder used as an absorbant to treat weeping wounds including ulcers.

Dermacort

Dermacort contains 0.1% hydrocortisone. It can be used sparingly to treat mild itchy skin conditions such as eczema and dermatitis. Overuse of steroids on the face can cause skin thinning, and skin infections of all sorts are made worse by steroids such as hydrocortisone.

Derminostat

A cream used as an antifungal treatment for fungal infections of the skin and nails.

Disadine DP

A powder spray used as an antiseptic for the prevention and treatment of infection in wounds such as burns, bed sores, varicose ulcers.

Side effects:
Caution: care in treating severe burns.
Not to be used for: patients suffering from non-toxic colloid goitre.
Caution needed with:

Dithrocream

A cream used as an antipsoriatic treatment for psoriasis.

Side effects: irritation, allergy.
Caution:
Not to be used for: patients suffering from acute psoriasis.
Caution needed with:

Dithrolan

An ointment used as an antipsoriatic and skin softener to treat psoriasis.

Dose: before going to bed, bath and then apply the ointment to the affected area.
Side effects: irritation, allergy.
Caution:
Not to be used for: patients suffering from acute psoriasis.
Caution needed with:

Dome-Acne

A cream used as a skin softener to treat acne.

Side effects: irritation, underactive thyroid gland.
Caution: keep out of the eyes, nose, and mouth.
Not to be used for: dark-skinned patients.
Caution needed with:

Drapolene

A cream used as an antiseptic to treat nappy rash.

Duofilm

A liquid used as a skin softener to treat warts.

Side effects:
Caution: do not apply to healthy skin.
Not to be used for: warts on the face or anal and genital areas.
Caution needed with:

E45

E45 cream contains lanolin, white soft paraffin, and light liquid paraffin. It is a good cream for use in children as both a skin softener or protector, for example, in nappy rash.

Ecostatin

A cream used as an antifungal treatment for fungal infections of the skin.

Efcortelan

Efcortelan cream or ointment contains 1% hydrocortisone and is therefore ten times stronger than Dermacort . Consequently, it should be treated with even more respect. It should not be used for children.

Eskamel

A cream used as a skin softener to treat acne.

Side effects: irritation.
Caution: in patients suffering from acute local infection; keep out of the eyes, nose, and mouth.
Not to be used for:
Caution needed with:

Exelderm

A cream used as an antifungal treatment for fungal infections of the skin.

Side effects:
Caution: keep out of the eyes; if the area becomes irritated, the treatment should be stopped.
Not to be used for:
Caution needed with:

Exolan

A cream used as an antipsoriatic treatment for psoriasis.

Side effects: irritation, allergy.
Caution:
Not to be used for: patients suffering from acute psoriasis.
Caution needed with:

Gelcosal

A gel used as an antipsoriatic and skin softener to treat psoriasis, dermatitis, when the condition is scaling.

Gelcotar

A gel used as an antipsoriatic treatment for psoriasis, dermatitis.

Side effects: irritation, sensitivity to light
Caution:
Not to be used for: patients suffering from acute psoriasis.
Caution needed with:

Genisol

A liquid used as an antipsioratic and anti-dandruff treatment

for psoriasis, dandruff, seborrhoeic inflammation of the scalp.

Side effects: irritation, sensitivity to light.
Caution:
Not to be used for: patients suffering from acute psoriasis.
Caution needed with:

Germolene

Germolene contains chlorhexidine, lanolin, paraffin, and salicylate and is available as a cream, ointment, or spray. It is a good general-purpose skin antiseptic useful for cleaning cuts and abrasions. Suitable for children.

Glutarol

A solution used as a virucidal, skin-drying agent to treat warts.

Side effects: staining of the skin.
Caution: do not apply to healthy skin.
Not to be used for: warts on the face or anal and genital areas.
Caution needed with:

Hibiscrub

A solution used as a disinfectant for cleansing and disinfecting skin and hands.

Hibisol

A solution used as a disinfectant for cleansing and disinfecting skin and hands.

Hibitane

A cream used as a disinfectant for cleansing and disinfecting hands and skin before surgery, and for prevention of infections in wounds, and after surgery.

Hioxyl

A cream used as a disinfectant to treat minor wounds, infections, bed sores, leg ulcers.

Hirudoid

Hirudoid contains heparin (blood-thinning) components and is useful in dissolving skin bruises and local clots of blood. It may also reduce the tenderness in varicose veins.

Ionax

A gel used as an abrasive, antibacterial preparation to clean the skin in the treatment of acne.

Side effects:
Caution:
Not to be used for: children under 12 years.
Caution needed with:

Ionil T

A shampoo used as an antipsoriatic treatment for seborrhoeic inflammation of the scalp.

Side effects: irritation, sensitivity to light.
Caution:
Not to be used for: patients suffering from acute psoriasis.
Caution needed with:

Keralyt

A gel used as a skin softener to treat thickened skin.

Side effects:
Caution: keep out of the eyes, nose, and mouth.
Not to be used for:
Caution needed with:

Lenium

An anti-dandruff preparation.

Side effects:
Caution: keep out of the eyes and any areas of broken skin; do not use within 48 hours of waving or colouring substances.
Not to be used for:
Caution needed with:

Malatex

A solution used as an anti-inflammatory preparation to treat varicose and indolent ulcers, bed sores, burns.

Manusept

A solution used as a disinfectant for cleansing and disinfecting skin and hands before surgery.

Side effects:
Caution: keep out of the eyes.
Not to be used for:
Caution needed with:

Meditar

A waxy stick used as an antipsoriatic treatment for psoriasis, eczema.

Side effects: irritation, sensitivity to light.
Caution:
Not to be used for: patients suffering from acute psoriasis.
Caution needed with:

Monphytol

A paint used as an antifungal treatment for athlete's foot.

Side effects:
Caution:
Not to be used for: children or pregnant women.
Caution needed with:

Nericur

A gel used as an antibacterial skin softener to treat acne.

Side effects: irritation, peeling.
Caution: keep out of the eyes, nose, mouth.
Not to be used for: children.
Caution needed with:

Panoxyl

A gel used as an antibacterial skin softener to treat acne.

Side effects: irritation, peeling.
Caution: keep out of the eyes, nose, mouth.
Not to be used for:
Caution needed with:

pHiso-Med

A solution used as a disinfectant to treat acne, and for disinfecting infants' skin, cleansing and disinfecting skin before surgery.

Side effects:
Caution: in newborn infants dilute 10 times.
Not to be used for:
Caution needed with:
Contains: chlorhexidine gluconate.

Phytex

A paint used as an antifungal treatment for skin and nail infections.

Side effects:
Caution:
Not to be used for: children under 5 years or pregnant women.
Caution needed with:

Phytocil

A cream used as an antifungal treatment for tinea infections.

Polytar Liquid

A liquid used as an antipsoriatic treatment for psoriasis of the scalp, dandruff, seborrhoea, eczema.

Ponoxylan

A gel used as an antibacterial treatment for infection and inflammation of the skin.

Posalfilin

An ointment used as a skin softener to treat warts.

Side effects: pain when the ointment is first applied.

Caution: do not use on healthy skin.
Not to be used for: pregnant women or on warts on the face or anal and genital areas.
Caution needed with:

Pragmatar

A cream used as an anti-itch, antiseptic, skin softener to treat scaly skin, scalp seborrhoea, and similar disorders.

Side effects: irritation.
Caution: dilute the cream first when using for infants.
Not to be used for:
Caution needed with:

Psoradrate

A gel used as an antipsoriatic, drying agent to treat psoriasis.

Side effects: irritation, hypersensitivity.
Caution:
Not to be used for: pustular psoriasis.
Caution needed with:

Psoriderm

An emulsion used as an antipsoriatic to treat psoriasis.

Side effects: irritation, sensitivity to light.
Caution:
Not to be used for: patients suffering from acute psoriasis.
Caution needed with:

Psorigel

A gel used as an antipsoriatic treatment for psoriasis.

Side effects: irritation, sensitivity to light.

Caution:
Not to be used for: patients suffering from acute psoriasis.
Caution needed with:

Psorin

An ointment used as an antipsoriatic skin softener to treat psoriasis, eczema.

Side effects:
Caution: keep out of the eyes, and avoid direct sunlight.
Not to be used for: patients suffering from unstable psoriasis.
Caution needed with:

Quinoderm Cream

A cream used as an antibacterial skin softener to treat acne, acne-like eruptions, inflammation of the follicles.

Side effects: irritation, peeling.
Caution: keep out of the eyes, nose, mouth.
Not to be used for:
Caution needed with:

Quinoped

A cream used as a steroid, antifungal, antibacterial treatment for skin disorders where there is also infection.

Side effects: fluid retention, suppression of adrenal glands, thinning of the skin may occur.
Caution: use for short periods of time only.
Not to be used for: patients suffering from acne or any other skin infections caused by tuberculosis, ringworm, viruses, or funguses, or continuously especially in pregnant women.
Caution needed with:

Roccal

A solution used as a disinfectant for cleansing and disinfecting the skin before surgery.

Rotersept

An aerosol used as a disinfectant for the prevention of mastitis, and to treat cracked nipples.

Side effects:
Caution:
Not to be used for: children.
Caution needed with:

Salactol

A paint used as a skin softener to treat warts.

Side effects:
Caution: do not apply to healthy skin.
Not to be used for: warts on the face or anal and genital areas.
Caution needed with:

Savloclens

A solution in a sachet used as a disinfectant for cleansing and disinfecting wounds and burns.

Savlodil

A solution in a sachet used as a disinfectant for cleansing and disinfecting wounds and burns.

Savlon

Savlon contains chlorhexidine and cetrimide and is available as a cream, liquid, barrier cream, nappy rash cream, sachets, and spray (containing povidine iodine). It is a useful antiseptic cream suitable for all age groups.

Savlon Hospital Concentrate
A solution used as a disinfectant and general antiseptic.

Selsun

A suspension used as an anti-dandruff treatment for dandruff, tinea versicolor (a scalp condition).

Side effects:
Caution: keep out of the eyes or broken skin; do not use within 48 hours of using waving or colouring substances.
Not to be used for:
Caution needed with:

Ster-Zac DC

A cream used as a disinfectant for cleansing and disinfecting the hands before surgery.

Side effects:
Caution: in children under 2 years.
Not to be used for:
Caution needed with:

Ster-Zac Powder

A powder used as a disinfectant for the prevention of infections in newborn infants, and to treat recurring skin infections.

Side effects:
Caution: in patients where the skin is broken.
Not to be used for:
Caution needed with:

Synogist

A shampoo used as an antifungal, antibacterial treatment for seborrhoea of the scalp.

Side effects:
Caution: keep out of the eyes.
Not to be used for:
Caution needed with:

TCP

TCP contains phenol and salicylate and is available as an antiseptic and lotion and ointment and throat pastilles containing blackcurrant, honey, and menthol or lemon. TCP is an efficient antiseptic which should be diluted with water to avoid too strong an astringent effect.

T Gel

A shampoo used as an antipsoriatic treatment for dandruff, seborrhoea, and psoriasis of the scalp.

Side effects: irritation.
Caution:
Not to be used for: patients suffering from acute psoriasis.
Caution needed with:

Theraderm

A gel used as an antibacterial skin softener to treat acne.

Side effects: irritation, peeling.
Caution: keep out of the eyes, nose, mouth.
Not to be used for:
Caution needed with:

Timoped

A cream used as an antifungal treatment for athlete's foot and similar skin infections.

Tineafax

An ointment used as an antifungal treatment for athlete's foot and similar skin infections.

Tisept

A solution in a sachet used as a disinfectant for cleansing and disinfecting wounds and burns, changing dressing, obstetrics.

Torbetol

A lotion used as an antibacterial treatment for acne.

Travasept 100

A solution used as an aminoglycocide antibiotic, antibacterial preparation for disinfecting wounds and burns.

Triclosept

A cream used as a disinfectant for cleansing and disinfecting

the hands and skin.

Unisept

A solution used as a disinfectant and general antiseptic.

Veracur

A gel used as a skin softener to treat warts.
Side effects:
Caution: do not apply to healthy skin.
Not to be used for: warts on the face or anal and genital areas.
Caution needed with:

Verrugon

An ointment with corn rings and plasters used as a skin softener to treat warts.

Side effects:
Caution: do not apply to healthy skin
Not to be used for: warts on the face or anal and genital regions.
Caution needed with:

Verucasep

A gel used as a virucidal, anhidrotic treatment for viral warts.

Side effects: stains the skin.
Caution: do not apply to healthy skin.
Not to be used for: warts on the face or anal and genital regions.
Caution needed with:

Videne Powder

A powder used as an antiseptic treatment for infections in wounds and burns.

Vita-E

An ointment used as an anti-oxidant to treat wounds, bed sores, burns, skin ulcers.

Side effects:
Caution:
Not to be used for: patients suffering from overactive thyroid gland.
Caution needed with: fish liver oils, digitalis, insulin.

Chapter 5

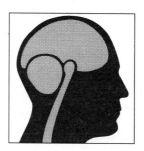

Nervous System

Please refer to 'Important Advice' on page 4 at the beginning of this book; and remember, if you are in any doubt, consult a physician.

Humans have highly developed nervous systems. The system is complex and involves a central nervous system of the spine and the brain, and a peripheral nervous system that supplies the muscles of the body as well as internal organs (a sympathetic and a parasympathetic nervous system). The brain itself is highly developed and separated into various parts with reasonably well-defined functions. The brain is very dependent on the rest of the body to supply it, however. Thus, it depends upon the cardiovascular system to supply it with blood and oxygen, and this system is delicate and prone to conditions such as stroke (CVA). The central nervous system is also unreasonably prone to trauma. Its complex structure makes it vulnerable to a number of degenerative conditions including dementia and Parkinson's disease. The origins of conditions such as multiple sclerosis are often not known although there may be a viral component.

Understanding the complex physiology of the central nervous system is a great challenge, but such an understanding will help us to treat a wide variety of neurological diseases that are currently untreatable.

Brain tumour

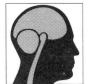

Brain tumours may be benign or malignant. In both cases, they cause their effects by local pressure rather than by spreading to other parts of the body. Very often, brain tumours are secondary to other cancers, such as lung cancer. Brain tumours may affect the main brain (cortex), lower brain (cerebellum), or spinal cord.

Symptoms

The symptoms of brain tumours are manifold because the tumour can mimic symptoms in any part of the body depending on where it sits in the brain or spinal column. The main symptoms of increased brain pressure are headache, nausea and vomiting, slowing of the pulse, loss of consciousness, or dementia. More specific symptoms include loss of speech, loss of vision, loss of hearing, loss of power, paralysis, loss of sensation, confusion, and disorientation. Epilepsy may also be a symptom of a brain tumour. The symptoms of brain tumours are persistent and worsening, whereas benign headache may come and go. Brain tumour symptoms seem to get worse gradually. Symptoms of raised brain pressure are worse in the morning.

Action

Where symptoms have persisted and where the patient is clearly deteriorating, medical attention is required. In the first place, you should try simple remedies for headaches, including analgesics such as aspirin or paracetamol.

Tests

The main tests for brain or spinal tumours are CT (computerized tomography) and MRI (magnetic resonance imaging) scans. Both of these scans give detailed pictures of internal organs. Tests, such as chest X-ray to look for for primary cancers, are important as are routine blood tests.

Medications and treatment

Dexamethasone is useful to reduce brain pressure. Brain tumours are treated by surgery, followed by chemo- and radiotherapy where appropriate for malignant tumours.

Further advice

Patients may suffer from post-operative epilepsy even if they did not have it before. This may require anticonvulsive medication.

Epilepsy and associated conditions ♥♥♥ including narcolepsy, petit mal epilepsy, grand mal epilepsy, and temporal lobe epilepsy

 Epilepsy is a condition caused by abnormal electrical patterns occurring within the brain which may trigger off a major seizure (grand mal) or brief loss of consciousness (petit mal). The cause of epilepsy is usually unknown but, apart from an association with family history, brain tumour, or other increases in brain pressure (e.g. abscess or haematoma) may trigger epilepsy. Epilepsy may be common when the blood sugar is low, such as after excess alcohol or premenstrually.

Main symptoms

Grand mal epilepsy: sudden collapse to the ground followed by spasm and then rhythmic jerking movements often of one side of the body. The seizure may be preceded by an aura or an unusual sensation or taste. Patients may often be incontinent or bite their tongues during a major attack and they may injure themselves in the fall. Petit mal epilepsy: perhaps just brief and repeated moments of loss of concentration and consciousness without collapse or jerky movements.
Temporal lobe epilepsy: the symptoms may be similar to grand mal epilepsy but they may also be accompanied by hallucinations,

particularly a sensation of smell. Narcolepsy: an irresistible desire and need to sleep.

Action
Where possible, a patient in grand mal epilepsy should be prevented from self-injury. Therefore, if a trained person is available, inserting something between the jaws to prevent biting the tongue may be helpful. It is important to maintain the patient's airway. For grand mal and for other types of epilepsy, you should seek medical assistance or advice as soon as possible.

Tests
These include electro-encephalograph (EEG), brain scan, and routine tests such as blood tests for precipitating factors.

Medications and treatment
There is a wide range of anticonvulsant medications including phenobarbitone, phenytoin, valproate, and carbamazepine. Examples: Ativan; clobazam; Epanutin; Epilim; Lamictal; Mysoline; Sabril; Valium; Zarontin. The practitioner will decide the dose and type of medication. Narcolepsy may respond to amphetamines.

Further advice
If you suffer from epilepsy, you should notify the driving authorities. You should also avoid excess alcohol and take precautions at times of greater risk. You may suffer from epilepsy only premenstrually or at night.

Migraine (and associated conditions, migrainous neuralgia and trigeminal neuralgia)

 Migraine is a condition where headache is associated with other symptoms described below. The cause of migraine is not known, but it is thought to be precipitated by certain factors such as emotional stress, physical stress, cold, eating

certain foods, e.g. cheese and chocolate.

Symptoms

The main symptom of migraine is a severe one-sided headache, but this is not always the typical presentation. The headache is associated with nausea and vomiting, prostration (need to lie down), visual disturbances (teichopsia) and occasionally weakness or numbness of parts of the body. These symptoms are caused by spasm of blood vessels in the brain. Migrainous neuralgia is a condition in which the headache may be associated with pain and watering in one eye (sometimes known as cluster headaches). Trigeminal neuralgia is similar in that there is facial pain on one side.

Action

If you are suffering from migraine, you should lie down in a darkened room and avoid stress or other precipitating factors. The symptoms may resolve spontaneously.

Tests

Nerve conduction studies may be appropriate, as are brain scan and EEG where symptoms are persistent and disabling.

Medications and treatment

Imigran is a relatively new but effective treatment for migraine. Otherwise, there are other ergot medications as well as over-the-counter preparations such as Migraleve. Trigeminal neuralgia and migrainous neuralgia may respond to carbamazepine. Examples: Betaloc; Blocadren; Cafergot; Corgard; Deseril; Dihydergot; Dixarit; Imigran; Inderal; Lingraine; Lopresor; Medihaler-Ergotamine; Midrid; Migraleve; Migravess; Migril; Paramax; Periactin; Sanomigran.

Further advice

Preventing attacks by avoiding precipitating factors may be helpful. Dietary maintenance is often effective.

Meningitis and encephalitis ♥♥♥♥♥

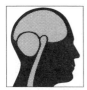

These serious conditions are caused by bacteria or viruses. Encephalitis is a rare late complication of measles. Meningitis may occasionally follow mumps infection but, often, it is a new infection passed around closed communities.

Symptoms

The symptoms of meningitis include fever, stiff neck, rigidity, rash on the body, deteriorating consciousness, unconsciousness, paralysis, and death. Encephalitis may appear similarly without the stiff neck characteristic of meningitis.

Action

As soon as these conditions are suspected, immediate medical attention is required to maintain the airway, and to begin diagnostic and therapeutic procedures.

Tests

Meningitis is diagnosed by lumbar puncture. Encephalitis may be harder to diagnose. Full blood tests, white count, sedimentation rates, chest X-ray, and skull X-ray are also part of the routine management of this condition. A high white count and raised sedimentation rate (ESR) are signs of infection.

Medications and treatment

Meningococcal meningitis responds to penicillin therapy. Viral meningitis does not respond to antibacterial therapy, and general supportive measures, including ventilation, may be required. Encephalitis is also usually a viral infection and the patient should be treated in hospital with general supportive measures.

Further advice

Meningitis contacts should be swabbed for carrier status. Vaccination is now available for certain types of meningitis.

Dementia, including presenile dementia ♥♥♥ (Alzheimer's disease)

 Dementia is a condition where brain function deteriorates gradually. It usually occurs in older people but certain forms may appear in the younger age group. It may be caused by hardening of the arteries (athero-sclerotic dementia), but, often, the cause is not known.

Main symptoms
Progressive deterioration in mental function, including loss of memory, particularly recent memory, whereas memory of an event that happened many years ago may remain intact. Patients repeat themselves in actions and words and may become very emotionally unstable because of their insecurity. As it progresses, dementia may cause patients to become dangers to themselves, e.g. they may turn on the gas but forget to light it. Patients may appear not to recognize close friends or relatives, including spouse.

Action
In the early stages, no action may be required but, where dementia is becoming difficult to live with, the patient and the carer may need counselling and support.

Tests
Investigations for general health, for example, heart and lung disease, are important. Therefore, chest X-ray, ECG, and routine blood tests should be part of the investigation of these patients. An ECG (electrocardiogram) is a test of the electrical impulses in the heart. It detects heart abnormalities that may relate to dementia. Conditions such as brain tumours may appear as dementia and these need to be excluded before definitive diagnosis of dementia or Alzheimer's disease can be made. Rarely brain biopsy may be performed.

Medications and treatment
Some agents are being developed for treating dementia. Treatment should be directed at heart disease and other causes where appropriate.

Further advice
Long-term planning is necessary for patients and for the carers to alleviate the effects of this distressing disease.

Associated conditions
Some conditions, such as Huntington's chorea (*see* below), may be associated with dementia.

Trauma/head injury ♥♥♥♥

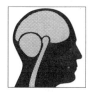 Head injury is common, particularly in road-traffic accidents, among motorcyclists, cyclists, and pedestrians. Some of the symptoms of head injury may be delayed.

Symptoms
Obvious trauma may be associated with bleeding from the ear or nose. Loss of consciousness may occur, and this is usually associated with more serious disease. Signs of raised brain pressure, e.g. headache, vomiting, deteriorating consciousness, require urgent attention. Blood clots in the brain, e.g. extradural or subdural haematomas, may cause delayed or very late symptoms which may appear with a slowly progressive dementia or epilepsy. Head injury may damage certain brain functions causing, for example, loss of smell, diabetes insipidus, loss of taste, loss of memory (anterograde or retrograde amnesia).

Action
Patients with obvious head injuries should be moved by skilled

medical or paramedical personnel only to prevent further damage, particularly to the spinal cord. Ventilation may be required.

Tests
Investigations include CT brain scan, MRI scans, skull X-rays, X-rays looking for injuries elsewhere, arteriography of brain blood vessels.

Medications and treatment
General supportive treatment, including the use of dexamethasone to reduce brain pressure, and antibiotics for infection, are included as part of the medical support for these patients.

Further advice
After a head injury, you may develop late symptoms, such as depression or epilepsy (*see* above).

Neuropathy, including peripheral ♥♥ neuropathy and nerve pressure symptoms, e.g. carpal tunnel syndrome and Bell's palsy

Neuropathy is a condition in which there is interference with, or damage to, the nerves, usually to the hands and feet. Neuropathy may be caused by certain types of vitamin deficiency, diabetes, certain drugs or toxins, and late manifestations of diseases such as syphilis.

Symptoms
The main symptoms of neuropathy are pain, tingling, or loss of sensation in certain areas of the body, usually in the hands and feet. Carpal tunnel syndrome is caused by pressure on a nerve at the wrists and this causes pain in the hands. Bell's palsy is caused by a

virus infection of the facial nerve, and this can cause paralysis of the muscles on one side of the face, mimicking a stroke. Patients may have walking difficulties, e.g. foot drop, or difficulty undoing or doing up buttons.

Action
Progressive neuropathy should be investigated and treated but it is not usually an emergency.

Tests
These include excluding vitamin deficiencies, diabetes, and other causes. Therefore, blood tests are carried out to check the blood sugar, anaemia, underactive thyroid gland and other possible causes. Nerve conduction studies are especially useful, e.g. in nerve compression syndrome such as the carpal tunnel syndrome.

Medications and treatment
The underlying causes should be treated specifically, e.g. antidiabetic agents for diabetes, vitamins for vitamin deficiency, and thyroxine for underactive thyroid.

Further advice
Pay particular attention to general health, e.g. alcohol intake and diet. You should exercise regularly.

Multiple sclerosis (disseminated sclerosis)

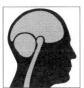 The cause of multiple sclerosis is not known for certain, although there is a suggestion that it is a degenerative and demyelinating disease triggered by earlier viral infection. The nerve tracts are affected by areas of loss of the fatty sheath (demyelination) which affects nerve conduction. Multiple

sclerosis is more common in mild climates and among people with a family history of the condition.

Symptoms

They may vary enormously. Typically, the symptoms are not noticed on both sides of the body at the same time, but they are patchy (i.e. disseminated). Temporary loss of vision may be an early symptom, as may be trigeminal neuralgia (*see* above). Pain or tingling sensations of heat, or pins and needles anywhere in the body, particularly in the limbs, may also be an early symptom. The symptoms may come and go in bursts with remissions and relapses. The disease progresses at different rates in different people and, while some patients progress inexorably to blindness and paralysis, others remain permanently stable after a brief display of symptoms. Mood changes, from depression to euphoria, may also be associated with the condition. Demyelination affecting the parasympathetic nervous system may cause bowel and bladder problems.

Action

You should seek specialist neurological opinion if your symptoms are alarming and persistent. Self-medication is generally not advisable because there are many unproven treatments available.

Tests

Lumbar puncture and biopsy are the tests which make the diagnosis of this condition. Suspicions may be made on clinical grounds alone. Brain scans, MRI scans, may show a very clear picture of demyelination.

Medications and treatment

While steroids may produce some benefit, and trials of interferon are under way, there are no recognized cures for multiple sclerosis, although general supportive measures are appropriate.

Further advice

Keeping yourself in good health and trying to maintain an optimistic outlook are essential in controlling this condition.

Parkinson's disease ♥♥♥

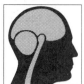

The cause of Parkinson's disease is not known. It results in loss of dopamine-producing nerve fibres in the brain. This causes the symptoms described below. Rarely, Parkinson's-type syndromes can occur after taking certain drugs, particularly phenothiazine types, and after virus infection (post-encephalitic parkinsonism).

Symptoms

These include tremor, usually of the hands, rigidity of the limbs and facial muscles. Patients have difficulty walking, writing, and, on some occasions, talking. For many patients, the rigidity is as serious a problem as the tremor. The disease is usually slowly progressive and affects both sides of the body simultaneously. The tremor occurs at rest and may affect the hands, legs, or head. It usually improves a little with movement (unlike cerebellar disease where the tremor worsens with movement — intension tremor). Rigidity of facial muscles may make the face appear expressionless. Rigidity of the limbs results in a characteristic shuffling gait. The tremor of the hands may be described as a pill-rolling tremor.

Action

There is no urgency to diagnose or to investigate this condition. Many people have benign familial tremors or shaking of the hands for other reasons.

Tests

A diagnosis is usually made clinically, but supported by brain scan and evidence of loss of dopaminergic nerve fibres.

Medications and treament

Dopamine-replacement drugs, such as Sinemet, and other anti-parkinsonian drugs, such as Eldepryl and Artane, are useful in this condition. Also: Akineton; Arpicolin, Celance; Cogentin; Disipal; Eldepryl; Kemadrin; Larodopa; Madopar; Nitoman; Parlodel; Pevaryl; Symmetrel; Tremonil.

Further advice

Maintaining a regular, gentle exercise pattern may reduce the rigidity that this condition causes. You should avoid chest infections which are often very severe because of the difficulty in moving chest muscles.

Associated conditions

Apart from benign tremors, there are other conditions which cause shaking, sometimes wild shaking (chorea). These include Tourette's syndrome and Huntington's chorea.

Motor neurone disease ♥♥♥♥♥ (also called amyotrophic lateral sclerosis)

 Motor neurone disease is a progressive neurological condition; its cause is not known. It affects the nerves supplying muscles, and so the symptoms are mainly related to movement rather than to sensation.

Symptoms

Slow, progressive weakness of muscles in certain parts of the body. These muscles may affect speech and swallowing (pseudo-bulbar palsy) or, more commonly, the hands. Weakness and wasting of muscles are characteristic with fibrillation. The condition worsens progressively, and eventually patients will die from the disease.

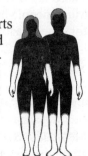

Action

Early diagnosis is important so that support systems can be established to maintain patients who may ultimately become paralysed and need supportive care.

Tests
Biopsy of nerve and muscle may be helpful in making the diagnosis but very often the disease is diagnosed clinically. MRI scan may be helpful.

Medications and treatment
There are no medications which are known to affect the progress of this disease, but treatment of infections, and general support are often required.

Cerebral vascular accident ♥♥♥♥♥ (CVA, Stroke, Cerebral vascular disease, Hardening of the arteries)

 CVAs and strokes are caused by thrombosis, i.e. blood clot in a vessel supplying blood and oxygen to pass to the brain, or by haemorrhage, i.e. breakdown of a major vessel which has the same ultimate effect of denying oxygen to the brain. Cerebral haemorrhage may occur as a result of trauma (*see* above) or rupture of a congenital aneurysm. Major catastrophic strokes may occur or the strokes may may be smaller and minor (including so-called transient ischaemic attacks – TIA – a brief and temporary loss of oxygen to the brain).

Symptoms
The symptoms of major stroke are sudden collapse with paralysis, often of one side of the body, loss of speech (if the right side of the body is involved). Patients may lapse into unconsciousness and may not

recover. More commonly, gradual recovery occurs with residual paralysis of one side of the body. Depending on the severity of the stroke, recovery may be rapid over a few days or may be more prolonged with spasticity of one half of the body, loss of bowel and bladder function, loss of speech, and loss of sensation. Although many cases resolve, some do not. This may be a cause of permanent paralysis of one side of the body (haemiparesis). The stroke may be secondary to a blood clot travelling through the body (embolus) which may arise after a heart attack. Therefore, patients suffering from a stroke may also show the symptoms of a heart attack.

Action

A stroke or CVA is a medical emergency and urgent medical attention is required. Transient ischaemic attacks, where brief loss of speech or brief tremor of the hand occurs, also need medical intervention because they could be caused by travelling blood clots.

Tests

Tests, such as ECG, chest X-ray, and blood tests for precipitating factors are important. Also tests for blood-clotting factors and for high blood pressure are valuable. Arteriography of brain circulation is helpful, particularly where there is an aneurysm which may be treatable surgically. Brain scan is also valuable in the diagnosis.

Medications and treatment

Anticoagulants are required for repeated thrombosis or embolus. Treating haemorrhagic disorders involves appropriate replacement therapy (e.g. factor 8 for haemophilia). Otherwise treatment and recovery from stroke include general supportive measures and treatment of high blood pressure or other precipitating factors.

Prescription Medicines

Akineton

A white, scored tablet supplied at a strength of 2 mg and used as an anticholinergic to treat Parkinson's disease.

Side effects: drowsiness, dry mouth, blurred vision.
Caution: in patients suffering from abnormal heart rhythm or heart attack, epilepsy, urinary obstruction.
Not to be used for: children or patients suffering from gastro-intestinal obstruction, glaucoma; pregnant women or nursing mothers.
Caution needed with: other anti-parkinson drugs, sedating drugs.

Arpicolin

A syrup supplied at strengths of 2.5 mg/5 ml, 5 mg/5 ml and used as an anticholinergic treatment for Parkinson's disease.

Side effects: anticholinergic effects, confusion at high doses.
Caution: in patients suffering from heart problems, gastro-intestinal obstruction, glaucoma, enlarged prostate. The dosage should be reduced gradually.
Not to be used for: children or patients suffering from tardive dyskinesia (a movement disorder).
Caution needed with: phenothiazines, antihistamines, antidepressants.

Artane

A white, scored tablet supplied at strengths of 2 mg, 5 mg and used as an anticholinergic treatment for Parkinson's disease, drug-induced Parkinson's disease.

Side effects: anticholinergic effects, confusion and agitation at high doses.
Caution: in patients suffering from heart, kidney, or liver disease, enlarged prostate, glaucoma, or gastro-intestinal obstruc-

tion. Dose should be reduced gradually.
Not to be used for: children.
Caution needed with: phenothiazines, antihistamines, antidepressants.

Ativan

A blue, oblong, scored tablet or a yellow, oblong, scored tablet according to strengths of 1 mg, 2.5 mg and used as a tranquillizer to treat anxiety.

Side effects: drowsiness, confusion, unsteadiness, stomach upset, low blood pressure, rash, changes in vision, changes in libido, retention of urine. Risk of addiction increases with dose and length of treatment. May impair judgement.
Caution: in the elderly, pregnant women, nursing mothers, in women during labour, and in patients suffering from lung disorders, kidney or liver disorders. Avoid long-term use and withdraw gradually.
Not to be used for: children, or for patients suffering from acute lung diseases, some chronic lung diseases, some obsessional and psychotic diseases.
Caution needed with: alcohol, other tranquillizers, anticonvulsants.

Blocadren

A blue, scored tablet supplied at a strength of 10 mg and used as a ß-blocker to treat angina, high blood pressure, migraine, and as a treatment following heart attack.

Side effects: cold hands and feet, sleep disturbances, slow heart rate, tiredness, wheezing, heart failure, stomach upset, dry eyes, rash.
Caution: in pregnant women, nursing mothers, and in patients suffering from diabetes, kidney or liver disorders. May need to be withdrawn before surgery. Withdraw gradually. Your doctor may advise additional treatment with digoxin and diuretics.

Not to be used for: children, or for patients suffering from heart block or failure, asthma.

Caution needed with: verapamil, clonidine withdrawal, some anti-arrhythmic drugs and anaesthetics, some antihypertensives, ergotamine, antidiabetics, cimetidine, sedatives, sympathomimetics, indomethacin.

Cafergot

A white tablet used as an ergot preparation to treat migraine.

Side effects: nausea, muscular pain, abdominal pain, reduced circulation, weak legs.
Caution:
Not to be used for: children, pregnant women, nursing mothers, or in patients suffering from coronary, peripheral, or occlusive vascular disease, severe high blood pressure, kidney or liver disease, sepsis.
Caution needed with: erythromycin, ß-blockers.

Celance

An ivory, green, or pink, rectangular, scored tablet according to strengths of 0.05 mg, 0.25 mg, 1 mg, and used as an antiparkinsonian drug as an additional treatment for Parkinson's disease.

Side effects: hallucinations, confusion, movement disorder, drowsiness, low blood pressure, heartbeat abnormalities, nausea, dyspepsia, inflammation of the nose, breathing difficulty, double vision.
Caution: in pregnant women, nursing mothers, and in patients suffering from heart disease, abnormal heart rhythm, or with a history of hallucinations. Treatment should be withdrawn gradually.
Not to be used for: children.
Caution needed with: other similar antiparkinsonian drugs, antihypertensives, anticoagulants.

Cogentin

A white, quarter-scored tablet supplied at a strength of 2 mg and used as an anticholinergic treatment for Parkinson's disease.

Side effects: anticholinergic effects, confusion, agitation, and rash at high doses.
Caution: in patients suffering from rapid heart rate, enlarged prostate, glaucoma, stomach blockage. Dose should be reduced gradually.
Not to be used for: infants under 3 years or for patients suffering from certain movement disorders.
Caution needed with: antihistamines, antidepressants, some tranquillizers.

Corgard

A pale-blue tablet supplied at strengths of 40 mg, 80 mg and used as a ß-blocker to treat heart rhythm disturbances, angina, high blood pressure, additional treatment in thyroid disease, migraine.

Side effects: cold hands and feet, sleep disturbances, slow heart rate, tiredness, wheezing, heart failure, stomach upset, dry eyes, rash.
Caution: in pregnant women, nursing mothers, and in patients suffering from diabetes, kidney or liver disorders, asthma. May need to be withdrawn before surgery. Withdraw gradually. Your doctor may advise additional treatment with diuretics or digoxin.
Not to be used for: children or for patients suffering from heart block or failure.
Caution needed with: verapamil, clonidine withdrawal, some anti-arrhythmic drugs and anaesthetics, reserpine, some antihypertensives, ergotamine, antidiabetics, cimetidine, sedatives, sympathomimetics, indomethacin.

Deseril

A white tablet supplied at a strength of 1 mg and used as an anti-spasmodic treatment for diarrhoea associated with carcinoid disease, migraine, severe headache.

Side effects: nausea and other stomach disturbances, drowsiness, dizziness, fluid retention, arterial spasm, retroperitonital, pleural, and heart valve fibrosis (membrane thickening), leg cramps, weight gain, rash, hair loss, disturbance of nervous system.
Caution: in patients suffering from or with a history of stomach ulcer.
Not to be used for: children, pregnant women, nursing mothers, or patients suffering from severe high blood pressure, collagen disorders, coronary, peripheral, or occlusive vascular disease, liver or kidney disease, weight loss, sepsis, lung disease.
Caution needed with: medicines affecting blood vessels, ergotamine.

Disipal

A yellow tablet supplied at a strength of 50 mg and used as an anticholinergic drug to treat Parkinson's disease.

Side effects: euphoria, anticholinergic effects, and confusion, agitation, and rash at high dose.
Caution: in patients suffering from heart problems or stomach obstruction. Reduce dose slowly.
Not to be used for: patients suffering from glaucoma, enlarged prostate, some movement disorders.
Caution needed with: phenothiazines, antihistamines, antidepressants.

Dixarit

A blue tablet supplied at a strength of 25 micrograms and used as a blood vessel antispasmodic drug to treat migraine, headache, menopausal flushing.

Side effects: sedation, dry mouth, dizziness, sleeplessness.
Caution: in nursing mothers or in patients suffering from depression.
Not to be used for: children.
Caution needed with: antihypertensives.

Eldepryl

A white, scored tablet supplied at strengths of 5 mg, 10 mg and used as an anti-parkinsonian treatment for Parkinson's disease.

Side effects: low blood pressure on standing, involuntary movements, nausea, confusion, mental disorders.
Caution:
Not to be used for: children.
Caution needed with:

Epanutin

A white/purple capsule, a white/pink capsule, or a white/orange capsule according to strengths of 25 mg, 50 mg, 100 mg and used as an anticonvulsant to treat epilepsy, neuralgia.

Side effects: stomach upset, sleeplessness, unsteadiness, allergies, gum swelling, hairiness and motor activity in young people, blood changes, lymph gland swelling, nystagmus (abnormal eye movements).
Caution: in pregnant women, nursing mothers, and in patients suffering from liver disease. Dose should be reduced gradually. Maintain adequate levels of vitamin D.
Not to be used for:
Caution needed with: coumarin anticoagulants, isoniazid, chloramphenicol, sulthiame, the contraceptive pill, doxycycline.

Epilim

A lilac tablet supplied at strengths of 200 mg, 500 mg and

used as an anticonvulsant to treat epilepsy.

Side effects: gain in weight, loss of hair, fluid retention, pancreatitis, liver failure, blood changes, neurological effects.
Caution: in pregnant women, in patients suffering from mental retardation, or who are undergoing major surgery.
Not to be used for: patients suffering from liver disease.
Caution needed with: antidepressants, other anticonvulsants, anticoagulants.

Imigran

A white, capsule-shaped tablet supplied at a strength of 100 mg and used to treat migraine.

Side effects: tiredness, dizziness, feelings of heaviness and weakness, throat symptoms, chest pain, raised blood pressure, liver disorder.
Caution: in pregnant women, nursing mothers, and in patients suffering from liver or kidney disorder.
Not to be used for: children, the elderly, or for patients suffering from heart disease or disorder, or uncontrolled high blood pressure.
Caution needed with: MAOIs, lithium, ergotamine, some antidepressants.

Inderal

A pink tablet supplied at strengths of 10 mg, 40 mg, 80 mg and used as a ß-blocker to treat angina, migraine, high blood pressure, anxiety, abnormal heart rhythm, other heart conditions, and as an additional treatment for thyrotoxicosis.

Side effects: cold hands and feet, sleep disturbance, slow heart rate, tiredness, wheezing, heart failure, stomach upset.
Caution: in pregnant women, nursing mothers, and in patients suffering from diabetes, kidney or liver disorders, asthma. May need to be withdrawn before surgery. Withdraw gradually. Your doctor may advise additional treatment with diuretics or digoxin.

Not to be used for: patients suffering from heart block or failure.
Caution needed with: verapamil, clonidine withdrawal, some
anti-arrhythmic drugs and anaesthetics, reserpine, cimetidine,
sedatives, sympathomimetics, indomethacin, antidiabetics,
ergotamine, some antihypertensives.

Kemadrin

**A white, scored tablet supplied at a strength of 5 mg and used
as an anticholinergic to treat Parkinson's disease.**

Side effects: anticholinergic effects, confusion at high doses.
Caution: in patients suffering from heart problems, stomach
obstruction, glaucoma, enlarged prostate. Reduce dose slowly.
Not to be used for: children or patients suffering from movement
disorders.
Caution needed with: phenothiazines, antihistamines, antidepressants, some tranquillizers.

Lamictal

**A yellow tablet supplied at strengths of 25 mg, 50 mg, 100 mg,
and used as an anticonvulsant to treat epilepsy.**

Side effects: rash, severe allergy, double or blurred vision,
dizziness, drowsiness, headache, stomach upset.
Caution: in pregnant women, nursing mothers, and in patients
suffering from rash, fever, influenza, drowsiness, or worsening of
symptoms. Must be withdrawn gradually.
Not to be used for: children, the elderly, or for patients suffering
from liver or kidney damage.
Caution needed with: phenytoin, carbamazepine, phenobarbitone, primidone, sodium valproate.

Larodopa

A white, quarter-scored tablet supplied at a strength of 500

mg and used as an anti-parkinsonian drug to treat Parkinson's disease.

Side effects: nausea, vomiting anorexia, low blood pressure on standing up, involuntary movments, heart and brain disturbances, discoloration of urine.
Caution: in pregnant women and in patients suffering from heart, liver, kidney, lung, or endocrine disease, stomach ulcer, and glaucoma. Your doctor may advise that blood and liver, kidney, and cardiovascular systems should be checked regularly.
Not to be used for: children, adults aged under 25, or for patients suffering from severe mental disorder, glaucoma, or a history of malignant melanoma.
Caution needed with: MAOIs, pyridoxine, antihypertensives, sympathomimetics, ferrous sulphate, some other similar drugs.

Lingraine

A green tablet supplied at a strength of 2 mg and used as an ergot preparation to treat migraine, headache.

Side effects: nausea, stomach pain, leg cramps.
Caution:
Not to be used for: children, pregnant women, nursing mothers, or for patients suffering from coronary, peripheral, or occlusive vascular disease, severe high blood pressure, kidney or liver disease, sepsis, overactive thyroid, porphyria (a rare blood disorder).
Caution needed with: erythromycin, ß-blockers.

Lopresor

A pink, scored tablet or a pale-blue, scored tablet according to strengths of 50 mg, 100 mg and used as a ß-blocker to treat angina, for the prevention of heart muscle damage, high blood pressure, and as an additional treatment in thyrotoxicosis, migraine.

Side effects: cold hands and feet, sleep disturbance, slow heart rate, tiredness, wheezing, heart failure, stomach upset, dry eyes, rash.

Caution: in pregnant women, nursing mothers, and in patients suffering from diabetes, kidney or liver disorders, asthma. May need to be withdrawn before surgery. Withdraw gradually. Your doctor may advise additional treatment with diuretics or digoxin.

Not to be used for: children, or for patients suffering from heart block or failure.

Caution needed with: verapamil, clonidine withdrawal, some anti-arrhythmic drugs and anaesthetics, reserpine, some antihypertensives, ergotamine, cimetidine, sedatives, antidiabetics, sympathomimetics, indomethacin.

Madopar

A blue/grey capsule, blue/pink capsule, or blue/caramel capsule according to strengths of 62.5 mg, 125 mg, 250 mg and used as an anti-parkinsonian combination to treat Parkinson's disease.

Side effects: nausea, vomiting, anorexia, low blood pressure on standing, involuntary movements, heart and brain disturbances, discoloration of urine, rarely haemolytic anaemia.

Caution: in patients suffering from cardiovascular, liver, lung, endocrine or kidney disease, stomach ulcer, mental disturbance, glaucoma, bone changes. Your doctor may advise that blood, liver, kidney, and cardiovascular systems should be checked regularly.

Not to be used for: children, adults under 25 years,pregnant women, nursing mothers, or for patients suffering from severe mental disorders, glaucoma, history of malignant melanoma.

Caution needed with: MAOIs, antihypertensives, sympathomimetics, ferrous sulphate, other similar drugs.

Medihaler-Ergotamine

An aerosol used to treat migraine.

Side effects: nausea, muscular pain.
Caution:
Not to be used for: children under 10 years, pregnant women, nursing mothers, or for patients suffering from coronary, peripheral, or occlusive vascular disease, severe high blood pressure, kidney or liver disease, or sepsis.
Caution needed with: erythromycin, ß-blockers.

Midrid

A red capsule used as an analgesic to treat migraine.

Side effects: dizziness.
Caution: in pregnant women and nursing mothers.
Not to be used for: children, or for patients suffering from severe kidney, liver, or heart disease, gastritis, severe high blood pressure, or glaucoma.
Caution needed with: MAOIs, other medicines containing paracetamol.

Migraleve

A pink tablet and a yellow tablet according to strength and contents and used as an analgesic, antihistamine treatment for migraine.

Side effects: drowsiness.
Caution: in patients suffering from kidney or liver disease.
Not to be used for: children under 10 years.
Caution needed with: other medicines containing paracetamol.

Migravess

A white, scored, effervescent tablet used as an anti-cmetic and analgesic to treat migraine.

Side effects: extrapyramidal reactions (shaking and rigidity), drowsiness, diarrhoea.

Caution: in pregnant women or in patients suffering from kidney or liver disease, asthma.

Not to be used for: children under 12 years or for patients suffering from stomach ulcer, haemophilia, or allergy to aspirin or anti-inflammatory drugs.

Caution needed with: anticholinergics, some sedatives, anticoagulants, antidiabetics and uric acid-lowering agents.

Migril

A white, scored tablet used as an ergot preparation to treat migraine.

Side effects: rebound headache, poor circulation, abdominal pain, drowsiness, dry mouth.

Caution: in patients suffering from sepsis, anaemia, overactive thyroid.

Not to be used for: children, pregnant women, nursing mothers, or for patients suffering from coronary, peripheral, or occlusive vascular disease, severe high blood pressure, kidney or liver disease.

Caution needed with: erythromycin, ß-blockers, sedatives.

Mysoline

A white, scored tablet supplied at a strength of 250 mg and used as an anticonvulsant to treat epilepsy

Side effects: drowsiness, hangover, dizziness, allergies, headache, confusion, excitement, anaemia.

Caution: in patients suffering from kidney, liver, or lung disease. Dependence (addiction) may develop.

Not to be used for: children, young adults, pregnant women, nursing mothers, the elderly, patients with a history of drug or alcohol abuse, or suffering from porphyria (a rare blood disorder), or in the management of pain.

Caution needed with: anticoagulants, alcohol, other tranquillizers, steroids, the contraceptive pill, griseofulvin, rifampicin, phenytoin, metronidazole, chloramphenicol.

Nitoman

A yellow/buff, scored tablet supplied at a strength of 25 mg and used as a sedative to treat Huntington's chorea, hemiballismus, senile chorea (movement disorders)

Side effects: drowsiness, depression, low blood presure on standing, tremor, rigidity.
Caution: in pregnant women.
Not to be used for: children or for nursing mothers.
Caution needed with: reserpine, levodopa, MAOIs.

Paramax

A white, scored tablet used as an analgesic, anti-emetic treatment for migraine.

Side effects: extrapyramidal reactions (shaking and rigidity), drowsiness, diarrhoea.
Caution: pregnant women, nursing mothers, and in patients suffering from liver or kidney disease.
Not to be used for: children under 12 years.
Caution needed with: anticholinergics, sedatives, other medicines containing paracetamol.

Parlodel

A white, scored tablet supplied at strengths of 1 mg, 2.5 mg and used as a hormone blocker to treat Parkinson's disease, inappropriate lactation, infertility, cyclical benign breast disease, elevated prolactin.

Side effects: low blood pressure on standing, brain and stomach disturbances, nausea, vomiting, constipation, headache, drowsiness, poor circulation, movement disorders, dry mouth, leg cramps, lung changes, dizziness, convulsions.

Caution: in women, patients suffering from a history of mental disorder, severe cardiovascular disease. Your doctor may advise regular examinations.
Not to be used for: children, women with complications of pregnancy, or for patients suffering from allergy to ergotamine.
Caution needed with: alcohol, eryhtromycin, ergotamine, drugs affecting blood pressure.

Periactin

A white, scored tablet supplied at a strength of 4 mg and used as an antihistamine, serotonin antagonist (hormone blocker) to improve appetite,and to treat allergies, itchy skin conditions, migraine.

Side effects: anticholinergic effects, reduced reactions, drowsiness.
Caution: in pregnant women and in patients suffering from bronchial asthma, raised eye pressure, overactive thyroid, cardiovascular disease, high blood pressure.
Not to be used for: children under 2 years, nursing mothers, the elderly, or patients suffering from glaucoma, enlarged prostate, bladder obstruction, retention of urine, stomach blockage, stomach ulcer, or debilitation.
Caution needed with: MAOIs, alcohol, sedatives.

Pevaryl

A cream used as an antifungal treatment for inflammation of the penis, inflammation of the vulva, thrush-like nappy rash, other skin infections such as tinea or nail infections.

Side effects: irritation.
Caution:
Not to be used for:
Caution needed with:

Sabril

A white, oval, scored tablet supplied at a strength of 500 mg and used to treat epilepsy.

Side effects: aggression, mental disturbance, tiredness, dizziness, nervousness, irritability, memory and visual disturbances, excitation, agitation, increased frequency of seizures.
Caution: in the elderly, and in patients with a history of mental or behavioural problems, or suffering from kidney damage. Your doctor may recommend regular examinations.
Not to be used for: children under 10 kg body weight, pregnant women, nursing mothers.
Caution needed with:

Sanomigran

An ivory, scored tablet supplied at strengths of 0.5 mg, 1.5 mg and used as a blood vessel stabilizer to treat migraine or headache.

Side effects: drowsiness, weight gain, excitement.
Caution: in patients suffering from glaucoma or retention of urine.
Not to be used for:
Caution needed with:

Sinemet

A blue, scored, oval tablet or a yellow, scored tablet according to strengths of LS 50/12.5 mg, 110 110/10 mg, Plus 100/25 mg, 275 250/25 mg and used as an anti-parkinsonian preparation to treat Parkinson's disease.

Side effects: nausea, vomiting, anorexia, low blood pressure on standing, involuntary movements, heart and brain disturbances, discoloration of urine.
Caution: in patients suffering from cardiovascular, liver, kidney, lung, or endocrine disease, stomach ulcer, or glaucoma. Your

doctor may advise that blood, liver, kidney, and cardiovascular system should be checked regularly.

Not to be used for: patients under 18 years, pregnant women, nursing mothers, or for patients suffering from severe mental disorders or glaucoma, or for patients with a history of malignant melanoma.

Caution needed with: drugs affecting brain peptides, MAOIs, antihypertensives, and sympathomimetics.

Symmetrel

A brownish-red capsule supplied at a strength of 100 mg and used as an anti-parkinsonian/antiviral drug to treat Parkinson's disease, virus infections.

Side effects: skin changes, fluid retention, rash, sight, brain and stomach disturbances.

Caution: in pregnant women, confused patients, and in patients suffering from liver or kidney disease or congestive heart failure.

Not to be used for: patients suffering from severe kidney disease or with a history of convulsions or stomach ulcers.

Caution needed with: anticholinergics, levodopa, stimulants.

Tremonil

A white, scored tablet supplied at a strength of 5 mg and used as an anticholinergic treatment for Parkinson's disease and senile tremor.

Side effects: anticholinergic effects, confusion at high doses, nausea, fatigue, stomach pain.

Caution: in patients with marked disease of the autonomic nervous system. Dose should be reduced slowly.

Not to be used for: children or for patients suffering from en-larged prostate, glaucoma, abnormal heart rhythm, intestinal slowness, tardive dyskinesia (a movement disorder), myasthenia gravis, urine retention.

Caution needed with: antihistamines, antidepressants, analgesics, alcohol, anticholinergics, some sedatives.

Valium

A white tablet, yellow tablet, or blue tablet according to strengths of 2 mg, 5 mg, 10 mg and used as a sedative to treat anxiety, acute alcohol withdrawal, and for the short-term treatment of sleeplessness where sedation during the day is not a difficulty, fear and sleepwalking at night in children, muscle spasm.

Side effects: drowsiness, reduced reactions, .
Caution: in the elderly, pregnant women, nursing mothers, and in patients suffering from chronic lung weakness, kidney or liver disease. Avoid long-term treament and withdraw gradually.
Not to be used for: patients with acute lung weakness, some mental disorders.
Caution needed with: alcohol, sedatives, anticonvulsants.

Zarontin

An orange capsule supplied at a strength of 250 mg and used as an anticonvulsant to treat epilepsy.

Side effects: stomach and brain disturbances, rash, blood changes, SLE (a multisystem disorder).
Caution: in pregnant women, nursing mothers, and in patients suffering from kidney or liver disease. Dose should be decreased gradually.
Not to be used for:
Caution needed with:

Antibiotics

Amoxil

A maroon/gold capsule supplied at a strength of 250 mg, 500

mg and used as a broad-spectrum penicillin to treat respiratory, ear, nose, and throat, urinary, venereal, and soft tissue infections. Also for dental abscess, and to prevent infection of the heart during dental procedures

Side effects: stomach upset, allergy.
Caution: in patients suffering from glandular fever.
Not to be used for: patients suffering from penicillin allergy.
Caution needed with:

Ciproxin

Tablets supplied at strengths of 250 mg, 500 mg, and used as an antibiotic to treat infections of the ear, nose, throat, urinary system, respiratory system, skin, soft tissues, bone, joints, stomach, and gonorrhoea (a venereal disease), and major infections.

Side effects: stomach and intestinal disturbances, dizziness, headache, tiredness, confusion, convulsions, rash, pain in the joints, changes in blood, liver, or kidneys, blurred vision, rapid heart rate.
Caution: in patients suffering from severe kidney disease or with a history of convulsions. Plenty of liquid should be drunk.
Not to be used for: children, growing youngsters unless absolutely necessary, and pregnant women or nursing mothers.
Caution needed with: theophylline, antacids, alcohol, anticoagulants, non-steroid anti-inflammatory drugs, cyclosporin.

Erythrocin

A white, oblong tablet supplied at strengths of 250 mg, 500 mg and used as an antibiotic to treat infections, including acne.

Side effects: stomach disturbances, allergies.
Caution: in patients suffering from liver disease.
Not to be used for: children.
Caution needed with: theophylline, anticoagulants taken by

mouth, carbamazepine, digoxin, terfenadine, astemizole.

Flagyl

An off-white tablet or an off-white, capsule-shaped tablet according to strengths of 200 mg, 400 mg and used as an antibacterial treatment for trichomoniasis, non-specific vaginitis, other infections, dysentery, abscess of the liver, ulcerative gingivitis (gum disease).

Side effects: stomach upset, furred tongue, unpleasant taste, allergy, rash, swelling, brain disturbances, dark-coloured urine, nerve changes, seizures, white cell changes.
Caution: in patients with brain disorder caused by liver disease. Short-term high-dose treatment should not be used for pregnant women or nursing mothers.
Not to be used for:
Caution needed with: alcohol, phenobarbitone, anticoagulants taken by mouth.

Floxapen

A black/caramel-coloured capsule supplied at strengths of 250 mg, 500 mg and used as a penicillin treatment for skin, soft tissue, ear, nose, and throat, and other infections.

Side effects: allergy, stomach disturbances.
Caution:
Not to be used for: patients suffering from penicillin allergy.
Caution needed with:

Keflex

A dark green/white capsule or dark green/light green capsule supplied at strengths of 250 mg, 500 mg and used as a cephalosporin antibiotic to treat respiratory, soft tissue, urine, and skin infections.

Side effects: allergic reactions, stomach disturbances.

Caution: in patients suffering from kidney disease or who are very sensitive to penicillin.
Not to be used for:
Caution needed with: loop diuretics.

Monotrim

A white, scored tablet supplied at strengths of 100 mg, 200 mg and used as an antibiotic to treat infections, urine infections.

Side effects: stomach disturbances, skin reactions.
Caution: in the elderly and in patients suffering from kidney disease from folate deficiency (vitamin deficiency). Your doctor may advise regular blood tests.
Not to be used for: infants under 6 weeks, pregnant women, or for patients suffering from severe kidney disease where regular blood tests cannot be made.
Caution needed with:

Negram

A pale-brown tablet supplied at a strength of 500 mg and used as an antiseptic to treat urinary and stomach infections.

Side effects: stomach upset, disturbed vision, rash, blood changes, seizures, sensitivity to light.
Caution: in pregnant women, nursing mothers and in patients suffering from liver or kidney disease. Keep out of the sunlight.
Not to be used for: infants under 3 months or for patients with a history of convulsions, porphyria (a rare blood disorder).
Caution needed with: anticoagulants, probenecid, antibacterials.

Penbritin

A black/red capsule supplied at strengths of 250 mg, 500 mg and used as a penicillin to treat respiratory, ear, nose, and throat infections, gonorrhoea, soft tissue infections, urinary

infections.

Side effects: allergy, stomach disturbances.
Caution: in patients suffering from glandular fever.
Not to be used for: patients suffering from penicillin allergy.
Caution needed with:

Septrin

A white tablet or an orange, dispersible tablet used as an antibiotic to treat respiratory, stomach, and skin infections.

Side effects: nausea, vomiting, tongue inflammation, rash, blood changes, folate (vitamin) deficiency, rarely skin changes.
Caution: in the elderly, nursing mothers, and in patients suffering from kidney disease. Your doctor may advise that patients undergoing prolonged treatment should have regular blood tests.
Not to be used for: pregnant women, new-born infants, or for patients suffering from severe kidney or liver disease, or blood changes.
Caution needed with: folate inhibitors, anticoagulants, anticonvulsants, antidiabetics.

Tetracycline Tablets

An orange tablet supplied at a strength of 250 mg and used as an antibiotic treatment for infections.

Side effects: stomach disturbances, allergy, additional infections.
Caution: in patients suffering from liver or kidney disease.
Not to be used for: children, nursing mothers, or women during the latter half of pregnancy.
Caution needed with: milk, antacids, mineral supplements, the contraceptive pill.

Vibramycin

A green capsule supplied at a strength of 100 mg and used as

a tetracycline treatment for pneumonia, respiratory, stomach, soft tissue, eye, and urinary infections.

Side effects: stomach disturbances, allergy, additional infections, oesophagitis, allergy, raised blood pressure in the brain.
Caution: in patients suffering from liver disease.
Not to be used for: children, nursing mothers, women in the last half of pregnancy, or even for pregnant women at all unless no other treatment is possible.
Caution needed with: antacids, mineral supplements, barbiturates, carbamazepine, phenytoin.

Zinnat

A white tablet supplied at strengths of 125 mg, 250 mg and used as a cephalosporin antibiotic to treat respiratory, ear, nose, and throat, skin, soft tissue, and urinary infections.

Side effects: stomach disturbances, allergy, colitis, blood changes, thrush, change in liver chemistry, headache, interference with some blood tests.
Caution: in pregnant women, nursing mothers, and in patients who are sensitive to penicillin.
Not to be used for:
Caution needed with:

Over-the-counter Medicines

aspirin

A white tablet supplied at a strength of 300 mg and used as an analgesic to relieve pain and reduce fever.

Side effects: stomach upsets, allergy, asthma.
Caution: in pregnant women, the elderly, or in patients with a history of allergy to aspirin, asthma, impaired kidney or liver function, indigestion.
Not to be used for: children, nursing mothers, or for patients

suffering from haemophilia or ulcers.
Caution needed with: anticoagulants (blood-thinning drugs), some antidiabetic drugs, anti-inflammatory agents, methotrexate, spironolactone, steroids, some antacids, some uric-acid lowering drugs.

Cafadol

A yellow, scored tablet used as an analgesic to relieve pain including period pain.

Side effects:
Caution: in patients with liver or kidney disease.
Not to be used for: children under 5 years.
Caution needed with:

Caprin

A pink tablet supplied at a strength of 324 mg and used as an analgesic to treat rheumatic and associated conditions.

Side effects: stomach upsets, allergy, asthma.
Caution: in pregnant women, the elderly, and in patients with a history of allergy to aspirin, asthma, impaired kidney or liver function, indigestion.
Not to be used for: children, nursing mothers, or for patients suffering from haemophilia or ulcers.
Caution needed with: anticoagulants (blood-thinning drugs), some antidiabetic drugs, anti-inflammatory agents, methotrexate, spironolactone, steroids, some antacids, some uric-acid lowering drugs.

Co-Codamol

A tablet used as an analgesic to relieve pain.

Side effects:
Caution: in patients suffering from kidney or liver disease.
Not to be used for: children under 7 years.
Caution needed with:

Co-Codaprin Dispersible

A dispersible tablet used as an analgesic to relieve pain.

Side effects: stomach upsets, allergy, asthma.
Caution: in pregnant women, the elderly, and in patients with a history of allergy to aspirin, asthma, impaired kidney or liver function, indigestion.
Not to be used for: children, nursing mothers, or for patients suffering from haemophilia or ulcers.
Caution needed with: anticoagulants (blood-thinning drugs), some antidiabetic drugs, anti-inflammatory agents, methotrexate, spironolactone, steroids, some antacids, some uric-acid lowering drugs.

Disprol Paed

A suspensions supplied at a strength of 120 mg/5 ml teaspoonful and used as an analgesic to relieve pain and fever in children.

Side effects:
Caution: in children suffering from liver or kidney disease.
Not to be used for:
Caution needed with:

Femerital

A white, scored tablet used as an antispasmodic and analgesic for the relief of period pain.

Side effects:
Caution: in patients suffering from liver or kidney disease.
Not to be used for: children.
Caution needed with:

Midrid

A red capsule used as an analgesic to treat migraine.

Side effects: dizziness.
Caution: in pregnant women and nursing mothers.
Not to be used for: children, or for patients suffering from severe kidney, liver, or heart disease, gastritis, severe high blood pressure, or glaucoma.
Caution needed with: MAOIs.

Migraleve

A pink tablet and a yellow tablet according to strength and contents and used as an analgesic, antihistamine treatment for migraine.

Side effects: drowsiness.
Caution: in patients suffering from liver or kidney disease.
Not to be used for: children under 10 years.
Caution needed with: .

Nurofen

A magenta-coloured, oval tablet supplied at strengths of 200 mg, 400 mg, 600 mg, and used as a non-steroid anti-inflammatory drug to treat pain, rheumatoid arthritis, ankylosing spondylitis, osteoarthritis, seronegative arthritis, peri-articular disorders, soft tissue injuries.

Side effects: dyspepsia, stomach bleeding, rash, rarely low blood platelet levels.
Caution: in pregnant women, and in patients suffering from asthma or allergy to aspirin or anti-inflammatory drugs.
Not to be used for: patients suffering from peptic ulcer.
Caution needed with:

Palaprin Forte

An orange, oval, scored tablet supplied at a strength of 600 mg and used as a non-steroid anti-inflammatory drug to treat rheumatoid arthritis, osteoarthritis, spondylitis.

Side effects: stomach upsets, allergy, asthma.
Caution: in pregnant women, the elderly, and in patients with a history of allergy to aspirin, asthma, impaired kidney or liver function, indigestion.
Not to be used for: children, nursing mothers, or for patients suffering from haemophilia or ulcers.
Caution needed with: anticoagulants (blood-thinning drugs), some antidiabetic drugs, anti-inflammatory agents, methotrexate, spironolactone, steroids, some antacids, some uric-acid lowering drugs.

---

paracetamol tablets

A tablet supplied at a strength of 500 mg and used as an analgesic to relieve pain and reduce fever.

Side effects:
Caution: in patients suffering from kidney or liver disease.
Not to be used for: children under 6 years.
Caution needed with:

Paracodol

A white, effervescent tablet used as an analgesic to relieve pain.

Side effects:
Caution: in patients suffering from kidney or liver disease, or who are on a limited consumption of salt.
Not to be used for: children under 6 years.
Caution needed with:

Parahypon

A pink, scored tablet used as an analgesic to relieve pain.

Side effects:
Caution: in patients suffering from kidney or liver disease.

Not to be used for: children under 6 years.
Caution needed with:

Parake

A white tablet used as an analgesic to relieve pain and reduce fever.

Side effects:
Caution: in patients suffering from kidney or liver disease.
Not to be used for: children.
Caution needed with:

Pardale

A white, scored tablet used as an analgesic to relieve head-ache, rheumatism, period pain.

Side effects:
Caution: in patients suffering from kidney or liver disease.
Not to be used for: children.
Caution needed with:

Paynocil

A white, scored tablet used as an analgesic to relieve pain, reduce fever, and to treat rheumatoid arthritis and other rheumatic conditions.

Side effects: stomach upsets, allergy, asthma.
Caution: in pregnant women, the elderly, or in patients with a history of allergy to aspirin, asthma, impaired kidney or liver function, indigestion.
Not to be used for: children, nursing mothers, or for patients suffering from haemophilia or ulcers.
Caution needed with: anticoagulants (blood-thinning drugs), some antidiabetic drugs, anti-inflammatory agents, methotrexate,

spironolactone, steroids, some antacids, some uric-acid lowering drugs.

Propain

A yellow, scored tablet used as an analgesic, antihistamine treatment for headache, migraine, muscle pain, period pain.

Side effects: drowsiness.
Caution: in patients suffering from liver or kidney disease.
Not to be used for: children.
Caution needed with: alcohol, sedatives.

Salzone

A syrup supplied at a strength of 120 mg/5 ml teaspoonful and used as an analgesic to relieve pain and reduce fever.

Side effects:
Caution: in children suffering from liver or kidney disease.
Not to be used for:
Caution needed with:

Solpadeine

A white, effervescent tablet used as an analgesic to relieve rheumatic, muscle, bone pain, headache, sinusitis, influenza.

Side effects: constipation.
Caution: in patients suffering from liver or kidney disease, or who have a restricted salt consumption.
Not to be used for: children under 7 years.
Caution needed with:

Solprin

A white, soluble tablet supplied at a strength of 300 mg used

as an analgesic to relieve pain and to treat rheumatic conditions.

Side effects:
Caution:
Not to be used for: children.
Caution needed with:

Syndol

A yellow, scored tablet used as an analgesic, antihistamine treatment for tension headache after dental or other surgery.

Side effects: drowsiness, constipation.
Caution: in patients suffering from liver or kidney disease.
Not to be used for: children.
Caution needed with: alcohol, sedatives.

Chapter 6

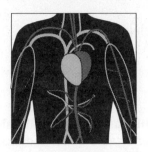

Blood Disorders

Please refer to 'Important Advice' on page 4 at the beginning of this book; and remember, if you are in any doubt, consult a physician.

The blood is the fluid of the circulatory system. It contains different cells to perform different functions. These include red blood cells for transporting oxygen and white blood cells which are part of the immunological and defence system. In addition, the plasma (the fluid in which blood cells circulate) itself is the vehicle for a number of nutrients and raw materials. The blood must also provide the circulatory system with a self-sealing, i.e. clotting, function. This is prone to imbalance and clotting may be excessive, or inadequate as in haemophilia. The association of the blood system with other defence mechanisms in the body in the lymphatic system is important because both are prone to malignant disease in the form of lymphomas and leukaemias. Inadequate blood, anaemia, is a common disorder.

Better nutrition and a better understanding of the defence mechanisms of the body will lead to improved prevention and treatment of blood disorders.

Anaemia

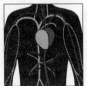 Anaemia is a condition caused by a deficiency of iron in the red blood cells (iron-deficiency anaemia). There are other types of anaemia caused by lack of vitamin B_{12} or folic acid, low thyroxine level, or anaemia may be caused by loss of blood through excessive bleeding. In addition, any chronic disorder may cause anaemia by affecting general health and bone marrow production of red blood cells. Any illness that invades the bone marrow, e.g. leukaemia (*see* below) can cause anaemia. Rarely the body will destroy its own red blood cells (auto-immune haemolytic anaemia).

Symptoms

Tiredness with associated pallor and some general weakness. Anaemia may be completely symptomless and picked up only on routine blood tests. Breathlessness on exercise and angina may also be symptoms of anaemia. There may be symptoms of the causes of anaemia, such as underactive thyroid gland, or excessive bleeding.

Action

Simple, mild anaemia may respond to self-medication but, where symptoms are severe, medical investigation is required.

Tests

Blood tests for haemoglobin red-cell count, iron level, iron binding capacity, vitamin B_{12}, folic acid, thyroxine, and other routine blood tests, such as kidney function (because kidney failure is another cause of anaemia due to lack of erythropoietin).

Medications and treatment

Medications, including iron and vitamins, are included at the end of this chapter. Thyroxine may be required in underactive thyroid patients, and erythropoietin in those with kidney failure. Blood transfusion may be required in severe cases of anaemia.

Further advice
Strict vegetarians may suffer from vitamin deficiency, particularly vitamin B_{12} deficiency. Iron deficiency may also occur when the diet is poor in meat. Dietary supplements may be required in children, the elderly, during pregnancy, and in vegetarians.

Associated conditions
Sickle-cell anaemia and thalassemia are conditions where changes in the haemoglobin cause anaemia or an anaemia-like syndrome. Iron should not be given to patients with thalassemia.

Haemophilia and other bleeding disorders ♥♥♥

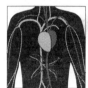 Haemophilia is an inherited condition where lack of a blood-clotting factor (factor 8) causes persistent bleeding. The condition is passed on from mother to son and carried by the daughters of patients with haemophilia. It presents almost exclusively in males, therefore. There are other bleeding disorders, such as von Willebrand's disease and Christmas disease which are similar to haemophilia. Lack of fibrinogen, particularly in severely ill patients in intensive care units, has a similar presentation. Bleeding may also be caused by abnormalities in the platelets, e.g. idiopathic thrombocytopenic purpura.

Symptoms
Persistent bleeding of wounds, bruising, but also internal bleeding, particularly into joints. Therefore, untreated patients or inadequately treated patients may get arthritis in joints such as the elbows and knees. Early symptoms of idiopathic thrombocytopenic pupura may include rash and bruising.

Action
Acute haemophiliac crises need urgent treatment under hospital supervision.

Tests
Blood tests for any bleeding disorder include clotting function and platelet function tests as well as genetic screening and tests for blood-clotting factors such as factor 8 and factor 9.

Medications and treatment
Haemophilia is treated with a concentrated extract of factor 8. In the past, some of these concentrates were contaminated with HIV virus, so haemophiliacs were infected with the virus and some have gone on to develop AIDS.

Further advice
Genetic counselling may be appropriate, and advice on prevention of trauma is invaluable to those suffering from haemophilia. Idiopathic thrombocytopenic purpura may respond to steroids or to removal of the spleen (splenectomy).

Leukaemias

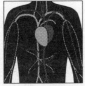 Leukaemias are conditions where excessive growth in the bone marrow of malignant white cells overwhelms the body's own normal cell production system. Leukaemia may be acute or chronic and may develop from the myeloid or lymphatic blood cell lines. Children usually develop acute lymphoblastic leukamia whereas the elderly may develop chronic myeloid or chronic lymphoblastic leukaemia.

Symptoms
Leukaemia may appear in a variety of ways: excessive bleeding; anaemia; bruising; enlarged glands; enlarged liver; enlarged spleen;

persistent infections, particularly shingles. Leukaemia may be detected by routine blood tests.

Action
Where suspected or diagnosed, leukaemia requires urgent specialist attention.

Tests
The tests for leukaemia include blood tests, bone marrow tests, scans of major organs, possible biopsies of lymph glands or spleen.

Medications and treatment
As well as general supportive medications, such as the treatment of anaemia and the use of steroids, specific cytotoxic (powerful cell-killing agents which destroy rapidly growing cells) chemotherapies are used for the treatment of leukaemias.

Further advice
Many types of leukaemia are now treatable and the long-term prognosis is very encouraging.

Associated conditions
There is a range of syndromes, including myelofibrosis (failure of the bone marrow) and polycythemia (excessive red blood cells), which are all related to the leukaemia syndromes.

Lymphomas (including Hodgkin's disease)

Lymphomas are malignant diseases of the lymph glands. There are various types including Hodgkin's disease and the so-called non-Hodgkin's lymphomas.

Symptoms

Lymphomas may appear with swelling of a lymph gland, or the liver or the spleen. Occasionally, the glands may be internal so that an enlarged and malignant gland may not be detectable. The condition may be picked up, therefore, on routine X-ray, e.g. chest X-ray, or other examination. As with other malignant diseases, lymphomas may appear with symptoms of anaemia, weakness, secondary infections such as shin- 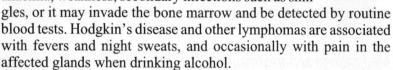 gles, or it may invade the bone marrow and be detected by routine blood tests. Hodgkin's disease and other lymphomas are associated with fevers and night sweats, and occasionally with pain in the affected glands when drinking alcohol.

Action

An enlarged lymph gland which is firm, rubbery, and not obviously infected requires investigation.

Tests

These include full blood count, routine liver and kidney tests, chest X-ray, scans of chest and abdomen, biopsy of affected or suspected glands.

Medications and treatment

As with the anaemias, supportive treatment, in the form of treatment of anaemia and use of steroids, is given in addition to cytotoxic chemotherapy and, where appropriate, radiotherapy.

Over-the-counter Medicines

Abidec

Drops used as a multivitamin preparation to treat vitamin deficiencies.

Side effects:

Caution:
Not to be used for:
Caution needed with: levodopa.

Allbee with C

A green/yellow capsule used as a multivitamin treatment for vitamin B and vitamin C deficiencies.

Side effects:
Caution:
Not to be used for:
Caution needed with: levodopa.

BC 500

An orange, oblong tablet used as a multivitamin preparation to treat vitamin B and vitamin C deficiencies, and to aid recovery from illness, long-term alcoholism, long-term antibiotic treatment.

Side effects:
Caution:
Not to be used for: children.
Caution needed with: levodopa.

BC 500 with Iron

A red tablet used as a vitamin and iron supplement to treat iron deficiency anaemia.

Side effects: nausea, constipation.
Caution:
Not to be used for: children.
Caution needed with: tetracyclines, levodopa.

Becosym

A brown tablet used as a source of B vitamins to treat vitamin B deficiencies.

Side effects:
Caution:
Not to be used for:
Caution needed with: levodopa.

Benerva

A white tablet supplied in strengths of 25 mg, 50 mg, 100 mg and used as a source of vitamin B_1 to treat beri-beri, neuritis.

Side effects:
Caution:
Not to be used for:
Caution needed with: levodopa.

Ce-Cobalin

A syrup used as a multivitamin preparation to treat anorexia, recovery from long-term illness.

Comploment Continus

A yellow tablet supplied at a strength of 100 mg and used as a source of vitamin B_6 to treat vitamin B_6 deficiency including that developed by the contraceptive pill.

Side effects:
Caution:
Not to be used for: children.
Caution needed with: levodopa.

Concavit

A capsule used as a multivitamin treatment for vitamin deficiencies.

Side effects:
Caution:
Not to be used for:
Caution needed with: levodopa.

Cytacon

A white tablet supplied at a strength of 50 micrograms and used as a source of vitamin B_{12} to treat undernourishment, vitamin deficiencies, some types of anaemia, vitamin B_{12} deficiency after stomach surgery.

Side effects: rarely allergy
Caution:
Not to be used for:
Caution needed with: para-aminosalicylic acid, methyldopa, colchicine, cholestyramine, neomycin, biguanides, potassium chloride, cimetidine.

Dalivit Drops

Drops used as a multivitamin preparation in the prevention and treatment of vitamin deficiency in children.

Side effects:
Caution:
Not to be used for:
Caution needed with: levodopa.

Fefol Spansule

A clear/green capsule used for the prevention of iron and folic acid deficiency in pregnancy.

Side effects: mild stomach upset.
Caution:
Not to be used for: children.
Caution needed with: tetracyclines.

Fefol Z Spansule

A clear/blue capsule used for the prevention of iron and folic acid deficiency in pregnancy where zinc supplement is also needed.

Side effects: mild stomach upset.
Caution: in patients suffering from kidney disease
Not to be used for: children.
Caution needed with: tetracyclines.

Fefol-Vit Spansule

A clear/white capsule used for the prevention of iron, folic acid, and vitamin deficiency in pregnancy.

Side effects: mild stomach upset.
Caution:
Not to be used for: children.
Caution needed with: tetracyclines.

Feospan Spansule

A clear/red capsule supplied at a strength of 150 mg and used as an iron supplement to treat iron deficiency, anaemia.

Side effects: mild stomach upset.
Caution:
Not to be used for: infants under 1 year.
Caution needed with: tetracyclines.

Fergon

A red tablet supplied at a strength of 300 mg and used as an iron supplement to treat iron deficiency, anaemia.

Side effects: nausea, constipation.
Caution:
Not to be used for: children under 6 years.
Caution needed with: tetracyclines.

Ferrocontin Continus

A red tablet supplied at a strength of 100 mg and used as an iron supplement to treat iron deficiency, anaemia.

Side effects:
Caution:
Not to be used for: children.
Caution needed with: tetracyclines.

Ferrograd

A red tablet supplied at a strength of 325 mg and used as an iron supplement to treat iron deficiency, anaemia.

Side effects:
Caution: in patients suffering from slow bowel actions.
Not to be used for: children, or for patients suffering from diverticular disease, blocked intestine.
Caution needed with: tetracyclines.

Ferrograd C

A red, oblong tablet used as an iron supplement to treat iron deficiency, anaemia where absorption is difficult.

Side effects:
Caution: in patients suffering from slow bowel action.
Not to be used for: children, or for patients suffering from diverticular

disease, blocked intestine.
Caution needed with: tetracyclines, Clinistix urine test.

Ferrograd Folic

A red yellow/tablet used as an iron supplement to treat anaemia in pregnancy.

Side effects:
Caution: in patients suffering from slow bowel movments.
Not to be used for: children, or for patients suffering from diverticular disease, intestinal blockage, vitamin B_{12} deficiency.
Caution needed with: tetracyclines.

Ferromyn

An elixir used as an iron supplement to treat iron deficiency anaemia.

Side effects: stomach upset.
Caution:
Not to be used for:
Caution needed with: tetracyclines, antacids.

Fersaday

A brown tablet supplied at a strength of 100 mg and used as an iron supplement to treat iron deficiency.

Side effects: stomach upset.
Caution: in patients with a history of peptic ulcer
Not to be used for: children.
Caution needed with: tetracyclines, antacids.

Fersamal

A brown tablet supplied at a strength of 65 mg and used as an

iron supplement to treat iron deficiency, anaemia.

Side effects: stomach upset.
Caution: in patients with a history of peptic ulcer.
Not to be used for:
Caution needed with: tetracyclines, antacids.

Fesovit Spansule

A yellow/clear capsule used as an iron and vitamin supplement to treat iron deficiency anaemia needing vitamins B and C.

Side effects: mild stomach upset.
Caution:
Not to be used for: infants under 1 year.
Caution needed with: tetracyclines.

Fesovit Z Spansule

An orange/clear capsule used as an iron, zinc, and vitamin supplement to treat iron deficiency anaemia where vitamins B and C and zinc are needed.

Side effects: mild stomach upset.
Caution: in patients suffering from kidney disease.
Not to be used for: infants under 1 year.
Caution needed with: tetracyclines.

Folex-350

A pink tablet used as an iron supplement for the prevention of iron and folic acid deficiency in pregnancy.

Side effects: nausea, constipation.
Caution:
Not to be used for: children, or for patients suffering from megaloblastic anaemia.
Caution needed with: tetracyclines.

Forceval

A brown/red capsule used as a source of multivitamins and minerals to treat vitamin and mineral deficiencies.

Side effects:
Caution:
Not to be used for: children under 5 years.
Caution needed with: levodopa.

Fosfor

A syrup used as a food supplement.

Galfer

A green/red capsule supplied at a strength of 290 mg and used as an iron supplement to treat iron deficiency anaemia.

Side effects: nausea, constipation.
Caution:
Not to be used for:
Caution needed with: tetracyclines.

Galfervit

An orange/maroon capsule used as an iron and vitamin supplement to treat iron deficiency anaemia where a vitamin supplement is also needed.

Side effects: nausea, constipation.
Caution:
Not to be used for:
Caution needed with: tetracyclines, levodopa.

Gevral

A brown capsule used as a source of multivitamins and

minerals to treat vitamin and mineral deficiencies.

Side effects:
Caution:
Not to be used for:
Caution needed with: levodopa.

Givitol

A maroon/red capsule used as an iron, folic acid, and vitamin supplement to treat iron and folic acid deficiences in pregnancy where vitamin supplements are also needed.

Side effects: nausea, constipation.
Caution:
Not to be used for: children.
Caution needed with: tatracyclines, levodopa.

Halycitrol

An emulsion used as a multivitamin preparation to treat vitamin A and vitamin D deficiencies.

Side effects: vitamin poisoning
Caution: in patients suffering from kidney disease, sarcoidosis (a chest disease that affects calcium levels).
Not to be used for:
Caution needed with:

Irofol C

A red, oblong tablet used as an iron, folic acid, and vitamin supplement for the prevention and treatment of iron and folic acid deficiency in pregnancy where vitamin supplement is also needed.

Side effects:
Caution: in patients suffering from slow bowel action.
Not to be used for: children or for patients suffering from

megaloblastic anaemia, diverticular disease, intestinal blockage.
Caution needed with: tetracyclines, Clinistix urine test.

Lipoflavonoid

A black/pink capsule used as a multivitamin treatment for vitamin B deficiency.

Side effects:
Caution:
Not to be used for: children.
Caution needed with:

Lipotriad

A clear/pink capsule used as a multivitamin treatment for vitamin B deficiency.

Side effects:
Caution:
Not to be used for: children.
Caution needed with: levodopa.

Minamino

A syrup used as a source of amino acids, B vitamins, and minerals to treat vitamin and mineral deficiences.

Side effects:
Caution:
Not to be used for:
Caution needed with: levodopa.

Multivite

A brown pellet used as a multivitamin treatment for vitamin deficiencies.

Niferex

An elixir used as an iron supplement to treat iron deficiency anaemia.

Side effects:
Caution: in patients with a history of peptic ulcer.
Not to be used for:
Caution needed with: tetracyclines.

Octovit

A maroon, oblong tablet used as a multivitamin treatment for vitamin and mineral deficiencies.

Side effects:
Caution:
Not to be used for: children
Caution needed with: tetracyclines, levodopa.

Orovite

A maroon tablet used as a source of multivitamins to aid recovery from feverish illness, infection or surgery, and to treat confusion in the elderly, mild alcoholic disorders, or for treatment after intravenous vitamin therapy.

Side effects:
Caution:
Not to be used for:
Caution needed with: levodopa.

Orovite 7

Granules in a sachet used as a multivitamin treatment for vitamin deficiencies.

Side effects:
Caution:

Not to be used for: children under 5 years.
Caution needed with: levodopa.

Plesmet

A syrup used as an iron supplement to treat iron-deficiency anaemia.

Side effects:
Caution:
Not to be used for:
Caution needed with: tetracyclines.

Polyvite

A red, oval capsule used as a multivitamin treatment for vitamin deficiencies.

Side effects:
Caution:
Not to be used for:
Caution needed with: levodopa.

Pregaday

A brownish-red tablet used as an iron and folic acid supplement in the prevention of iron and folic acid deficiency in pregnancy.

Side effects: stomach upset, allergy.
Caution: in patients with a history of peptic ulcer or who are in the first three months of pregnancy..
Not to be used for: patients suffering from vitamin B_{12} deficiency.
Caution needed with: tetracyclines, antacids, anticonvulsant drugs, co-trimoxazole.

Pregnavite Forte F

A lilac-coloured tablet used as an iron, folic acid, and vitamin supplement to treat iron and vitamin deficiencies.

Side effects: stomach upset.
Caution:
Not to be used for: children or for patients suffering from megaloblastic anaemia.
Caution needed with: tetracyclines, levodopa.

Redoxon

A white tablet supplied at strengths of 25 mg, 50 mg, 200 mg, and used as a vitamin C treatment for scurvy, and as an additional treatment for wounds and infections.

Side effects: diarrhoea.
Caution:
Not to be used for:
Caution needed with:

Slow-Fe

An off-white tablet supplied at a strength of 160 mg and used as an iron supplement to treat iron-deficiency anaemia.

Side effects: nausea, constipation.
Caution:
Not to be used for: children under 6 years.
Caution needed with: tetracyclines.

Slow-K

An orange tablet supplied at a strength of 600 mg and used as a potassium supplement to treat potassium deficiency.

Side effects: blocked or ulcerated small bowel.
Caution: in patients suffering from kidney disease or peptic ulcer.

Not to be used for: patients suffering from advanced kidney disease.
Caution needed with:

Solvazinc

An off-white effervescent tablet supplied at a strength of 200 mg and used as a zinc supplement to treat zinc deficiency.

Side effects: stomach upset.
Caution: in patients suffering from kidney failure.
Not to be used for:
Caution needed with: tetracyclines.

Surbex T

An orange, oval tablet used as a multivitamin treatment for vitamin B and vitamin C deficiencies.

Side effects:
Caution:
Not to be used for: children under 6 years.
Caution needed with: levodopa.

Sytron

An elixir used as an iron supplement to treat iron-deficiency anaemia.

Side effects: nausea, diarrhoea.
Caution:
Not to be used for:
Caution needed with: tetracyclines.

Tonivitan

A brown capsule used as a multivitamin treatment for vitamin deficiencies.

Side effects:
Caution:
Not to be used for:
Caution needed with:

Tonivitan A & D

A syrup used as a source of vitamins A and D and minerals, and used as a tonic.

Side effects:
Caution:
Not to be used for:
Caution needed with:

Tonivitan B

A syrup used as a source of vitamin B and minerals, and used as a tonic.

Side effects:
Caution:
Not to be used for:
Caution needed with: levodopa.

Verdiviton

A liquid used as a source of vitamin B complex for maintaining vitamin B complex levels.

Side effects:
Caution:
Not to be used for: children, or for patients suffering from hepatitis, alcoholism
Caution needed with: levodopa

Chapter 7

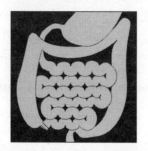

The Digestive System

Please refer to 'Important Advice' on page 4 at the beginning of this book; and remember, if you are in any doubt, consult a physician.

The digestive system is in many ways the most complex part of the human body. It must convert food from the external environment into absorbable raw materials and deliver those materials to the blood stream. It must also provide the systems for storage and release of materials. The oesophagus, stomach, and intestines are designed to ingest and break down food which is then delivered to other organs such as the liver. Each part of this complex system is prone to assaults of various kinds, including infections, tumours, overproduction of acid (particularly in the stomach and duodenum), and blockage.

Other organs, such as the gall bladder, exist merely to help with fat digestion, yet they are prone to various conditions including gall stones. The pancreas gland serves a double function, as a digestive gland and also as an endocrine gland to provide insulin. It, too, is vulnerable to infections and malignancies. The digestive system's vulnerability to malignancy is probably because of its exposure to external toxins and because of its rapid cell turnover in that rapidly dividing cells are more likely to become cancerous.

Because it functions as a blood filter, the liver is particularly susceptible to toxins such as alcohol and to viruses such as hepatitis.

Peptic ulcer ♥♥
(including gastric ulcer and duodenal ulcer)

 These ulcerous conditions are caused by burning of the lining of the stomach, usually by excess acid. The acid creates a crater or ulcer which is painful. Excess acid may be caused by an inherited overproduction of acid, an overproduction of acid caused by an excess production of hormones such as gastrin, excess alcohol and nicotine. Stress also causes increased acid production. Precursors of ulcers include gastritis and hiatus hernia, where acid is released from the stomach into the oesophagus (reflux), particularly on bending or when lying flat.

Symptoms
The symptoms of ulcers, gastritis, and hiatus hernia include abdominal pain. Typically, duodenal ulcer pain is worse after a meal and the pain is to the right side of the abdomen. Gastric ulcer pain is often relieved by food, as is gastritis. Hiatus hernia usually causes symptoms when increased abdominal pressure — during pregnancy or when bending, for example — pushes acid up into the stomach (reflux). In general, these symptoms can be bracketed under the heading of indigestion. Nausea, vomiting, vomiting of blood, loss of weight, diarrhoea and constipation, chest pain, back pain, pain radiating through from the stomach to the back, may all be symptoms of indigestion, gastritis, and ulcer disease.

Action
Self-medication is usually appropriate in the early stages of this treatment but, where serious symptoms occur, e.g. vomiting blood, suggestions of obstruction, passing blood or altered blood out of the back passage (melaena or black stools) the patient should be investigated.

Tests
Routine blood and liver-function tests are needed as well as investigations of the stomach, including barium meal and endoscopy. Biopsies should normally be taken during an endoscopy where the ulcer is looked at directly.

Medications and treatment
Antacid remedies may relieve symptoms of gastritis or hiatus hernia, but more severe symptoms need more potent drugs, such as cimetidine, ranitidine, or omeprazole. Algicon; Algitec; Alumix; Asilone; Axid; Caved S; Colofac; Colpermin; Cytotec; Gastrocote; Gastrozepin; Gaviscon; Kolanticon; Maalox; Mucaine; Nacton; Pepcid; Piptal; Prepulsid; Pyrogastrone; Roter; Topal are all used to treat and relieve gastric disorders.

Further advice
If you suffer from indigestion, acid symptoms, or ulcers, you should eat a healthy diet low in spicy foods, reduce alcohol intake, reduce smoking, and, where possible, reduce stress.

Associated conditions
Rarely, a tear of the oesophagus can cause pain and vomiting of blood. Oesophagitis is inflammation of the oesophagus and may occur as part of hiatus hernia. Ulcers may progress to become stomach cancer (*see* below).

Stomach cancer

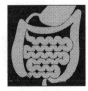 Stomach cancer is decreasing in frequency but it remains a common cause of death, particularly among men. It may develop from previous ulcer disease although this is uncertain. Certainly high spirit intakc and nicotinc may provokc stomach cancer.

Symptoms
There may be no symptoms of stomach cancer. Alternatively, it may

proceed insidiously with slight indigestion, loss of weight, anaemia, and symptoms of peptic ulcer. Vomiting blood, or passing blood, or altered blood (melaena) in the stools may be a symptom of this condition. Symptoms may also appear from secondary spread to the lungs, bone, or liver.

Action
Persistent indigestion should be investigated if it does not respond to self-medication.

Tests
The best test to exclude stomach cancer is endoscopy (telescope into the stomach) and biopsy. It is important, therefore, that this is done before treating ulcers because anti-ulcer treatment may take away the symptoms of stomach cancer. Blood tests, liver-function tests, and chest X-ray are all used to investigate this condition.

Medications and treatment
Stomach cancer is treated surgically with the addition of chemotherapy and radiotherapy where appropriate. Supportive treatment is required.

Further advice
Prevention of stomach cancer is best achieved by attention to diet, alcohol, and nicotine intake.

Associated conditions
Cancer of the oesophagus is similar and will appear with dysphagia (difficulty in swallowing). Cancer of the small intestine is unusual. For cancer of the colon or rectum *see* below.

Intestinal obstruction including inflammatory diseases of the bowel, appendicitis, peritonitis, diverticulitis ♥♥♥

 Bowel obstruction may be caused by a number of conditions, including appendicitis and diverticulitis, either of which may lead to inflammation of the surrounding sac, i.e. peritonitis. Intestinal obstruction may also occur through cancer, inflamed ulcer with stenosis of the pyloris (pyloric stenosis), perforation of the bowel, including perforated duodenal ulcer which leads to peritonitis and intestinal collapse mimicking intestinal obstruction. Diverticulitis and appendicitis are caused by inflammation of material within the gut.

Symptoms

The classic symptoms of intestinal obstruction are vomiting, abdominal pain, and complete constipation, i.e. absence of passing faeces or wind. Bowel perforation, as in perforated ulcer, presents suddenly and dramatically with collapse and abdominal rigidity. The rigidity is caused by peritonitis which can also occur with ruptured appendix or ruptured diverticulum. Appendicitis itself usually presents with central abdominal pain, which shifts down towards the right hip, followed by vomiting and constipation although, occasionally, there may be diarrhoea. Abdominal muscle tension causes guarding (involuntary tension of abdominal muscles) on examination and also complete rigidity of the stomach.

Action

These conditions are surgical emergencies and medical attention should be sought as soon as possible.

Tests

Clinical examination may reveal classical signs, e.g. guarding and rigidity. Plain X-ray of the abdomen may show fluid levels characteristic of bowel obstruction. Ultrasound examination may be useful, and occasionally limited barium studies may help in making the diagnosis. Air in the peritoneum, seen on the abdominal X-ray, signifies perforation with release of air into the peritoneum. Chest X-ray should always be carried out because conditions such as pneumonia may appear with abdominal pain. Blood tests for haemoglobin, urea and electrolytes, liver function, and kidney function should also be performed. White cell count is a good indicator of the presence of infection if it is elevated.

Medications and treatment
These conditions are usually treated surgically, although some conditions recover with high doses of antibiotics while awaiting the definitive diagnosis. There is some dispute about the reality of chronic appendicitis because it is usually an acute condition.

Further advice
If you have suffered from diverticulitis, you should eat a high-fibre diet to prevent further pouches developing and becoming infected.

Associated conditions
For gastro-enteritis (bowel infections) *see* below. Similarly, there may be acute abdominal symptoms with disorders such as cholera, typhoid, or worms.

Liver disorders including hepatitis A, ♥♥♥♥ hepatitis B, non-A non-B hepatitis, cirrhosis of the liver, cancer of the liver

The liver is the largest organ of the body and is responsible for the removal of toxic substances and the storage of other substances, such as glucose. The liver can be affected by viruses such as glandular fever, hepatitis A or hepatitis B, or a third virus known as non-A non-B hepatitis. There is also a hepatitis C. Hepatitis A is usually contracted by drinking infected water whereas hepatitis B is contracted by receiving infected blood or sexually transmitted disease. Cirrhosis of the liver is a thickening and degeneration of the liver which may occur as a late result of virus infection or due to alcohol. Liver cancers are usually secondary from the bowel, but primary liver cancer may also occur.

Symptoms
The main symptoms of liver disease are jaundice, i.e. yellowness of the skin and eyes caused by an elevated level of bilirubin. Enlarge- ment of the liver may occur such that the liver may be felt below the rib cage. A collection of fluid in the peritoneum (ascites) and the development of haemorrhoids are also signs of liver failure. Blood vessel swelling may also occur around the oesophagus resulting in vomiting of blood. Prolonged liver failure may eventually lead to coma and death. The jaundice that occurs with hepatitis or glandular fever is usually transient, disappearing after a short time. Long-term effects may include depression and sensitivity to alcohol. The spleen may also be enlarged and can be felt under the left rib cage.

Tests
Liver function tests including antibodies for hepatitis viruses and glandular fever viruses are important. Ultrasound or CT scan of the liver will reveal the possibility of cirrhosis or cancer. Endoscopy may be required.

Treatment
Occasionally steroids may be used to treat hepatitis, but the usual treatment is isolation and allowing the virus to settle. Interferon has been used with some success. Rarely, liver cancers may be treated surgically or with chemotherapy. Cirrhosis requires the removal of alcohol from the system and a gradual recovery.

Further advice
Avoiding fatty foods may be helpful for some time after liver infections and cirrhosis. Avoiding alcohol is valuable in all liver diseases because the liver may be particularly sensitive.

Associated conditions

Gilbert's syndrome is a condition which is benign where there is an elevation of bilirubin. Haemachromatosis is a condition where there are deposits of iron in the liver which may cause cirrhosis. There are other types of cirrhosis which are not related to alcohol, e.g. primary biliary cirrhosis.

Gall bladder disorders including gallstones, cholecystitis (inflamed gall bladder)

 The gall bladder is an organ that stores bile which helps to digest fats. The gland itself can become inflamed (cholecystitis) or the bile may gather into various types of stones (gallstones). The stones may cause inflammation or they may block the bile duct causing biliary colic.

Symptoms

Biliary colic is an extremely painful condition usually affecting the right side of the body under the ribs. It may be associated with jaundice (yellowness of the skin and eyes) and vomiting. Similarly, the presence of gallstones or cholecystitis will be associated with pain on the right side of the upper abdomen with nausea and vomiting, and possibly fever. The pain may radiate through to the back or to the groin. An obstructive jaundice would cause the urine to be dark and the stools to be pale.

Action

Severe acute obstructive jaundice is an emergency which must be treated urgently. Milder inflammation of the gall bladder may settle down and not require urgent attention.

Tests

Ultrasound of the gall bladder, liver scan, full blood count, sedimentation rate, white count, liver function tests, and tests for hepatitis are all part of the investigation of this condition. Endoscopy, perhaps with the use of special dyes, may be helpful, and laparoscopic investigation of the gall bladder may also be valuable. Cholecystography and cholangiography are investigations which look at the biliary tree, i.e. the tubes taking bile from the gall bladder and liver to the intestines. Cholecystitis may rarely be associated with pancreatitis.

Medications and treatment

These conditions are usually treated surgically, although there are some medications which dissolve gallstones, and antibiotics may be valuable in treating infection of the gall bladder.

Further advice

Where possible, avoid fatty food which usually provokes gall bladder diseases.

Associated conditions

Jaundice due to gall bladder disease may mimic hepatitis so the causes of jaundice should be investigated.

Disorders of the pancreas ♥♥♥
including acute and chronic pancreatitis and cancer of the pancreas (for diabetes mellitus see Chapter 16)

 The pancreas gland is a digestive organ which may be involved in acute inflammation (acute pancreatitis) or slower inflammation (chronic pancreatitis). Both these conditions may be related to a high alcohol intake, and pancreatitis may occur as part of a virus disease including the mumps virus.

Cancer of the pancreas is an unusual cancer.

Symptoms

Acute pancreatitis: severe upper abdominal pain with associated peritonitis (*see* above).

Chronic pancreatitis and cancer of the pancreas: possibly low-grade upper abdominal pain and associated jaundice. Any of these conditions may provoke diabetes (*see* below) because of destruction of the islet cells in the pancreas gland. The upper abdominal pain may radiate through to the back and may be indistinguishable from gall bladder disease, indigestion, or even heart disease.

Action

Acute pancreatitis with collapse is a medical emergency. Any patient with low-grade upper abdominal pain and jaundice needs to be considered for chronic pancreatitis or cancer of the pancreas, and investigated accordingly.

Tests

Ultrasound examinations of the pancreas, CT scan, and endoscopy with the use of special dyes all help to diagnose pancreatic disease. Blood tests of amylase are very useful in making the diagnosis of pancreatitis.

Medications and treatment

Aprotinin may be useful in acute pancreatic disorders. Surgical investigation is rarely used although surgery may sometimes be attempted for pancreatic disorders. Acute pancreatitis is normally treated by rehydration and nasogastric tube and by awaiting spontaneous recovery.

Associated conditions

Mumps or gallstones may be associated with pancreatitis. Severe drop in calcium levels can occur with acute pancreatitis as can bruising over the stomach.

Inflammatory bowel disorders: ♥♥ ulcerative colitis and Crohn's disease

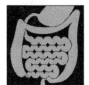 These are distinct conditions which occasionally overlap. Ulcerative colitis normally affects the colon whereas Crohn's disease normally affects the small bowel. There are mixed variants of these conditions, however. Neither disease has a known cause. They are thought to be associated with a family history and with stress.

Symptoms

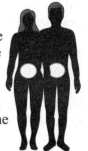 Abdominal pain, passing blood or mucus from the back passage, weight loss, and diarrhoea. Ulcerative colitis may be associated with more profuse bleeding whereas Crohn's disease is often associated with abdominal pain and the formation of fistulae and abscesses including anal fistulae. Patients may become thin and anaemic.

Action

Persistent bloody diarrhoea should be referred for investigation. Short-term symptoms, such as diarrhoea with or without blood, may be caused by gastro-enteritis (*see* below).

Tests

Endoscopy and biopsy are often required as are barium enema or barium meal with follow-through barium to the small bowel. Blood tests for anaemia, liver-function tests, raised sedimentation rate, raised white-cell count, and other signs of auto-immune disease may help in making the diagnosis.

Medications and treatment

Steroids, either in tablet form or enema (Predsol), may be useful as are drugs such as Salazopyrin or mesalazine. The objective is to control symptoms with the minimum dose of steroids. Drugs such as Salazopyrin need to be continued on a long-term basis. Surgical treatment should be avoided where possible but, occasionally, removal of part of the bowel may be necessary. Also: Anusol HC; Asacol; Colifoam; Dipentum; Salofalk; Scheriproct.

Further advice
Keeping to a low-roughage diet and low stress levels may be helpful in the management of these conditions.

Associated conditions
Diverticulitis (*see* above) is different from these conditions and responds to antibiotic therapy and high roughage diet. Ulcerative colitis may rarely be associated with a condition resembling ankylosing spondylitis with involvement of the joints in the back and inflammation of the eyes. Skin rashes may also occur. Fistulae in ano or anal tear may be associated with ulcerative colitis or Crohn's disease.

Irritable bowel syndrome ♥

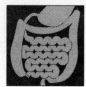
Irritable bowel syndrome is caused by spasm of the small or large bowel and is often related to stress.

Symptoms
The symptoms of irritable bowel syndrome are intermittent abdominal pain with the passing of diarrhoea with or without mucus. Occasionally blood may be seen but this is not usually a feature in this condition. The patient is often tender in the abdomen close to the left hip or in the groin.

Action
Irritable bowel syndrome may respond to self-medication.

Tests

Prolonged symptoms may lead to investigation for other conditions. The investigations would include blood tests and possible endoscopy, and barium meal or barium enema.

Medications and treatment

Peppermint oils, such as Colpermin, or drugs such as Colofac may be helpful in the management of this condition.

Further advice

Reducing stress and eating a high-roughage diet may improve the symptoms of irritable bowel syndrome.

Associated conditions

This condition is also sometimes known as spastic colon.

Bowel infections including gastro-enteritis

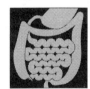 Bowel infections are often caused by bacterial infection, e.g. staphylococcus, salmonella, and more rarely by cholera and typhoid. They are usually caused by eating infected food or drinking infected water. Occasionally, gastro-enteritis may be caused by a virus infection.

Symptoms

Abdominal pain and diarrhoea, often associated with vomiting. Staphylococcal gastro-enteritis usually occurs within a few hours whereas salmonella may take between 12 and 24 hours to present itself. The abdominal pain may be very severe and is usually centred around the umbilicus. The vomiting may continue for some time until eventually bile is being vomited.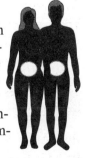

Action

These conditions usually respond to starving and to maintaining fluid intake where possible. If patients are unable to keep fluids down for 24 hours then medical advice is usually required.

Tests

Blood tests and cultures of bowel material should be taken to check whether the patient has salmonella, cholera, or typhoid. Blood tests should also be checked to see if there is dehydration or change in electrolytes such as sodium and potassium.

Medications and treatment

Fluid replacement, possibly using intravenous fluid, may be required. Antinausea drugs, such as Stemetil or Maxolon, may be used and can be given by injection. Imodium or Lomotil can be used for diarrhoea. Antibiotics may be required.

Further advice

Gastro-enteritis may be prevented by strict hygiene, particularly when travelling abroad. Certain foods, particularly seafoods, may have grown in infected water.

Associated conditions

Tapeworm or threadworm infections may also be included in this category, and specific antiworm preparations are available for their treatment. Examples: Alcopar; Avloclor; Combantrin; Eskazole; Flagyl; Mintezol; Pripsen; Vermox; Zadstat.

Bowel cancer
(including cancer of the rectum)

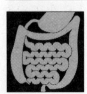
Bowel cancer is a common form of cancer and is separate from stomach cancer.

Symptoms

The symptoms of bowel cancer may be difficult to detect. Alteration in bowel habit, e.g. changing from constipation to diarrhoea or vice versa, may be the only sign. The condition may be symptomless and picked up on routine examination either by rectal examination or on fuller sigmoidoscopy or colonoscopy. Certain patients with polyps may be more prone to this condition and will need regular investigation. Passing blood, or altered blood with or without mucus may also be a sign of bowel cancer. Occasionally, the condition presents with intestinal obstruction because the tumour fills the bowel. Fatigue, anaemia, and weight loss may also be features of bowel cancer.

Action

Any persistent alteration in bowel habits should be reported to a physician for investigation.

Tests

Sigmoidoscopy, colonoscopy, barium enema, blood tests (including tests for the CEA which is specific for bowel cancer) are all part of the investigations for this condition. Biopsies should be taken.

Medications and treatment

Generally, this condition is treated surgically, and cytotoxic chemotherapy with drugs such as 5FU may be useful.

Further advice

Eating a high-roughage diet will help to prevent bowel cancer.

Associated conditions

Cancer of the rectum and anus are rare. Cancer of the small bowel is very unusual. Bowel cancer often spreads to the liver and may appear with evidence of liver enlargement or liver failure (*see* above).

Haemorrhoids (piles) ♥

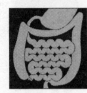 Haemorrhoids are caused by swelling of veins at the end of the digestive passage around the anus. They may be associated with liver failure.

Symptoms
Bleeding on passing motions, feeling of a lump around the back passage, painful itchy sensation, and pain on opening bowels.

Action
Most haemorrhoids respond to self-medication but, if they persist, you should seek medical advice.

Tests
There are no tests for the investigation of haemorrhoids other than tests for liver failure and possibly barium enema. Sigmoidoscopy (telescope into the colon) may be required.

Medications and treatment
Haemorrhoids are usually treated surgically if necessary, but itchiness and soreness can be controlled by ointments including Anacal, Anugesic HC, Anusol, Proctosedyl, Scheriproct, Ultraproct, Uniroid, Xyloproct.

Further advice
Eating a high-roughage diet may prevent or control haemorrhoids.

Associated conditions
Anal fissure may cause pain on opening the bowels. It is caused by a small tear in the anus.

Hernia ♥♥

 A hernia is a swelling of the intestine which protrudes out through abdominal muscle. Hernias may occur in the groin (inguinal or femoral hernia) or where there is a scar (incisional hernia) or around the navel (umbilical hernia). Hiatus hernia (*see* above) is a condition where part of the stomach slides up into the chest and causes indigestion.

Symptoms
The presence of a lump, usually in the groin and occasionally (in men) descending into the scrotum causing an enlarged scrotum. Occasionally these swellings will be painful, particularly where the hernia strangulates or where the blood supply of the hernia is cut off. Strangulated hernia is a surgical emergency. The hernia most commonly appears after heavy lifting, straining, or coughing, and disappears on lying down. Therefore, the lump usually appears at the end of the day and is not present first thing in the morning.

Action
There is usually no urgency, but a persistent or enlarging hernia needs a medical opinion. The painful hernia may be strangulated and, therefore, could be an emergency.

Tests
Plain abdominal X-ray to check there is no strangulated hernia and thus bowel obstruction. Pre-operative investigations include chest X-ray and full blood count.

Treatment
Hernias are treated by surgery. Wearing a truss is a temporary measure.

Coeliac disease

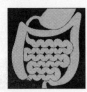

Coeliac disease is caused by an allergy to gluten which is used for making bread, pasta, etc. It is probably an inherited disease.

Symptoms
The symptoms of coeliac disease usually occur in childhood but may appear in adults. These include diarrhoea, weight loss, fatty stools (steatorrhea). Malabsorption of various vitamins and minerals with associated weakness, bone thinning, and even rickets. There may be some liver enlargement.

Action
Where coeliac disease is suspected, investigation is required and the patient should go on a gluten-free diet.

Tests
Measurement of the fat content of stools, blood counts, vitamin levels in the blood, and biopsy of the intestinal mucosa are required in a full investigation of this condition.

Treatment
A gluten-free diet.

Further advice
If gluten is reintroduced into the diet, there will be a relapse.

Associated conditions
Tropical sprue and bowel infections may cause a malabsorption state. Overuse of antibiotics can produce similar results.

Prescription Medicines

Algicon

A white tablet used as an antacid to treat heartburn, hiatus hernia, indigestion.

Side effects: few; constipation or diarrhoea.
Caution: patients suffering from diabetes owing to sucrose content.
Not to be used for: children, or in kidney failure or severe debilitation.
Caution needed with: tetracycline antibiotics, tablets which are specially coated to protect the stomach.

Algitec *see* Tagamet

Anacal

An ointment used as a soothing, anti-inflammatory treatment for haemorrhoids, anal fissure, anal itch.

Side effects:
Caution:
Not to be used for: children under 5 years.
Caution needed with:

Anugesic-HC

A cream used as a soothing, antiseptic, steroid treatment for haemorrhoids, anal itch, and other rectal disorders.

Side effects: systemic corticosteroid effects: weight gain, hypertension, thinning of the skin, stretch marks.
Caution: do not use for prolonged periods; special care is required for pregnant women.
Not to be used for: children or for patients suffering from tuber-

culous, fungal, and viral infections.
Caution needed with:

Anusol

A suppository used as a soothing, antiseptic, astringent treatment for haemorrhoids, anal itch, and other rectal and anal disorders.

Side effects:
Caution:
Not to be used for: children.
Caution needed with:

Anusol HC

A suppository used as a steroid, antiseptic, astringent treatment for haemorrhoids and inflammation of the anus and rectum.

Side effects: systemic corticosteroid effects: weight gain, hypertension, thinning of the skin, stretch marks.
Caution: in pregnant women; do not use for prolonged periods.
Not to be used for: children or for patients suffering from tuberculous, fungal, and viral infections.
Caution needed with:

Asacol

A red, coated, oblong tablet supplied at a strength of 400 mg and used as a salicylate to treat ulcerative colitis.

Side effects: stomach disturbances, headache.
Caution: in patients suffering from kidney disease, raised blood urea, protein in the urine, and in pregnant women.
Not to be used for: children.
Caution needed with: lactulose or any preparations that increase the acidity of the motions.

Asilone

A white liquid used as an antacid, anti-wind preparation to treat gastritis, ulcers, dyspepsia, wind.

Side effects: occasionally constipation.
Caution:
Not to be used for: infants and children.
Caution needed with: tablets which are coated to protect the stomach.

Axid

A pale-yellow/ dark-yellow capsule supplied at a strength of 150 mg and 300 mg and used for treatment and prevention of ulcers and to treat gastro-oesophageal reflux.

Side effects: headache, chest pain, muscle ache, fatigue, dreams, runny nose, sore throat, cough, itch, sweating, changes in liver enzymes.
Caution: in pregnant women and nursing mothers, and in patients suffering from impaired kidney and liver functions.
Not to be used for: children.
Caution needed with:

Biogastrone

A white, scored tablet supplied at a strength of 50 mg and used as an anti-ulcer treatment for stomach ulcers.

Side effects: fluid retention, low potassium levels, high blood pressure.
Caution: in patients suffering from sodium or water retention.
Not to be used for: children, the elderly, pregnant women, or for patients with heart, kidney, or liver problems or low potassium levels.
Caution needed with: digoxin, diuretics.

Caved-S

A brown tablet used as a cell-surface protector and antacid to treat peptic ulcer.

Side effects: few; occasionally constipation.
Caution:
Not to be used for: children.
Caution needed with: tetracycline antibiotics.

Colifoam

Foam supplied in an aerosol and used as a steroid treatment for ulcerative colitis and other bowel inflammations.

Side effects: high blood sugar, thin bones, mood changes, ulcers.
Caution: in pregnant women and in patients suffering from severe ulcerative disease. Do not use for prolonged periods.
Not to be used for: children or for patients suffering from obstruction, abscess, fresh intestinal surgery, tuberculous, fungal or viral infections.
Caution needed with:

Colofac

A white tablet supplied at a strength of 135 mg and used as an anti-spasm treatment for bowel spasm.

Colpermin

A blue capsule used as an antispasm treatment for irritable bowel syndrome.

Side effects: heartburn, allergy, rash, headache, irregular heartbeat, tremor, loss of co-ordination.
Caution: must not be broken or chewed.
Not to be used for: children.
Caution needed with:

Cystrin

A white tablet supplied at strengths of 3 mg, 5 mg and used as an antispasmodic and anticholinergic treatment for incontinence, urgency or frequency of urination, or night-time incontinence in children.

Side effects: anticholinergic effects, flushing of the face.
Caution: in pregnant women, and in patients suffering from liver or kidney disease, heart disorders, overactive thyroid, enlarged prostate, hiatus hernia or existing disturbance of normal bodily functions.
Not to be used for: children under 5 years, nursing mothers, or for patients suffering from blockage in the bowel or bladder, severe ulcerative colitis, other intestinal disorders, myaesthenia gravis, or glaucoma.
Caution needed with: sedatives, amantadine, levodopa, digoxin, tricyclic antidepressants, other anticholinergics.

Cytotec

A white, hexagonal tablet supplied at a strength of 200 micrograms and used as a prostaglandin for the prevention and treatment of ulcers caused by anti-inflammatory drugs.

Side effects: diarrhoea, abdominal pain, stomach upset, menstrual disturbance, vaginal bleeding, rash, dizziness.
Caution: in patients suffering from circulatory disorders of the brain, heart, or peripheral vessels. Women of child-bearing age must use contraception.
Not to be used for: nursing mothers, pregnant women, or those planning a pregnancy.
Caution needed with:

Dipentum

A caramel-coloured capsule supplied at a strength of 250 mg used as a salicylate to treat ulcerative colitis.

Side effects: stomach upset, rash, headache, joint pains.
Caution:
Not to be used for: children, pregnant women, or for patients
suffering from aspirin allergy or kidney disease.
Caution needed with:

Gastrocote

**A white tablet used as an antacid and reflux suppressant to
treat dyspepsia, hiatus hernia, oesophagitis**

Side effects: occasionally constipation.
Caution:
Not to be used for: children under 6 years.
Caution needed with: tetracycline antibiotics, tablets which are
coated to protect the stomach.

Gastrozepin

**A white tablet used as an antispasm, anticholinergic treat-
ment for gastric and duodenal ulcers.**

Side effects: blurred vision, confusion, dry mouth.
Caution:
Not to be used for: children, or for patients with glaucoma,
inflammatory bowel disease, intestinal obstruction, or enlarged
prostate.
Caution needed with:

Gaviscon

**A white tablet or pink liquid used as an antacid and reflux
suppressant to treat reflux symptoms.**

Side effects: occasionally constipation.
Caution: in pregnant women, and in patients suffering from high
blood pressure, heart or kidney failure.
Not to be used for:

Caution needed with: tetracycline antibiotics, tablets which are coated to protect the stomach.

Imodium

A dark green/grey capsule supplied at a strength of 2 mg and used to treat diarrhoea.

Side effects: rash.
Caution: in patients suffering from severe ulcerative colitis.
Not to be used for: children under 4 years.
Caution needed with:

Kolanticon

A gel used as an antacid, antispasm, and anticholinergic treatment for bowel/stomach spasm, acidity, wind, ulcers.

Side effects: occasionally constipation, blurred vision, confusion, dry mouth.
Caution:
Not to be used for: children or for patients suffering from glaucoma, inflammatory bowel disease, intestinal obstruction, or enlarged prostate.
Caution needed with: tetracycline antibiotics and tablets which are coated to protect the stomach.

Lomotil

A white tablet used to slow down intestinal contents and as an anticholinergic to treat diarrhoea.

Side effects: allergy, stomach upset, anticholinergic effects, disturbance of brain and spinal cord.
Caution: in pregnant women, nursing mothers, or in patients suffering from liver disorder, dehydration, body fluid imbalance.
Not to be used for: children under 4 years, or for patients suffering from blockage in the intestine, jaundice, colitis.

Caution needed with: MAOIs, sedatives

Losec

A pink/brown capsule tablet supplied at a strength of 20 mg and used as an anti-ulcer drug for ulcers which are difficult to treat, and as a treatment for reflux oesophagitis.

Side effects: constipation, diarrhoea, headache, nausea, rashes.
Caution: your doctor may advise endoscopic checks of the stomach.
Not to be used for: pregnant women or nursing mothers.
Caution needed with: diazepam, phenytoin, warfarin.

Maalox

A white tablet used as an antacid to treat gastric and duodenal ulcer, gastritis, heartburn, acidity.

Side effects: occasionally constipation.
Caution:
Not to be used for: children.
Caution needed with: tetracycline antibiotics, tablets which are coated to protect the stomach.

Maxolon

A white tablet supplied at a strength of 10 mg and used as an anti-sickness (anti-dopaminergic), antispasm drug to treat nausea, vomiting, dyspepsia, wind, heartburn, and other symptoms related to stomach and bowels, intolerance to cytotoxic drugs, congestive heart failure, after operations, deep X-ray or cobalt treatment.

Side effects: occasionally parkinsonian-type symptoms, extrapyramidal reactions (tremor, rigidity).
Caution: in pregnant women, nursing mothers, and in patients suffering from liver and kidney problems or epilepsy.

Not to be used for: where recent gastric or bowel surgery has occurred. Some rare tumours such as phaeochromocytoma (a disease of the adrenal glands) or prolactin-dependent breast cancers.

Caution needed with: anticholinergics, some sedatives, tranquillizers and antidepressants.

Mucaine

A white liquid used as an antacid plus local anaesthetic to treat oesophagitis and hiatus hernia.

Side effects: occasional constipation.
Caution:
Not to be used for: children.
Caution needed with: tetracycline antibiotics.

Nacton Forte

An orange tablet supplied at a strength of 4 mg and used as an anti-spasm, anticholinergic treatment for spasm, acidity, ulcers.

Side effects: blurred vision, confusion, dry mouth.
Caution: in patients suffering from rapid heart rate, glaucoma, or difficulty in passing urine.
Not to be used for: children.
Caution needed with:

Pentasa *see* Asacol

Pepcid

A brown, square tablet supplied at strengths of 20 mg, 40 mg and used as an H_2 blocker in the prevention and treatment of duodenal and gastric ulcers, Zollinger-Ellison syndrome

(high acid production).

Side effects: headache, dizziness, constipation, diarrhoea, dry mouth, nausea, rash, bowel discomfort, loss of appetite, fatigue.
Caution: in pregnant women, nursing mothers, and in patients suffering from impaired kidney function. Stomach cancer should be excluded as a diagnosis.
Not to be used for: children.
Caution needed with:

Piptal

An orange tablet supplied at a strength of 5 mg and used as an anti-spasm, anticholinergic treatment for excess stomach acid, overactive intestine.

Side effects: blurred vision, confusion, dry mouth, nausea, sleeplessness, constipation, urinary retention, rapid heart rate, dizziness.
Caution: in patients suffering from glaucoma, enlarged prostate, urinary retention.
Not to be used for: children, pregnant women, nursing mothers, or for patients suffering from inflammatory bowel disease, intestinal obstruction, other gastro-intestinal disorders, rapid heart rate, untreated angina, liver or kidney disease, myaesthenia gravis.
Caution needed with: tricyclic antidepressants, some sedatives, antihistamines.

Predsol Enema

An enema supplied at a strength of 20 mg and used as a steroid treatment for ulcerative colitis.

Side effects: systemic corticosteroid effects: weight gain, hypertension, thinning of the skin, stretch marks.
Caution: in pregnant women. Do not use for prolonged periods.
Not to be used for: children.
Caution needed with:

Prepulsid

A white tablet supplied at a strength of 10 mg and used as a stomach-emptying drug to treat gastric reflux and to encourage emptying of the stomach in conditions where the nerve supply is impaired.

Side effects: abdominal cramps, stomach rumbling, diarrhoea, occasionally headaches and convulsions.
Caution: in the elderly, nursing mothers, and in patients suffering from kidney or liver impairment.
Not to be used for: pregnant women or for patients suffering from stomach block, perforation, or bleeding.
Caution needed with: sedatives, anticoagulants, anticholinergics.

Proctosedyl

Suppositories used as a steroid, local anaesthetic treatment for haemorrhoids, anal fissure, inflammation, itch.

Side effects: systemic corticosteroid effects: weight gain, hypertension, thinning of the skin, stretch marks.
Caution: in pregnant women; do not use for prolonged periods.
Not to be used for: patients suffering from tuberculous, fungal or viral infections.
Caution needed with:

Pyrogastrone *see* Biogastrone

Roter

A pink tablet used as an antacid and antibulking agent to treat stomach ulcers, gastritis.

Side effects: constipation, nerve damage.
Caution:
Not to be used for: for children.
Caution needed with: tetracycline antibiotics, tablets which are

coated to protect the stomach.

Salofalk *see* Asacol

Scheriproct

An ointment used as a steroid, local anaesthetic treatment for haemorrhoids, anal fissure, itch, bowel inflammation.

Side effects: systemic corticosteroid effects: weight gain, hypertension, thinning of the skin, stretch marks.
Caution: in pregnant women; do not use for prolonged periods.
Not to be used for: patients suffering from tuberculous, fungal, or viral infections
Caution needed with:

Stemetil

A cream tablet or a cream, scored tablet according to strengths of 5 mg, 25 mg and used as a anti-sickness medication for minor mental and emotional problems, schizophrenia and other mental disorders, vertigo caused by Ménière's disease, severe nausea, vomiting.

Side effects: brain disturbances, anticholinergic effects, ECG and hormone changes, allergies, reduced judgement and abilities, rarely extrapyramidal effects, jaundice, blood disorder.
Caution: in the elderly, nursing mothers, and in patients suffering from cardiovascular disease, undiagnosed or prolonged vomiting.
Not to be used for: patients in an unconscious state, pregnant women, or patients suffering from bone marrow depression, liver or kidney disease, Parkinson's disease.
Caution needed with: sedatives, alcohol, analgesics, antihypertensives, antidepressants, anticholinergics, anticonvulsants, antidiabetics.

Tagamet

A green tablet supplied at strengths of 200 mg, 400 mg, 800 mg and used as an H$_2$ blocker to treat duodenal and gastric ulcers, hiatus hernia, dyspepsia, oesophageal reflux.

Side effects: diarrhoea, rash, tiredness, dizziness, liver changes, confusion, breast swelling; rarely kidney, pancreas, bone marrow, joint, and muscle problems; headache.
Caution: in pregnant women, nursing mothers and in patients suffering from impaired kidney function. Ensure cancer has not been missed as a diagnosis. Monitor patients on long-term therapy.
Not to be used for:
Caution needed with: oral anticoagulants, phenytoin, theophylline.

Topal

A cream tablet used as an antacid to treat oesophagitis, heartburn, gastritis, dyspepsia, reflux oesophagitis.

Side effects:
Caution:
Not to be used for: infants.
Caution needed with: tetracycline antibiotics, tablets which are coated to protect the stomach.

Ultraproct

A suppository supplied at a strength of 1 mg and used as a steroid, local anaesthetic, antihistamine treatment for haemorrhoids, anal fissure, proctitis, anal itch.

Side effects: systemic corticosteroid effects: weight gain, hypertension, thinning of the skin, stretch marks.
Caution: do not use for prolonged periods; care in pregnant women.
Not to be used for: children, or for patients suffering from tuber-

culous, fungal, or viral infections.
Caution needed with:

Uniroid-HC

An ointment used as a steroid and local anaeesthetic treatment for pain, irritation, and itching associated with haemorrhoids and other itchy anal conditions.

Side effects: allergy, systemic corticosteroid effects: weight gain, hypertension, thinning of the skin, stretch marks.
Caution:
Not to be used for: children under 12 years, pregnant women, nursing mothers, or for patients suffering from tuberculous, fungal, or viral infections, or allergy to any ingredient.
Caution needed with:

Xyloproct

A suppository used as a local anaesthetic and steroid treatment for haemorrhoids, anal itch, anal fissure and fistula.

Side effects: systemic corticosteroid effects: weight gain, hypertension, thinning of the skin, stretch marks.
Caution: do not use for prolonged periods; care in pregnant women.
Not to be used for: patients suffering from tuberculous, fungal, or viral infections
Caution needed with:

Zantac

A peach or white tablet supplied at strengths of 150 mg, 300 mg and used as an H_2 blocker to treat duodenal and gastric ulcers, oesophagitis, dyspepsia, reduction of gastric acid.

Side effects: headache, dizziness, occasionally hepatitis, low platelet counts, low white blood cell counts, allergy, confusion,

breast symptoms.
Caution: exclude malignant disease. Care in pregnant women, nursing mothers, and in patients suffering from impaired kidney function.
Not to be used for:
Caution needed with:

Antibiotics

Amoxil

A maroon/gold capsule supplied at a strength of 250 mg, 500 mg and used as a broad-spectrum penicillin to treat respiratory, ear, nose, and throat, urinary, venereal, and soft tissue infections. Also for dental abscess, and to prevent infection of the heart during dental procedures

Side effects: stomach upset, allergy.
Caution: in patients suffering from glandular fever.
Not to be used for: patients suffering from penicillin allergy.
Caution needed with:

Ciproxin

Tablets supplied at strengths of 250 mg, 500 mg, and used as an antibiotic to treat infections of the ear, nose, throat, urinary system, respiratory system, skin, soft tissues, bone, joints, stomach, and gonorrhoea (a venereal disease), and major infections.

Side effects: stomach and intestinal disturbances, dizziness, headache, tiredness, confusion, convulsions, rash, pain in the joints, changes in blood, liver, or kidneys, blurred vision, rapid heart rate.
Caution: in patients suffering from severe kidney disease or with a history of convulsions. Plenty of liquid should be drunk.
Not to be used for: children, growing youngsters unless absolutely necessary, and pregnant women or nursing mothers.

Caution needed with: theophylline, antacids, alcohol, anticoagulants, non-steroid anti-inflammatory drugs, cyclosporin.

Erythrocin

A white, oblong tablet supplied at strengths of 250 mg, 500 mg and used as an antibiotic to treat infections, including acne.

Side effects: stomach disturbances, allergies.
Caution: in patients suffering from liver disease.
Not to be used for: children.
Caution needed with: theophylline, anticoagulants taken by mouth, carbamazepine, digoxin, terfenadine, astemizole.

Flagyl

An off-white tablet or an off-white, capsule-shaped tablet according to strengths of 200 mg, 400 mg and used as an antibacterial treatment for trichomoniasis, non-specific vaginitis, other infections, dysentery, abscess of the liver, ulcerative gingivitis (gum disease).

Side effects: stomach upset, furred tongue, unpleasant taste, allergy, rash, swelling, brain disturbances, dark-coloured urine, nerve changes, seizures, white cell changes.
Caution: in patients with brain disorder caused by liver disease. Short-term high-dose treatment should not be used for pregnant women or nursing mothers.
Not to be used for:
Caution needed with: alcohol, phenobarbitone, anticoagulants taken by mouth.

Floxapen

A black/caramel-coloured capsule supplied at strengths of 250 mg, 500 mg and used as a penicillin treatment for skin,

soft tissue, ear, nose, and throat, and other infections.

Side effects: allergy, stomach disturbances.
Caution:
Not to be used for: patients suffering from penicillin allergy.
Caution needed with:

Keflex

A dark green/white capsule or dark green/light green capsule supplied at strengths of 250 mg, 500 mg and used as a cephalosporin antibiotic to treat respiratory, soft tissue, urine, and skin infections.

Side effects: allergic reactions, stomach disturbances.
Caution: in patients suffering from kidney disease or who are very sensitive to penicillin.
Not to be used for:
Caution needed with: loop diuretics.

Monotrim

A white, scored tablet supplied at strengths of 100 mg, 200 mg and used as an antibiotic to treat infections, urine infections.

Side effects: stomach disturbances, skin reactions.
Caution: in the elderly and in patients suffering from kidney disease from folate deficiency (vitamin deficiency). Your doctor may advise regular blood tests.
Not to be used for: infants under 6 weeks, pregnant women, or for patients suffering from severe kidney disease where regular blood tests cannot be made.
Caution needed with:

Negram

A pale-brown tablet supplied at a strength of 500 mg and

used as an antiseptic to treat urinary and stomach infections.

Side effects: stomach upset, disturbed vision, rash, blood changes, seizures, sensitivity to light.
Caution: in pregnant women, nursing mothers and in patients suffering from liver or kidney disease. Keep out of the sunlight.
Not to be used for: infants under 3 months or for patients with a history of convulsions, porphyria (a rare blood disorder).
Caution needed with: anticoagulants, probenecid, antibacterials.

Penbritin

A black/red capsule supplied at strengths of 250 mg, 500 mg and used as a penicillin to treat respiratory, ear, nose, and throat infections, gonorrhoea, soft tissue infections, urinary infections.

Side effects: allergy, stomach disturbances.
Caution: in patients suffering from glandular fever.
Not to be used for: patients suffering from penicillin allergy.
Caution needed with:

Septrin

A white tablet or an orange, dispersible tablet used as an antibiotic to treat respiratory, stomach, and skin infections.

Side effects: nausea, vomiting, tongue inflammation, rash, blood changes, folate (vitamin) deficiency, rarely skin changes.
Caution: in the elderly, nursing mothers, and in patients suffering from kidney disease. Your doctor may advise that patients undergoing prolonged treatment should have regular blood tests.
Not to be used for: pregnant women, new-born infants, or for patients suffering from severe kidney or liver disease, or blood changes.
Caution needed with: folate inhibitors, anticoagulants, anticonvulsants, antidiabetics.

Tetracycline Tablets

An orange tablet supplied at a strength of 250 mg and used as an antibiotic treatment for infections.

Side effects: stomach disturbances, allergy, additional infections.
Caution: in patients suffering from liver or kidney disease.
Not to be used for: children, nursing mothers, or women during the latter half of pregnancy.
Caution needed with: milk, antacids, mineral supplements, the contraceptive pill.

Vibramycin

A green capsule supplied at a strength of 100 mg and used as a tetracycline treatment for pneumonia, respiratory, stomach, soft tissue, eye, and urinary infections.

Side effects: stomach disturbances, allergy, additional infections, oesophagitis, allergy, raised blood pressure in the brain.
Caution: in patients suffering from liver disease.
Not to be used for: children, nursing mothers, women in the last half of pregnancy, or even for pregnant women at all unless no other treatment is possible.
Caution needed with: antacids, mineral supplements, barbiturates, carbamazepine, phenytoin.

Zinnat

A white tablet supplied at strengths of 125 mg, 250 mg and used as a cephalosporin antibiotic to treat respiratory, ear, nose, and throat, skin, soft tissue, and urinary infections.

Side effects: stomach disturbances, allergy, colitis, blood changes, thrush, change in liver chemistry, headache, interference with some blood tests.
Caution: in pregnant women, nursing mothers, and in patients who are sensitive to penicillin.
Not to be used for:

Caution needed with:

Over-the-counter Medicines

Actal

A white tablet supplied at a strength of 360 mg and used as an antacid to treat indigestion, dyspepsia.

Side effects: few; sodium overload is possible.
Caution:
Not to be used for: children.
Not to be used with: tetracycline antibiotics.

Actonorm

A white liquid supplied in 200 ml bottles and used as an antacid to treat indigestion, wind.

Side effects: few; occasionally constipation or diarrhoea.
Caution:
Not to be used for: children.
Not to be used with: tetracycline antibiotics.

Agarol

An emulsion used as a lubricant and stimulant to treat constipation.

Side effects: allergies to phenolphthalein, blood or protein in the urine.
Caution:
Not to be used for: children under 5 years.
Not to be used with:

Algicon

A white tablet used as an antacid to treat heartburn, hiatus

hernia indigestion.

Side effects: few; constipation or diarrhoea.
Caution: in patients suffering from diabetes because of sucrose content.
Not to be used for: children, or in patients suffering from kidney failure or severe debilitation.
Not to be used with: tetracycline antibiotics.

Alka Seltzer

Alka Seltzer contains aspirin, citric acid, and sodium bicarbonate. Although the sodium bicarbonate is an alkali, the combination with aspirin means that this preparation is not suitable for those with ulcer disease, because aspirin makes ulcers bleed. Alka Seltzer can be used for mild headache and indigestion combined, for example in those with a hangover.

Alophen

A brown pill used as a stimulant and anticholinergic to treat constipation.

Side effects: allergies to phenolphthalein, skin rash, protein in the urine.
Caution:
Not to be used for: children or for patients suffering from glaucoma or inflammatory bowel disease.
Not to be used with:

Altacite Plus

A white liquid supplied in 500 ml bottles and used as an antacid and anti-wind preparation to treat wind, indigestion, dyspepsia, and gastric ulcers.

Side effects: few; occasional diarrhoea and constipation.
Caution:

Not to be used for: children under 8 years.
Not to be used with: tetracycline antibiotics.

Alu-Cap

A green/red capsule supplied at a strength of 475 mg and used as an antacid to treat hyperacidity.

Side effects: few; occasional bowel disorder such as constipation.
Caution:
Not to be used for: children.
Not to be used with: tetracycline antibiotics.

Aluhyde

A white scored tablet used as an antispasmodic and antacid to treat hyperacidity and intestinal spasm.

Side effects: occasionally constipation and blurred vision.
Caution: in patients suffering from prostate enlargement.
Not to be used for: children or for patients suffering from glaucoma.
Not to be used with: tetracycline antibiotics.

Andursil

A white liquid supplied in 100 ml bottles and used as an antacid and anti-wind preparation to treat dyspepsia, heartburn, peptic ulcer.

Side effects: few; possibly constipation or diarrhoea.
Caution:
Not to be used for: children.
Not to be used with: tetracycline antibiotics.

Arret

A capsule used to treat diarrhoea.

Side effects: rashes
Caution: in severe colitis.
Not to be used for: children.
Not to be used with:

Asilone

A white liquid used as an antacid, anti-wind preparation to treat gastritis, ulcers, dyspepsia, wind.

Side effects: few; occasionally constipation.
Caution:
Not to be used for: infants.
Not to be used with:

Bellocarb

A beige tablet used as an antacid and anti-spasm treatment for bowel spasm, ulcers, dyspepsia.

Side effects: few; occasional constipation.
Caution: in patients suffering from enlarge prostate, heart, kidney, or liver problems.
Not to be used for: patients suffereing from glaucoma.
Not to be used with:

Carbellon

A black tablet used as an anti-spasm, anti-wind, antacid preparation to treat acidity, ulcers, food poisoning.

Side effects: few; occasionally constipation.
Caution:
Not to be used for: patients suffering from glaucoma, pyloric stenosis, enlarged prostate.
Not to be used with:

Caved-S

A brown tablet used as a cell-surface protector and antacid to treat peptic ulcer.

Side effects: few; occasionally constipation.
Caution:
Not to be used for: infants.
Not to be used with: tetracycline antibiotics.

Colpermin

A blue capsule used as an anti-spasm treatment for irritable bowel syndrome.

Side effects:
Caution:
Not to be used for: children.
Not to be used with:

De-Nol

A white liquid used as a cell-surface protector to treat gastric and duodenal ulcer.

Side effects: black colour to tongue and stools.
Caution:
Not to be used for: children of for patients suffering from kidney failure.
Not to be used with:

Dioralyte

Cherry- or pineapple-flavoured powder supplied as sachets and used as a fluid and electrolyte replacement to treat acute watery diarrhoea including gastro-enteritis.

Diovol

A white suspension used as an antacid and anti-wind preparation to treat ulcers, hiatus hernias, wind, and acidity.

Side effects: few; occasionally constipation.
Caution:
Not to be used for: infants.
Not to be used with: tetracycline antibiotics.

Droxalin

A white tablet used as an antacid to treat acidity, dyspepsia, and hiatus hernia.

Side effects: few; occasionally constipation.
Caution:
Not to be used for: infants.
Not to be used with: tetracycline antibiotics.

Dulcolax

A yellow tablet supplied at a strength of 5 mg and used as a stimulant to treat constipation and for evacuation of the bowels before surgery.

Duphalac

A syrup used as a laxative to treat constipation, brain disease due to liver problems.

Side effects:
Caution:
Not to be used for: patients suffering from galactosaemia (an inherited disorder).
Not to be used with:

ENO

ENO contains sodium bicarbonate, tartaric acid, and citric acid and is useful as an effervescent antacid. Care should be taken to avoid sodium overload. In contrast, Andrew's (Sterling Health) contains magnesium sulphate and acts as both an antacid and laxative. Andrew's Answer is another hangover remedy which contains paracetamol, caffeine, sodium bicarbonate, and citric acid.

Exlax

Exlax contains phenolphthalein which is a powerful laxative only to be used when other simple remedies have failed.

Fybranta

A mottled, pale-brown, chewable 2 g tablet used as a bulking agent in the treatment of diverticular disease, irritable colon syndrome, constipation through a diet lacking in fibre.

Gastrocote

A white tablet used as an antacid and reflux suppressant to treat dyspepsia, hiatus hernia, oesophagitis.

Side effects: few; occasionally constipation.
Caution:
Not to be used for: infants.
Not to be used with: tetracycline antibiotics.

Gastron

A white tablet used as an antacid and reflux suppressant to treat reflux symptom.

Side effects: few; occasionally constipation.
Caution: in pregnant women and in patients suffering from high blood pressure, heart or kidney failure.
Not to be used for: infants.
Not to be used with: tetracycline antibiotics.

Gaviscon

A white tablet used as an antacid and reflux suppressant to treat reflux.

Side effects: few; occasionally constipation.
Caution: in pregnant women, and in patients suffering from high blood pressure, heart or kidney failure.
Not to be used for: infants.
Not to be used with: tetracycline antibiotics.

Gelusil

A white tablet used as an antacid to treat dyspepsia, heart-burn.

Side effects: few; occasionally constipation.
Caution:
Not to be used for: infants.
Not to be used with: tetracycline antibiotics.

kaolin

Kaolin preparations are useful for mild diarrhoea; they are not absorbed into the body and so have limited side effects. Products containing kaolin include Kaopectate, Kaodene, Enterosan (with belladonna and morphine), and Collis Browne's (with morphine, peppermint oil, and calcium carbonate).

Kolanticon

A gel used as an antacid, anti-spasm, and anticholinergic preparation to treat bowel/stomach spasm, acidity, wind, ulcers.

Side effects: occasionally constipation, blurred vision, confusion, dry mouth.
Caution:
Not to be used for: infants or for patients suffering from glaucoma, inflammatory bowel disease, intestinal obstruction, or enlarged prostate.
Not to be used with: tetracycline antibiotics.

Loasid

A white tablet used as an antacid and anti-wind preparation to treat ulcers, oesophagitis, gastritis, hiatus hernia, heart-burn.

Side effects: few; occasionally constipation.
Caution: in patients suffereing from kidney failure.
Not to be used for: infants.
Not to be used with: tetracycline antibiotics.

Maalox

A white tablet used as an antacid to treat gastric and duode-nal ulcer, hiatus hernias, wind, and acidity.

Side effects: few; occasionally constipation.
Caution:
Not to be used for: infants.
Not to be used with: tetracycline antibiotics.

Malinal

A scored, white chewable tablet supplied at a strength of 500

mg and used as an antacid to treat indigestion, ulcers, hyperacidity.

Side effects:
Caution:
Not to be used for: children.
Not to be used with: tetracycline antibiotics.

Milk of Magnesia

Milk of Magnesia contains magnesium hydroxide and is available in liquid and tablet form, as well as in combination with paraffin as Milpar.

Mintec

A green/ivory capsule used as an anti-spasm treatment for irritable bowel syndrome, spastic colon.

Nulacin

A beige tablet used as an antacid to treat dyspepsia, acidity, oesophagitis, hiatus hernia.

Side effects: diarrhoea.
Caution: in patients suffering from kidney impairment.
Not to be used for: children, or for patients suffering from coeliac disease.
Not to be used with: tetracycline antibiotics.

Peptobismol

Peptobismol contains bismuth salicylate (see also De-Nol). Bismuth may colour the stools black and should be used with caution in patients suffering from kidney disease.

Roter

A pink tablet used as an antacid and antibulking agent to treat peptic ulcer, gastritis.

Side effects: constipation, nerve damage.
Caution:
Not to be used for: infants.
Not to be used with: tetracycline antibiotics.

---

senna tablets

A tablet supplied at a strength of 7.5 mg and used as a stimulant laxative to treat constipation.

Side effects:
Caution:
Not to be used for: pregnant women, children under 6 years.
Not to be used with:

Senokot

A brown tablet supplied at a strength of 7.5 mg and used as a stimulant to treat constipation.

Side effects:
Caution:
Not to be used for: infants under 2 years.
Not to be used with:

Setlers

Setlers contain calcium carbonate, magnesium carbonate and hydroxide, and aluminium hydroxide. Setlers Tums contain calcium carbonate only. Various strength and flavours are available and there are liquid and tablet preparations.

Spasmonal

A blue/grey capsule supplied at a strength of 60 mg and used as an anti-spasmodic treatment for irritable bowel syndrome.

Side effects: blurred vision, confusion, dry mouth.
Caution:
Not to be used for: children or for patients suffering from glaucoma, inflammatory bowel disease, intestinal obstruction, enlarged prostate.
Not to be used with:

Topal

A cream tablet used as an antacid to treat oesophagitis, heartburn, gastritis.

Side effects: occasionally constipation.
Caution:
Not to be used for: infants.
Not to be used with: tetracycline antibiotics.

Chapter 8

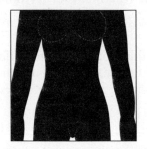

Reproductive System including Breasts

Please refer to 'Important Advice' on page 4 at the beginning of this book; and remember, if you are in any doubt, consult a physician.

Because of the complex nature of reproduction, and its need to be delicately managed by hormones, the reproductive system and the breasts are prone to slight imbalances caused by these hormones. Thus, many breast tumours are hormone dependent, as are other gynaecological tumours. Similarly, men are vulnerable to tumours of the testicles. The other major cause of diseases in the reproductive system is exposure to infections, and some of these infections may be pre-malignant. By its very nature, the womb, which must expand during pregnancy, provides a ready nest for infections and abnormalities of bleeding. Menstrual disorders and uterine disease are, therefore, common. This seems to be the price we must pay for the achievement of reproduction.

Gametes are produced in the testes and in the ovary, and they meet in the uterus during copulation. The fallopian tubes conduct the ovum from the ovaries to the uterus. All of this is under the hormonal control of the pituitary gland. Any of these organs can be affected by infection, malignancy, or benign tumour. In particular, the uterus is prone to fibroids. Dramatic hormonal changes also affect the mood as in premenstrual tension, for example.

The breasts must be able to provide milk to a suckling infant and are, therefore, vulnerable to infection and mastitis.

The menopause occurs at an age when women would normally have been expected to die in prehistoric times. It is, therefore, physiological in one sense, although not one for which the human body is adequately equipped. Treatment of the menopause and adequate control of infection are the major challenges in the treatment of diseases of the reproductive system for the future.

Diseases of the breast ♥♥♥♥♥ including breast cysts, breast abscess, fibroadenosis, and breast cancer

 The breast is an organ which is highly susceptible to hormonal changes, and various conditions may appear as a lump in a breast. Most breast lumps are benign but breast cancer is one of the commonest diseases in women. Rarely, breast cancer may occur in men.

Symptoms
Usually the presence of a lump in the breast. A painful lump usually indicates breast abscess whereas a collection of painful lumps may indicate fibroadenosis or mastitis. Mastitis or breast tenderness is usually worse before a period. Breast tenderness also occurs during pregnancy. A single painless lump may well be a cyst, but it may also be breast cancer. Breast cancer may additionally be complicated by changes to the nipple, including nipple retraction, changes to the skin above the lump giving it an orange-peel type texture. Lumps may appear elsewhere including in the armpit and other breast. Symptomatically, it may be difficult to diagnose breast cancer and further investigation may be required.

Action
If you find a new lump in a breast, then you should seek medical advice immediately.

Tests
Clinical examination and special investigations, including aspiration of cysts, aspiration biopsy, mammography, and breast ultrasound, are all part of the investigation of lumps in the breast. Full clinical examination may also include bone scans, liver scans, and brain scans. Routine blood tests, such as full blood count, ESR, alkaline phosphatase, and liver function tests may also be included.

Medications and treatment

Breast lumps are usually treated by surgery. Severe fibroadenosis and premenstrual syndromes may respond to various hormonal treatments, however. Breast abscesses need to be treated with antibiotics or by drainage. Breast cysts may be treated by aspiration.

Further advice

Regular self-monitoring of breasts for lumps is a good way to identify changes in the breast. Breast abscesses may occur during lactation when bacteria enter through a crack in the nipple. Improved nipple hygiene may prevent this occurring.

Diseases of the testes ♥♥♥♥♥
including cancer of the testes (seminoma or teratoma), epididymitis, torsion of the testicle, orchitis, and varicocoele

 Scrotal lumps may be due to lumps in the testis itself which may be benign or malignant; or enlargement of the epididymis, either an epididymal cyst or an inflamed epididymis (epididymitis). Enlarged veins in the scrotum may appear as a varicocoele which is rather like varicose veins. Inflammation of the testes may occur, for example after mumps infection, resulting in orchitis.

Symptoms

The presence of a painful or painless lump in the scrotum may be alarming. Pain usually indicates infection, e.g. orchitis, epididymitis, or torsion of the testicle. A painless lump is more likely to be a cyst of the epididymis or possibly a malignancy, e.g. seminoma or teratoma. Infections may also appear with urinary symptoms such as pain on passing urine. Blood in the semen may also be a symptom of these conditions.

Action
Torsion of the testicle, where the blood supply may be cut off, is an emergency, and, if this is suspected, medical advice should be sought urgently.

Tests
Clinical examination, ultrasound of the testicles, routine X-ray, bone scan, analysis of semen and urine may be included in the investigation of these conditions.

Medications and treatment
Infections are treated with antibiotics. Suspicion of malignancy requires biopsy. Epididymal cysts may be drained, and torsion of the testis requires immediate interventionist surgery. Varicocoele requires surgical operation to correct the presence of veins.

Further advice
Men should examine themselves to detect and prevent these conditions.

Associated conditions
Undescended testicle may occur where the testis is on a short cord and fails to descend directly into the scrotum. Surgery is required in these conditions. Inguinal hernias may enter the scrotum and produce a scrotal lump (*see* above).

Pregnancy and its complications

The main complications of early to mid-pregnancy are ectopic pregnancy and antepartum haemorrhage. In addition, threatened miscarriage (threatened abortion) is also a symptom of pregnancy.

Symptoms

Ectopic pregnancy usually presents with abdominal pain and some vaginal bleeding. Threatened abortion will also appear with pain and bleeding. Later in pregnancy antepartum, haemorrhage may appear with catastrophic abdominal pain and bleeding. All of these conditions may mimic other acute surgical abdominal emergencies.

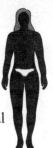

Action

Patients should lie down, and medical attention should be sought immediately.

Tests

Abdominal ultrasound, vaginal examination, tests for haemoglobin, and other routine blood tests may be included in the investigation of these conditions.

Medications and treatment

Ectopic pregnancy is treated by surgery. Threatened abortion may settle but may progress such that a dilatation and curettage is required. Antepartum haemorrhage may also settle but may be catastrophic or require surgical intervention.

Further advice

Some of these conditions may be prevented by reducing activity, e.g. by avoiding driving or air travel during pregnancy. The use of the IUCD may lead to ectopic pregnancies.

Associated conditions

Chorio-carcinoma and hydatidiform mole are conditions where pregnancy may be mimicked and may appear with bleeding and abdominal pain.

Diseases of the uterus and cervix   ♥♥♥♥♥

Diseases of the uterus and cervix include cancer of the womb, cancer of the cervix, fibroids, cervical erosions, and pelvic inflammatory disease.

Symptoms

These conditions may be symptomless. Inflammatory disease may appear with chronic pelvic pain and vaginal discharge. Fibroids may appear with heavy periods and abdominal pain. Cancer of the cervix may be picked up on routine cervical smear but it may also appear as post-coital bleeding. Cervical erosions, warts of the cervix, and other disorders of the cervix may also appear with post-coital bleeding.

Action

Investigation of pelvic pain, abnormal bleeding, or abnormal discharge should be carried out under medical supervision.

Tests

Vaginal swabs, low and high, abdominal ultrasound, pelvic examination, and routine blood tests may be included in the investigation of these conditions.

Medications and treatment

Pelvic inflammatory disease should be treated with antibiotics. Disorders of the cervix may require cautery or surgical treatments such as cone biopsy. Malignancies will require biopsy and further surgery including hysterectomy on occasions. Further treatment with chemo- and radiotherapy may also be required. Fibroids may respond to hormonal treatment but often hysterectomy is required. Fibroids may be removed leaving the womb intact (myomectomy).

Further advice

Women should have regular cervical smears and any problems should be investigated immediately.

Associated conditions

Womb infections are likely to occur after childbirth, particularly if there are retained products of conception.

Menstrual disorders ♥♥
including heavy bleeding (menorrhagia), intermenstrual bleeding, painful bleeding (dysmenorrhea), dysfunctional uterine bleeding

 Abnormalities of menstruation are very common and, although they may herald diseases of the womb, such as fibroids (*see* above), they may be related to hormonal fluctuations, and it is often difficult to establish a true causative factor.

Symptoms
Abnormally heavy bleeding, periods which are either too short or too long, cycles which are too short or too long, bleeding between periods (intermenstrual bleeding), bleeding after intercourse (post-coital bleeding), painful menstruation (dysmenorrhea).

Action
Persistent abnormalities in the menstrual cycle should be investigated.

Tests
Clinical examination, ultrasound examination, tests of hormonal function including tests for the menopause should all be carried out.

Medications and treatment
Clinical examination and diagnostic dilatation and curettage (D & C) are part of the management of this condition. The use of hormones may re-establish a normal cycle. Intermenstrual bleeding

or post-coital bleeding may be caused by abnormalities of the womb or cervix (*see* above). Very often the D & C is both investigative and curative, and restarts the normal cycles. The menopause may need to be treated with hormone replacement therapy, including Cycloprogynova, Duphaston, Estraderm, Estrapak, Harmogen, Hormonin, Ortho Dienoestrol, Ortho-Gynest, Ovestin, Premarin, Prempak, Trisequens, Vagifem.

Further advice
The IUCD may cause heavy periods, while taking the oral contraceptive pill may cause particularly light periods.

Vaginal diseases and infections

 This class of diseases includes cystitis, fungus infections (thrush), discharges from the vagina, trichomonal vaginitis, vaginismus, and overlaps with pelvic infections (*see above* diseases of the uterus and cervix). Bartholin cysts are present as a lump in the vagina.

Symptoms
Usually vaginal discharge. Vaginismus presents as a spasm of the vagina on examination or during or after intercourse. Cystitis presents as pain on passing urine, sometimes with blood and cloudy, infected urine.

Action
These conditions should be investigated as soon as possible.

Tests
Low vaginal and high vaginal swab for microbiology are useful, as is a midstream urine specimen for diagnosis of cystitis. Abdominal ultrasound may be required to look for deeper pelvic infections.

Medications and treatment

Trichomonas infections respond to metronidazole. Thrush usually responds to an antifungal cream. Cystitis will require antibiotics, and deeper pelvic infections may require prolonged courses of antibiotics. Vaginismus or muscular spasm may require both physical and psychological intervention.

Further advice

Trichomonas may be a venereal disease (*see* below), and the partner may also need treatment. Thrush is more common in those on the contraceptive pill and after taking broad-spectrum antibiotics. Thrush and cystitis may also be more common in people with diabetes.

Diseases of the ovary

The ovary may develop cysts and tumours. Polycystic ovaries are a rare cause of amenorrhoea, excess hair, and infertility (*see* below).

Symptoms

Ovarian disease may be symptomless but, occasionally, there may be abnormal menstrual bleeding, abdominal swelling, and pain. Ovarian cysts may rupture or bleed and this may be an acutely painful condition.

Action

If ovarian disease is suspected, urgent investigation is required.

Tests

Abdominal ultrasound should detect the presence of ovarian disease. Clinical examination and further CT scans may be required.

Medications and treatment

Usually surgery.

Associated conditions

Amenorrhoea may also be a symptom of pregnancy or other uterine disease (*see* above dysfunctional uterine bleeding). It also occurs as part of the anorexia syndrome (*see* below) and may occur at times of emotional stress (e.g. during travel or after moving away from home).

Premenstrual tension

 PMT is a hormonal condition which is found in women of all age groups. PMT symptoms may merge into, and overlap with, menopausal symptoms in the older age groups. Symptoms of premenstrual tension include fluid retention, breast tenderness, mental irritability, insomnia, hypersomnia, hyperphagia (excessive eating), and frank depression.

Action

Persistent premenstrual tension should be investigated.

Tests

Hormonal tests may reveal imbalances between oestrogen and progesterone that may be responsive to medication.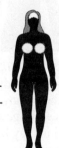

Medications and treatment

Diuretics, vitamin B_6, evening primrose oil, and hormones such as oestrogen and progesterone. The contraceptive pill may improve the symptoms of PMT.

Further advice

Avoiding alcohol and improving diet is said by some to reduce the symptoms of PMT.

Uterine prolapse

Prolapse of the womb occurs through loss of ligamentous support of the womb, and occurs after childbirth, particularly after multiple childbirth or difficult childbirth.

Symptoms
A feeling of having a swelling in the genital area, frequent urinary infections, stress incontinence (release of urine on coughing, sneezing, or laughing), heavy menstrual bleeding, and a dragging sensation.

Action
Symptoms may resolve, particularly if they have been there for a short time after pregnancy. Pelvic floor exercises may improve the symptoms.

Tests
Tests for bladder function including urine tests for infection (cystometry), investigations using dyes, and flow rates of urine may be helpful.

Medications and treatment
Prolapse may respond to the insertion of a vaginal ring to support the womb. Greater degrees of prolapse may require surgery.

Further advice
Continuing pelvic floor exercises can prevent and treat prolapse, particularly after pregnancy.

Venereal diseases

The range of venereal diseases includes non-specific urethritis, trichomonas vaginitis, gonorrhoea, syphilis, hepatitis B, and HIV infection. All of these may be sexually transmitted.

Symptoms

The symptoms of gonorrhoea or urethritis include discharge from the urethra in men or vagina in women. Syphilis may appear as a hard lump (chancre) on the penis or in the vagina. Genital warts appear with the presence of painless warts around the vagina, anus, or on the penis. Herpes presents with sores inside or outside the genitalia. Hepatitis B infection usually presents with jaundice while HIV infection presents after many years with immune deficiency – AIDS – (*see* General Conditions). Minor conditions, such as trichomonas vaginitis, appear with a white vaginal discharge. These conditions may all be asymptomatic, i.e. they may be carried by a person who does not have symptoms but can still infect others.

Action

If any of these symptoms appear, you should seek medical advice immediately.

Tests

Blood tests to check for infectious agents, swabs of vagina or urethra and cervix to check for bacteria; smears may see changes due to warts or viruses.

Medications and treatment

Trichomonas infections usually respond to metronidazole. Urethritis, gonorrhoea, and syphilis respond to antibiotics. Virus infections such as HIV, herpes, and warts may require specific antiviral therapy, such as acyclovir; e.g. Zovirax. Warts may respond to interferon.

Associated conditions

HIV infections may be transmitted nonsexually, e.g. by blood transfusion or accidentally by contamination among health-workers. Similarly, hepatitis B can be transmitted accidentally.

The menopause

The menopause occurs at about the age of 50 years in women and is brought on by a gradual failure of the ovaries to produce hormones. The main hormone involved is oestrogen, and lack of it affects several organs in the body.

Symptoms

Flushing due to excess pituitary hormone, hot sweats, loss of calcium from bone, bone pain and fractures, irritability, unwanted hair growth, dryness of the vagina, and loss of libido. Menstruation becomes irregular and bleeding lighter. Menstruation eventually ceases altogether.

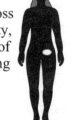

Action

The menopause is a natural process and many women believe that no further action needs to be taken.

Tests

Testing for the menopause, which may begin in the mid- to late thirties, involves hormone tests of oestrogen, progesterone and FSH. Cervical smears may give an indication of the amount of oestrogen present.

Medications and treatment

Hormone replacement therapy using skin patches, vaginal pessaries, hormonal implants, or oral tablets may all be valuable in reversing the menopause. Where a woman has had a hysterectomy, unopposed oestrogen may be used, but otherwise oestrogen and progestogens are given together. These cause re-establishment of menstruation. Examples include: Cycloprogynova, Duphaston, Estraderm, Estrapak, Harmogen, Hormonin, Ortho Dienoestrol, Ortho-Gynest, Ovestin, Premarin, Prempak, Trisequens, Vagifem.

Further advice

Hormone replacement therapy may slightly increase the risk of breast cancer but probably reduces the risk of heart disease and fractures of the bones, particularly the hip. Worsening premenstrual symptoms may be a sign of the menopause (*see* premenstrual tension above).

Infertility and endometriosis ♥♥

Infertility is inability to conceive and may have many causes. Endometriosis may be one of those causes, which is a condition where the lining of the womb may become displaced into other parts of the pelvis and cause disruption of fertility.

Symptoms

Inability to conceive after regular intercourse over a period of 12 months. Infertility may also appear as repeated miscarriage (spontaneous abortion). Endometriosis may appear as infertility or as painful menstruation with pains spreading all over the abdomen and pelvis.

Action

Infertility may require medical advice and intervention if it persists. Endometriosis may settle down but may also require medical intervention.

Tests

Investigation of infertility includes plotting a temperature chart, hormonal tests to check for ovulation, analysis of sperm, post-coital analysis of sperm, immunology tests to check for antibody production, pelvic ultrasound to check for ovarian cysts and to prove ovulation. Laparoscopy may involve the removing of ova and preparations for in-vitro fertilization.

Medications and treatment

Endometriosis may respond to hormonal blockers such as bromocriptine. Various hormonal supplements, such as oestrogen, LHRH, or progesterone, may be used to treat infertility depending on where the hormone defect is. LHRH is used to control and stimulate ovulation.

Further advice

Women trying to conceive should take regular exercise, eat a healthy diet, avoid nicotine and alcohol. Endometriosis may resolve on pregnancy.

Associated conditions

The presence of uterine fibroids may cause infertility as may any congenital abnormalities of the womb. Repeated miscarriages may occur with incompetence of the uterine cervix which may respond to suturing. Infertility may also be caused by genetic abnormalities.

Prescription Medicines

Comploment Continus

A yellow tablet supplied at a strength of 100 mg and used as a source of vitamin B_6 to treat vitamin B_6 deficiency including that developed by the contraceptive pill.

Side effects:
Caution:
Not to be used for: children.
Caution needed with: levodopa.

Dianette

A beige tablet used as an anti-androgen and oestrogen to

treat severe acne in women, hairiness.

Side effects: enlarged breasts, bloating and fluid retention, cramps, leg pains, mood change, reduction in sexual desire, headaches, nausea, vaginal erosion, discharge, and bleeding, weight gain, skin changes. The tablet also functions as an oral contraceptive.

Caution: in patients suffering from high blood pressure, diabetes, vascular disorders, asthma, depression, kidney disease, multiple sclerosis, womb diseases. Your doctor may advise you not to smoke, to have regular examinations. You should stop treatment at the first sign of serious symptoms such as severe headache or jaundice. Treatment should be stopped before surgery.

Not to be used for: children, males, pregnant women, or for patients suffering from sickle-cell anaemia, history of heart disease or thrombosis, liver disorders, some cancers, undiagnosed vaginal bleeding, some ear, skin, and kidney disorders.

Caution needed with: rifampicin, tetracyclines, griseofulvin, barbiturates, phenytoin, primidone, carbamazepine, ethosuximide, chloral hydrate, dichloralphenazone.

Duphaston

A white, scored tablet supplied at a strength of 10 mg and used as a progestogen to treat period pain, habitual and threatened abortion, endometriosis (a womb disorder), infertility, premenstrual syndrome, and as an additional treatment to oestrogen in hormone replacement.

Side effects: irregular bleeding, breast discomfort, acne, headache.

Caution: in patients suffering from high blood pressure or tendency to thrombosis, migraine, liver abnormalities, ovarian cysts.

Not to be used for: children, pregnant women, women having suffered a previous ectopic pregnancy, or for patients suffering from severe heart or kidney disease, benign liver tumours, undiagnosed vaginal bleeding.

Caution needed with: barbiturates, phenytoin, pyridone,

carbamazepine, chloral hydrate, dichloralphenazone, ethosuximide, rifampicin, chlorphenesin, meprobamate, griseofulvin.

Estraderm

A patch supplied at strengths of 25 micrograms, 50 micrograms, 100 micrograms and used as an oestrogen in oestrogen replacement therapy during the menopause. (Estraderm 50 used to prevent osteoporosis.)

Side effects: headache, nausea, tender breasts, redness at the site of the patch, rashes, skin changes, liver function disorders, sodium retention.

Caution: in patients suffering from high blood pressure, kidney or heart disease, asthma, varicose veins, epilepsy, diabetes, thyroid disease, womb disease. Your doctor may advise that your blood pressure, breasts, pelvic organs should be checked regularly.

Not to be used for: pregnant women, nursing mothers, or for patients suffering from severe liver or kidney disease, breast, genital tract, or other oestrogen-dependent cancers, genital bleeding, some ear disorders, or a history of or tendency towards thrombophlebitis, thromoboembolic diseases, cerebrovascular disease, sickle cell anaemia, porphyria, (a rare blood disorder).

Caution needed with: liver enzyme-inducing drugs (such as barbiturates, anti-epileptics), diuretics, antihypertensives.

Estrapak

A patch plus a red tablet supplied at strengths of 50 microgram and 1 mg respectively and used as oestrogen and progestogen in hormone replacement.

Side effects: headache, nausea, tender breasts, redness at site of patch, rashes, skin changes, liver function disorders, sodium retention.

Caution: in patients with breast disease or a family history of breast cancer, high blood pressure, cholelithiasis (gallstones), kidney or heart disease, asthma, varicose veins, epilepsy, migraine, diabetes, thyroid disease, womb disease. Your doctor may advise that your blood pressure, breasts, pelvic organs should be checked regularly.

Not to be used for: children, pregnant women, nursing mothers or for patients suffering from severe liver or kidney disease, breast, genital tract, or other oestrogen-dependent cancers, genital bleeding, some ear disorders, or a history of or tendency towards thrombophlebitis, thromboembolic disorders, or cerebrovascular disease, sickle cell anaemia, porphyria (a rare blood disorder).

Caution needed with: liver enzyme-inducing drugs (such as barbiturates, anti-epileptics), diuretics, antihypertensives.

Harmogen

An orange, oval, scored tablet supplied at a strength of 1.5 mg and used as an oestrogen to treat menopausal oestrogen deficiency.

Side effects: enlarged breasts, fluid retention, nausea, vaginal bleeding, weight gain, skin changes, liver disorders, jaundice, rashes, vomiting, headaches.

Caution: in patients suffering from high blood pressure, diabetes, heart disease, vascular disorders, asthma, kidney disease, epilepsy, migraine, womb diseases, thyroid disorder. Your doctor may advise you to have regular examinations.

Not to be used for: pregnant women, nursing mothers, or for patients suffering from sickle-cell anaemia, thrombosis, liver disorders, some cancers, undiagnosed vaginal bleeding, some ear, skin, and kidney disorders, jaundice, porphyria (a rare blood disorder), brain blood vessel disease.

Caution needed with: diuretics, antihypertensives, drugs which induce liver enzymes (eg barbiturates, carbamazepine, phenytoin, rifampicim).

Hormonin

A pink, scored tablet used as an oestrogen treatment for symptoms associate with the menopause.

Side effects: enlarged breasts, fluid retention, headaches, nausea, vaginal bleeding, weight gain, skin changes, rashes, liver disorders, jaundice, vomiting.

Caution: in patients suffering from high blood pressure, diabetes, heart disease, vascular disorders, asthma, kidney disease, epilepsy, womb diseases, migraine, thyroid disorder. Your doctor may advise you to have regular examinations.

Not to be used for: pregnant women, nursing mothers, or for patients suffering from sickle-cell anaemia, thrombosis, liver disorders, some cancers, undiagnosed vaginal bleeding, some ear, skin, and kidney disorders, jaundice, porphyria (a rare blood disorder), brain blood vessel disease.

Caution needed with: diuretics, antihypertensives, drugs which induce liver enzymes (eg barbiturates, phenytoin, carbamazepine, rifampicin).

Navidrex

A white, scored tablet supplied at a strength of 0.5 mg and used as a diuretic to treat heart failure, fluid retention, high blood pressure.

Side effects: rash, sensitivity to light, blood changes, stomach upset, pancreatitis, headache, dizziness, tingling sensation, electrolyte and metabolic disturbances, lung and liver changes.

Caution: the elderly, and in patients suffering from diabetes, kidney or liver disease, gout, high blood lipid levels. Potassium supplements may be needed.

Not to be used for: pregnant women, nursing mothers, or for patients suffering from inability to produce urine or severe kidney failure, low sodium or potassium levels, Addison's disease, high calcium or uric acid levels.

Caution needed with: digoxin, lithium, antihypertensives, non-steroid anti-inflammatory drugs.

Ortho Dienoestrol

A cream with applicator used as an oestrogen treatment for atrophic inflammation of the vagina, other disease of the vulva or painful intercourse.

Side effects: tender breasts, headaches, nausea, vaginal bleeding, weight gain, skin changes, rashes, liver function disorders, sodium retention, vomiting.

Caution: in patients suffering from high blood pressure, diabetes, vascular disorders, asthma, kidney disease, heart disease, epilepsy, migraine, thyrotoxicosis, womb diseases. Your doctor may advise you to have regular examinations.

Not to be used for: children, pregnant women, nursing mothers, or for patients suffering from sickle-cell anaemia, thrombosis, liver disorders, some cancers, undiagnosed vaginal bleeding, some ear, skin, and kidney disorders, porphyria (a rare blood disorder), brain blood vessel disease.

Caution needed with: diuretics, antihypertensives, and drugs that change liver enzymes (eg barbiturates, carbamazepine, phenytoin).

Ortho-Gynest

A pessary supplied at a strength of 0.5 mg and used as an oestrogen treatment for atrophic inflammation of the vagina, other disease of the vulva or painful intercourse.

Side effects: tender breasts, fluid retention, headaches, nausea, vaginal bleeding, weight gain, skin changes, rashes, liver function disorders, sodium retention, vomiting.

Caution: in patients suffering from high blood pressure, diabetes, vascular disorders, asthma, kidney disease, heart disease, epilepsy, migraine, thyrotoxicosis, womb diseases. Your doctor may advise you to have regular examinations.

Not to be used for: children, pregnant women, nursing mothers, or for patients suffering from sickle-cell anaemia, thrombosis, liver disorders, some cancers, undiagnosed vaginal bleeding, some ear, skin, and kidney disorders, porphyria (a rare blood disorder), brain blood vessel disease.

Caution needed with: diuretics, antihypertensives, and drugs that change liver enzymes (eg barbiturates, carbamazepine, phenytoin).

Ovestin

A white tablet supplied at a strength of 0.25 mg, and used as an oestrogen for treating genital or urinary complaints caused by oestrogen deficiency, and some cases of infertility.

Side effects: enlarged breasts, fluid retention, headaches, nausea, vaginal bleeding, weight gain, skin changes, rash, liver disorder, jaundice, vomiting.

Caution: in patients suffering from high blood pressure, heart disease, diabetes, vascular disorders, asthma, kidney disease, womb disease, migraine, thyroid disorder, epilepsy.

Not to be used for: pregnant women, nursing mothers, or for patients suffering from sickle-cell anaemia, thrombosis, liver disorders, some cancers, undiagnosed vaginal bleeding, some ear, skin, and kidney disordrs, brain blood vessel dissea, porphyria (a rare bood disorder).

Caution needed with: diuretics, antihypertensives, drugs which induce liver enzymes (eg barbiturates, carbamazepine, phenytoin, primidone, rifampicin).

Ovestin Cream

A cream used as an oestrogen treatment for atrophic inflam-mation of the vagina, itch, as a treatment before vaginal surgery, other diseases of the vulva.

Side effects: tender breasts, fluid retention, headaches, nausea, vaginal bleeding, weight gain, skin changes, rashes, vomiting, sodium retention, liver disorder, jaundice.

Caution: in patients suffering from high blood pressure, diabetes, vascular disorders, asthma, kidney disease, womb diseases, heart disease, epilepsy, migraine. Your doctor may advise you to have regular examinations.

Not to be used for: children, pregnant women, nursing mothers, or for patients suffering from sickle-cell anaemia, brain blood vessel disease, thrombosis, liver disorders, some cancers, undiagnosed vaginal bleeding, some ear, skin, and kidney disorders, porphyria (a rare blood disorder).

Caution needed with: diuretics, antihypertensives, and drugs that change liver enzymes (eg barbiturates, carbamazepine, phenytoin).

Premarin

A maroon, oval tablet, yellow, oval tablet, or purple, oval tablet according to strengths of 0.625 mg, 1.25 mg, 2.5 mg and used as an oestrogen for hormone replacement during and after the menopause, and to treat atrophic inflammation of the vagina, inflammation of the urethra, certain kinds of breast cancer, and to prevent thinning of the bones.

Side effects: enlarged breasts, fluid retention, nausea, vaginal bleeding, weight gain, skin changes, liver disorders, jaundice, rashes, vomiting.

Caution: in patients suffering from high blood pressure, diabetes, heart disease, vascular disorders, asthma, kidney disease, epilepsy, womb diseases, thyroid disorder. Your doctor may advise you to have regular examinations.

Not to be used for: children, pregnant women, nursing mothers or for patients suffering from sickle-cell anaemia, thrombosis, liver disorders, some cancers, undiagnosed vaginal bleeding, some ear, skin, and kidney disorders, jaundice, porphyria (a rare blood disorder), brain blood vessel disease.

Caution needed with: diuretics, antihypertensives, and drugs that change liver enzymes (eg barbiturates, carbamazepine, phenytoin).

Prempak-C

A maroon, oval tablet or yellow, oval tablet according to

strengths of 0.625 mg, 1.25 mg plus a brown tablet 0.15 mg and used as an oestrogen, progestogen for hormone replacement during and after the menopause, and treatment of post-menopausal osteoporosis, atrophic inflammation of the vagina, inflammation of the urethra.

Side effects: enlarged breasts, bloating and fluid retention, cramps, leg pains, mood change, reduction in sexual desire, headaches, nausea, vaginal erosion, discharge, and bleeding, weight gain, skin changes.

Caution: in patients suffering from high blood pressure, diabetes, vascular disorders, asthma, depression, kidney disease, multiple sclerosis, womb diseases. Your doctor may advise you not to smoke, to have regular examinations. You should stop treatment at the first sign of serious symptoms such as severe headache or jaundice. Treatment should be stopped before surgery.

Not to be used for: children, pregnant women, or for patients suffering from sickle-cell anaemia, history of heart disease or thrombosis, liver disorders, some cancers, undiagnosed vaginal bleeding, some ear, skin, and kidney disorders.

Caution needed with: rifampicin, griseofulvin, barbiturates, phenytoin, primidone, carbamazepine, ethosuximide, chloral hydrate, dichloralphenazone.

Trisequens

Twelve blue tablets, 10 white tablets, and 6 red tablets used as a oestrogen, progestogen treatment for menopausal symptoms, and to prevent bone thinning after the menopause.

Side effects: enlarged breasts, bloating and fluid retention, cramps, leg pains, mood change, reduction in sexual desire, headaches, nausea, vaginal erosion, discharge, and bleeding, weight gain, skin changes.

Caution: in patients suffering from high blood pressure, diabetes, vascular disorders, asthma, depression, kidney disease, multiple sclerosis, womb diseases. Your doctor may advise you not to smoke, to have regular examinations. You should stop treatment at the first sign of serious symptoms such as severe headache or

jaundice. Treatment should be stopped before surgery.
Not to be used for: children, pregnant women, or for patients suffering from sickle-cell anaemia, history of heart disease or thrombosis, liver disorders, some cancers, undiagnosed vaginal bleeding, some ear, skin, and kidney disorders.
Caution needed with: diuretics, antihypertensives, and drugs that change liver enzymes, rifampicin, tetracyclines, griseofulvin, barbiturates, phenytoin, primidone, carbamazepine, ethosuximide, chloral hydrate, dichloralphenazone.

Vagifem

Pessaries supplied with applicators, and used as an oestrogen treatment for atrophic inflammation of the vagina.

Side effects: enlarged breasts, fluid retention, headaches, nausea, vaginal bleeding, weight gain, skin changes, liver disorders, jaundice, rashes, vomiting.
Caution: in patients suffering from high blood pressure, diabetes, heart disease, vascular disorders, asthma, kidney disease, epilepsy, migraine, womb disease, thyroid disorder. Your doctor may advise you to have regular examinations.
Not to be used for: pregnant women, nursing mothers, or for patients suffering from sickle-cell anaemia, history of heart disease or thrombosis, liver disorders, some cancers, undiagnosed vaginal bleeding, some ear, skin and kidney disorders, jaundice, porphyria (a rare blood disease), brain blood vessel disorder.
Caution needed with: diuretics, antihypertensives, drugs which induce liver enzymes (eg barbiturates, carbamazepine, phenytoin, primidone, rifampicin).

Zovirax

A blue, shield-shaped tablet supplied at strengths of 200 mg, 400 mg, 800 mg and used as an antiviral treatment for genital herpes, other skin herpes, shingles.

Side effects: irritation (local use).

Caution: in patients suffering from kidney damage; drink plenty of fluids.
Not to be used for:
Caution needed with: probenecid.

Antibiotics

Amoxil

A maroon/gold capsule supplied at a strength of 250 mg, 500 mg and used as a broad-spectrum penicillin to treat respiratory, ear, nose, and throat, urinary, venereal, and soft tissue infections. Also for dental abscess, and to prevent infection of the heart during dental procedures

Side effects: stomach upset, allergy.
Caution: in patients suffering from glandular fever.
Not to be used for: patients suffering from penicillin allergy.
Caution needed with:

Ciproxin

Tablets supplied at strengths of 250 mg, 500 mg, and used as an antibiotic to treat infections of the ear, nose, throat, urinary system, respiratory system, skin, soft tissues, bone, joints, stomach, and gonorrhoea (a venereal disease), and major infections.

Side effects: stomach and intestinal disturbances, dizziness, headache, tiredness, confusion, convulsions, rash, pain in the joints, changes in blood, liver, or kidneys, blurred vision, rapid heart rate.
Caution: in patients suffering from severe kidney disease or with a history of convulsions. Plenty of liquid should be drunk.
Not to be used for: children, growing youngsters unless absolutely necessary, and pregnant women or nursing mothers.
Caution needed with: theophylline, antacids, alcohol, anticoagu-

lants, non-steroid anti-inflammatory drugs, cyclosporin.

Erythrocin

A white, oblong tablet supplied at strengths of 250 mg, 500 mg and used as an antibiotic to treat infections, including acne.

Side effects: stomach disturbances, allergies.
Caution: in patients suffering from liver disease.
Not to be used for: children.
Caution needed with: theophylline, anticoagulants taken by mouth, carbamazepine, digoxin, terfenadine, astemizole.

Flagyl

An off-white tablet or an off-white, capsule-shaped tablet according to strengths of 200 mg, 400 mg and used as an antibacterial treatment for trichomoniasis, non-specific vaginitis, other infections, dysentery, abscess of the liver, ulcerative gingivitis (gum disease).

Side effects: stomach upset, furred tongue, unpleasant taste, allergy, rash, swelling, brain disturbances, dark-coloured urine, nerve changes, seizures, white cell changes.
Caution: in patients with brain disorder caused by liver disease. Short-term high-dose treatment should not be used for pregnant women or nursing mothers.
Not to be used for:
Caution needed with: alcohol, phenobarbitone, anticoagulants taken by mouth.

Floxapen

A black/caramel-coloured capsule supplied at strengths of 250 mg, 500 mg and used as a penicillin treatment for skin, soft tissue, ear, nose, and throat, and other infections.

Side effects: allergy, stomach disturbances.
Caution:
Not to be used for: patients suffering from penicillin allergy.
Caution needed with:

Keflex

A dark green/white capsule or dark green/light green capsule supplied at strengths of 250 mg, 500 mg and used as a cephalosporin antibiotic to treat respiratory, soft tissue, urine, and skin infections.

Side effects: allergic reactions, stomach disturbances.
Caution: in patients suffering from kidney disease or who are very sensitive to penicillin.
Not to be used for:
Caution needed with: loop diuretics.

Monotrim

A white, scored tablet supplied at strengths of 100 mg, 200 mg and used as an antibiotic to treat infections, urine infections.

Side effects: stomach disturbances, skin reactions.
Caution: in the elderly and in patients suffering from kidney disease from folate deficiency (vitamin deficiency). Your doctor may advise regular blood tests.
Not to be used for: infants under 6 weeks, pregnant women, or for patients suffering from severe kidney disease where regular blood tests cannot be made.
Caution needed with:

Negram

A pale-brown tablet supplied at a strength of 500 mg and used as an antiseptic to treat urinary and stomach infections.

Side effects: stomach upset, disturbed vision, rash, blood changes, seizures, sensitivity to light.
Caution: in pregnant women, nursing mothers and in patients suffering from liver or kidney disease. Keep out of the sunlight.
Not to be used for: infants under 3 months or for patients with a history of convulsions, porphyria (a rare blood disorder).
Caution needed with: anticoagulants, probenecid, antibacterials.

Penbritin

A black/red capsule supplied at strengths of 250 mg, 500 mg and used as a penicillin to treat respiratory, ear, nose, and throat infections, gonorrhoea, soft tissue infections, urinary infections.

Side effects: allergy, stomach disturbances.
Caution: in patients suffering from glandular fever.
Not to be used for: patients suffering from penicillin allergy.
Caution needed with:

Septrin

A white tablet or an orange, dispersible tablet used as an antibiotic to treat respiratory, stomach, and skin infections.

Side effects: nausea, vomiting, tongue inflammation, rash, blood changes, folate (vitamin) deficiency, rarely skin changes.
Caution: in the elderly, nursing mothers, and in patients suffering from kidney disease. Your doctor may advise that patients undergoing prolonged treatment should have regular blood tests.
Not to be used for: pregnant women, new-born infants, or for patients suffering from severe kidney or liver disease, or blood changes.
Caution needed with: folate inhibitors, anticoagulants, anticonvulsants, antidiabetics.

Tetracycline Tablets

An orange tablet supplied at a strength of 250 mg and used as an antibiotic treatment for infections.

Side effects: stomach disturbances, allergy, additional infections.
Caution: in patients suffering from liver or kidney disease.
Not to be used for: children, nursing mothers, or women during the latter half of pregnancy.
Caution needed with: milk, antacids, mineral supplements, the contraceptive pill.

Vibramycin

A green capsule supplied at a strength of 100 mg and used as a tetracycline treatment for pneumonia, respiratory, stomach, soft tissue, eye, and urinary infections.

Side effects: stomach disturbances, allergy, additional infections, oesophagitis, allergy, raised blood pressure in the brain.
Caution: in patients suffering from liver disease.
Not to be used for: children, nursing mothers, women in the last half of pregnancy, or even for pregnant women at all unless no other treatment is possible.
Caution needed with: antacids, mineral supplements, barbiturates, carbamazepine, phenytoin.

Zinnat

A white tablet supplied at strengths of 125 mg, 250 mg and used as a cephalosporin antibiotic to treat respiratory, ear, nose, and throat, skin, soft tissue, and urinary infections.

Side effects: stomach disturbances, allergy, colitis, blood changes, thrush, change in liver chemistry, headache, interference with some blood tests.
Caution: in pregnant women, nursing mothers, and in patients who are sensitive to penicillin.
Not to be used for:
Caution needed with:

Over-the-counter Medicines

Aci-Jel

A jelly with applicator used as an antiseptic to treat non-specific vaginal infection.
Side effects: irritation and inflammation.
Caution:
Not to be used for: children.
Not to be used with:

Betadine

A pessary and applicator supplied at a strength of 200 mg and used as an antiseptic to treat inflammation of the vagina.

Side effects: irritation and sensitivity.
Caution:
Not to be used for: children.
Not to be used with:

Effercitrate

A white effervescent tablet used as an alkalizing agent to treat cystitis.

Side effects: raised potassium levels, stomach irritation, mild diuresis.
Caution: in patients suffering from kidney disease.
Not to be used for: infants under 1 year or for patients suffering from ulcerated or blocked small bowel.
Not to be used with: potassium-sparing diuretics.

Furadantin

A yellow, pentagonal, scored tablet supplied at strengths of 50 mg, 100 mg, and used as an antiseptic to treat infection of the urinary tract.

Side effects: stomach upset, allergy, jaundice, nerve inflammation, blood changes, possible liver damage.
Caution:
Not to be used for: infants under 1 month or for patients suffering from kidney problems resulting in reduced urine output.
Not to be used with:

Hiprex

A white, oblong, scored tablet supplied at a strength of 1 g and used as an antibacterial treatment for infections of the urinary tract.

Side effects: stomach upset, rash, bladder irritation.
Caution:
Not to be used for: patients suffering from severe dehydration, severe kidney failure, or electrolyte changes.
Not to be used with: sulphonamides, alkalizing agents.

Pevaryl

A cream used as an antifungal treatment for inflammation of the penis, inflammation of the vulva, thrush-like nappy rash, other skin infections such as tinea or nail infections.

Side effects: irritation.
Caution:
Not to be used for:
Not to be used with:

Urisal

Orange-flavoured granules in sachets of 4 g used as an alkalizing agent to relieve the pain of cystitis.

Side effects:
Caution: in patients suffereing from kidney disease.
Not to be used for: children, pregnant women, or for patients

suffering from heart disease, high blood pressure, or with a history of kidney disease.

Not to be used with:

Chapter 9

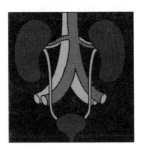

Kidneys and Excretion

Please refer to 'Important Advice' on page 4 at the beginning of this book; and remember, if you are in any doubt, consult a physician.

The kidneys function as a filtering system to remove from the body toxins which have not been removed by the liver. Beyond the kidney is an elaborate plumbing system involving the ureter, bladder, and urethra, and in men the prostate gland. Primarily, the kidney is the major organ of this system and, like other major organs, it is prone to tumours and to infection. Its special position in the filtering system may leave it vulnerable to external toxins. Similarly, the bladder connects with the outside world, and is liable to infections such as cystitis. Abnormal precipitation within the urinary tract causes stones. Control of infections is still a major challenge for the treatment of the genito-urinary system.

Cancer of the kidney and bladder ♥♥♥♥

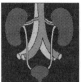

The urinary tract may be affected by malignancy, and the organs usually involved are the kidney and the bladder. Some children suffer from a rare type of kidney tumour, but more commonly it occurs in adults.

Symptoms

Passing blood in the urine. This may not be obvious and may only be detectable on routine urine testing (microscopic haematuria). Pain on passing urine or pain in the loins or flank may indicate the presence of a tumour. The symptoms may be similar to those of renal colic (*see* below).

Associated symptoms

Symptoms of malignancy, such as fever and weight loss, may also be present.

Action

Urgent investigation of any of these symptoms is required.

Tests

Urine analysis, cystoscopy, intravenous pyelogram, biopsy, ultrasound examination of the kidneys, and routine blood tests to look for anaemia.

Medications and treatment

Tumours of the kidney or bladder need to be removed surgically. Radiotherapy may be helpful, and interferon and interleukin may also be used.

Further advice

Tumours of the genito-urinary tract are more common in smokers.

Associated conditions

Warts or papillomas of the bladder may be benign but they may convert to malignant tumours.

Diseases of the prostate

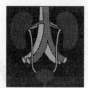

The prostate gland is found at the neck of the bladder in men. It is likely to become enlarged (benign prostatic hypotrophy) or to develop tumours (carcinoma of the prostate). Both of these occur more frequently as men get older.

Symptoms

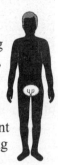

The symptoms of prostate disease are difficulty passing urine, poor stream of urine, difficulty starting urination, difficulty stopping urination, dribbling after urination, and incontinence. Retention of urine, with total inability to pass urine may occur. Cancer of the prostate may additionally appear with other symptoms of malignant disease such as secondary metastases to the bones causing bone pain.

Action

Symptoms may come and go in the early stages, and may be made worse when there is urine infection. If the symptoms persist for more than a month, you should seek medical advice.

Tests

Tests include routine blood tests, tests for evidence of tumours in the bone (alkaline phosphatase), tests for prostatic cancer (acid phosphatase), and also prostate-specific antigen. Physical examination, as well as cystoscopy, intravenous pyelography, and studies of bladder function may also be included.

Medications and treatment

Benign prostatic hypotrophy is usually treated by surgery, although recently Proscar tablets have been made available, and these can reduce the size of the prostate gland. Prostatic cancer may respond to hormonal treatment, and rarely castration is advised to slow down the progress of the disease because the cancer grows in the presence of androgens (male hormones).

Further advice
After prostate surgery, you may suffer from impotence and incontinence.

Kidney failure

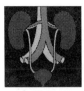 The kidneys are organs of excretion, and there are several causes of failure. These include acute sudden failure as in glomerulonephritis which may occur after streptococcal infection. Damage to the kidneys through repeated infection, hypertension, or diabetes (diabetic nephropathy) may also cause kidney failure. Congenital abnormalities of the kidneys or polycystic kidneys may also lead to kidney failure.

Symptoms
These include fluid retention, nausea, weight gain, pale skin and anaemia, swelling of the ankles and abdomen, the passing of excess urine or failure to pass urine at all, the passing of blood in the urine (haematuria), breathing problems, heart problems (due to changes in potassium levels), and death.

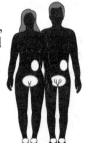

Action
Suspected kidney failure must be treated as a medical emergency.

Tests
Investigations include routine blood tests to look for causes of kidney failure, concentrating particularly on urea, potassium, creatinine and creatinine clearance. Patients are often anaemic, and this should also be investigated and treated.

Medications and treatment
Treatment of kidney failure includes attention to the cause of the kidney failure, peritoneal dialysis, haemo-dialysis, or kidney trans-

plant. Drugs such as erythropoietin may be useful to treat the anaemia caused by kidney failure.

Further advice

If you are suffering from chronic kidney failure, you may need to go on special diets which are low in potassium and protein. Special foods are available.

Kidney stones (renal calculus)

 Kidney stones are formed from calcium oxidate or uric acid and they can appear anywhere in the urinary tract from the kidney down to the bladder and urethra. Their appearance may be related to dehydration or conditions where there is an increased calcium level in the blood, hypocalcemia due to overactive parathyroid glands, increased calcium intake with alkalis, or where there is disease of the bones, including malignancy, which releases calcium from bones. Some people have raised calcium in the urine for unknown reasons (idiopathic hypercalciuria).

Symptoms

There may be none. Occasionally, patients may pass bits of gravel, or blood may be detected. Renal colic is a seriously painful condition where a stone becomes trapped in the ureter. Spasm of the ureter, which is trying to expel the stone, results in pain which is continuous and may worsen acutely. The pain may radiate from loin down to the groin and into the genitalia. It may be associated with passing blood or gravel. Late presentation of kidney stones may be with kidney failure. Stones in the bladder may cause irritable bladder and haematuria.

Action

Severe renal colic is a medical emergency. Detection of stones in the urinary tract should always be fully investigated.

Tests

Investigations include cystoscopy, urine measurements for infection, blood, and crystals, intravenous pyelogram (IVP), ultrasound studies, blood tests for calcium and uric acid.

Medications and treatment

The pain of renal colic may resolve with narcotic analgesics. High fluid intake is usually encouraged for the stone to pass naturally. Stones which do not pass naturally may require surgical intervention to remove them.

Further advice

In hot climates, especially, you should drink plenty of non-alcoholic fluids to prevent a high concentration of calcium in the urine.

Associated conditions

Bladder stones may be present without kidney stones. These may form around other bladder abnormalities, e.g. papilloma.

Infections of the renal tract (pyelonephritis and cystitis)

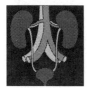 Cystitis (infection of the bladder) has been dealt with in Chapter 8 above.

Serious infection of the kidney (pyelonephritis) can occur when cystitis remains untreated and the infection ascends, or due to metastatic spread of bacteria.

Symptoms

Fever, pains in the loin or bladder, passing of infected urine or bloody urine.

Action

Minor urinary tract infections may respond to a high fluid intake, urine alkalinizers, and bedrest and hot-water bottle. More serious infections require medical intervention.

Tests

Tests include examination of the urine and culture for infection, routine blood tests for infection, intravenous pyelography, ultrasound studies particularly where kidney abscess is suspected.

Medications and treatment

Infections will normally respond to antibiotics. Severe, recurrent kidney infections may require surgical intervention to remove the damaged kidney or to correct a urinary tract abnormality which may be congenital.

Further advice

You should drink plenty of non-alcoholic fluids to prevent and treat urinary tract infections.

Associated conditions

Kidney cysts or abscesses may be present, and these may need to be treated separately.

Functional disorders of the bladder ♥

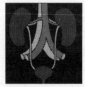

The bladder functions to expel urine and is under the control of the parasympathetic nervous system. Various conditions may affect bladder function, including multiple sclerosis, paralysis, or simply prolapse.

Symptoms

Stress incontinence has been dealt with above. Difficulty passing urine, a poor stream of urine, frequency of urination, passing of small volumes of urine with blood, and incontinence – particularly nocturnal incontinence.

Action
Where symptoms are distressing and persistent, they should be fully investigated.

Tests
Specialized tests involving cystometry, cystoscopy, measurement of flow rates of urine, testing for infection, and examination for prolapse are all part of the investigation of the neurogenic bladder. ·

Medications and treatment
A number of medications, such as Cystrin, may be helpful in this condition. Occasionally surgery may be required to improve sphincter function.

Further advice
Chronic low-grade infection may appear with symptoms similar to neurogenic bladder.

Prescription Medicines

Cystrin

A white tablet supplied at strengths of 3 mg, 5 mg and used as an antispasmodic and anticholinergic treatment for incontinence, urgency or frequency of urination, or night-time incontinence in children.

Side effects: anticholinergic effects, flushing of the face.
Caution: in pregnant women, and in patients suffering from liver or kidney disease, heart disorders, overactive thyroid, enlarged prostate, hiatus hernia or existing disturbance of normal bodily functions.
Not to be used for: children under 5 years, nursing mothers, or for patients suffering from blockage in the bowel or bladder,

severe ulcerative colitis, other intestinal disorders, myaesthenia gravis, or glaucoma.
Caution needed with: sedatives, amantadine, levodopa, digoxin, tricyclic antidepressants, other anticholinergics.

Proscar

A blue, apple-shaped tablet supplied at a strength of 5 mg and used to treat enlarged prostate gland.

Side effects: impotence, decreased libido, decreased volume of ejaculate.
Caution: in patients suffering from urine outflow obstruction or prostate cancer. Your doctor may advise regular tests before and during treatment. Female partners of patients being treated who are or who may become pregnant should not handle the tablets and avoid exposure to semen by using a condom.
Not to be used for: children.
Caution needed with:

Antibiotics

Amoxil

A maroon/gold capsule supplied at a strength of 250 mg, 500 mg and used as a broad-spectrum penicillin to treat respiratory, ear, nose, and throat, urinary, venereal, and soft tissue infections. Also for dental abscess, and to prevent infection of the heart during dental procedures

Side effects: stomach upset, allergy.
Caution: in patients suffering from glandular fever.
Not to be used for: patients suffering from penicillin allergy.
Caution needed with:

Ciproxin

Tablets supplied at strengths of 250 mg, 500 mg, and used as

an antibiotic to treat infections of the ear, nose, throat, urinary system, respiratory system, skin, soft tissues, bone, joints, stomach, and gonorrhoea (a venereal disease), and major infections.

Side effects: stomach and intestinal disturbances, dizziness, headache, tiredness, confusion, convulsions, rash, pain in the joints, changes in blood, liver, or kidneys, blurred vision, rapid heart rate.

Caution: in patients suffering from severe kidney disease or with a history of convulsions. Plenty of liquid should be drunk.

Not to be used for: children, growing youngsters unless absolutely necessary, and pregnant women or nursing mothers.

Caution needed with: theophylline, antacids, alcohol, anticoagulants, non-steroid anti-inflammatory drugs, cyclosporin.

Erythrocin

A white, oblong tablet supplied at strengths of 250 mg, 500 mg and used as an antibiotic to treat infections, including acne.

Side effects: stomach disturbances, allergies.

Caution: in patients suffering from liver disease.

Not to be used for: children.

Caution needed with: theophylline, anticoagulants taken by mouth, carbamazepine, digoxin, terfenadine, astemizole.

Flagyl

An off-white tablet or an off-white, capsule-shaped tablet according to strengths of 200 mg, 400 mg and used as an antibacterial treatment for trichomoniasis, non-specific vaginitis, other infections, dysentery, abscess of the liver, ulcerative gingivitis (gum disease).

Side effects: stomach upset, furred tongue, unpleasant taste, allergy, rash, swelling, brain disturbances, dark-coloured urine, nerve changes, seizures, white cell changes.

Caution: in patients with brain disorder caused by liver disease. Short-term high-dose treatment should not be used for pregnant women or nursing mothers.
Not to be used for:
Caution needed with: alcohol, phenobarbitone, anticoagulants taken by mouth.

Floxapen

A black/caramel-coloured capsule supplied at strengths of 250 mg, 500 mg and used as a penicillin treatment for skin, soft tissue, ear, nose, and throat, and other infections.

Side effects: allergy, stomach disturbances.
Caution:
Not to be used for: patients suffering from penicillin allergy.
Caution needed with:

Keflex

A dark green/white capsule or dark green/light green capsule supplied at strengths of 250 mg, 500 mg and used as a cephalosporin antibiotic to treat respiratory, soft tissue, urine, and skin infections.

Side effects: allergic reactions, stomach disturbances.
Caution: in patients suffering from kidney disease or who are very sensitive to penicillin.
Not to be used for:
Caution needed with: loop diuretics.

Monotrim

A white, scored tablet supplied at strengths of 100 mg, 200 mg and used as an antibiotic to treat infections, urine infections.

Side effects: stomach disturbances, skin reactions.

Caution: in the elderly and in patients suffering from kidney disease from folate deficiency (vitamin deficiency). Your doctor may advise regular blood tests.

Not to be used for: infants under 6 weeks, pregnant women, or for patients suffering from severe kidney disease where regular blood tests cannot be made.

Caution needed with:

Negram

A pale-brown tablet supplied at a strength of 500 mg and used as an antiseptic to treat urinary and stomach infections.

Side effects: stomach upset, disturbed vision, rash, blood changes, seizures, sensitivity to light.

Caution: in pregnant women, nursing mothers and in patients suffering from liver or kidney disease. Keep out of the sunlight.

Not to be used for: infants under 3 months or for patients with a history of convulsions, porphyria (a rare blood disorder).

Caution needed with: anticoagulants, probenecid, antibacterials.

Penbritin

A black/red capsule supplied at strengths of 250 mg, 500 mg and used as a penicillin to treat respiratory, ear, nose, and throat infections, gonorrhoea, soft tissue infections, urinary infections.

Side effects: allergy, stomach disturbances.

Caution: in patients suffering from glandular fever.

Not to be used for: patients suffering from penicillin allergy.

Caution needed with:

Septrin

A white tablet or an orange, dispersible tablet used as an antibiotic to treat respiratory, stomach, and skin infections.

Side effects: nausea, vomiting, tongue inflammation, rash, blood changes, folate (vitamin) deficiency, rarely skin changes.
Caution: in the elderly, nursing mothers, and in patients suffering from kidney disease. Your doctor may advise that patients undergoing prolonged treatment should have regular blood tests.
Not to be used for: pregnant women, new-born infants, or for patients suffering from severe kidney or liver disease, or blood changes.
Caution needed with: folate inhibitors, anticoagulants, anticonvulsants, antidiabetics.

Tetracycline Tablets

An orange tablet supplied at a strength of 250 mg and used as an antibiotic treatment for infections.

Side effects: stomach disturbances, allergy, additional infections.
Caution: in patients suffering from liver or kidney disease.
Not to be used for: children, nursing mothers, or women during the latter half of pregnancy.
Caution needed with: milk, antacids, mineral supplements, the contraceptive pill.

Vibramycin

A green capsule supplied at a strength of 100 mg and used as a tetracycline treatment for pneumonia, respiratory, stomach, soft tissue, eye, and urinary infections.

Side effects: stomach disturbances, allergy, additional infections, oesophagitis, allergy, raised blood pressure in the brain.
Caution: in patients suffering from liver disease.
Not to be used for: children, nursing mothers, women in the last half of pregnancy, or even for pregnant women at all unless no other treatment is possible.
Caution needed with: antacids, mineral supplements, barbiturates, carbamazepine, phenytoin.

Zinnat

A white tablet supplied at strengths of 125 mg, 250 mg and used as a cephalosporin antibiotic to treat respiratory, ear, nose, and throat, skin, soft tissue, and urinary infections.

Side effects: stomach disturbances, allergy, colitis, blood changes, thrush, change in liver chemistry, headache, interference with some blood tests.

Caution: in pregnant women, nursing mothers, and in patients who are sensitive to penicillin.

Not to be used for:

Caution needed with:

Chapter 10

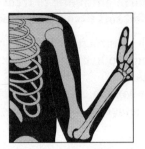

Bones, Joints, and Muscles

Please refer to 'Important Advice' on page 4 at the beginning of this book; and remember, if you are in any doubt, consult a physician.

The function of the skeletal system is to support the remainder of the body and to enable movement or locomotion. Thus, muscles are attached to bones, and bones articulate with one another via joints; the muscles are under nervous control. Because this is an ancient and internal system with little need for rapid cell changeover, malignant disease is rare. In other words, unlike the gut, for example, bones are not exposed to a potentially hostile environment, nor do the cells divide often so there is little chance for cancerous division. Most problems are caused by trauma, especially sports injuries and those illnesses resulting from degeneration, particularly loss of calcium in the bone leading to osteoporosis and the common condition of backache.

Muscles are functionally well established – that is, they are well defined and have limited actions – and have no need to communicate with the outside world. Thus they are not vulnerable to the afflictions, such as infections, of other organs.

We have evolved from animals that walked on all fours for much of the time, and one of the legacies of our vertical posture is that abnormal strain has been thrown upon the spine, hips and knees. It is not surprising that these joints are most commonly affected in most of the diseases of the locomotory system. The major challenges for the future are to prevent and treat osteoporosis, and to manage sports injuries, particularly to the knee, more effectively.

Sports injuries and trauma ♥

 There is a wide range of sports injuries, from tennis elbow to torn cartilage conditions. Repetitive strain injury falls into this category and may affect the fingers in typists and keyboard operatives, for example. Bone fractures may also be caused by sports injuries, and fracture is usually easily diagnosed. Tendon and cartilage injuries, particularly in the knee, are very common in sports. Inflammation of the bursa, or sac of fluid, causes conditions such as tennis elbow or golfer's elbow where there is pain particularly on gripping or movement. A similar condition is the carpal tunnel syndrome where there is pressure on the nerve in the wrist.

Symptoms
Symptoms of a fracture include severe pain, swelling, inability to move, and occasionally cracking or crepitus. When bone breaks through the skin surface, it is known as a compound fracture. Cartilage injuries, particularly in the knee, appear with locking of the knee, pain and swelling, and discomfort on exercise. Tennis elbow and other conditions, such as bursitis, appear with pain on gripping or moving the affected joint. Carpal tunnel syndrome presents with pins and needles in the hand (usually excluding the little finger) particularly at night and in women during pregnancy and at the time of the menopause. Repetitive strain injury presents with pain and stiffness in the fingers. Any joint may be affected by a sports injury, and others commonly affected are the shoulder and ankle. Neck ache and stiff neck may result from certain types of injury.

Action
Most sports injuries respond to rest and treatment with ice. Failure to respond after a short time will require medical intervention.

Tests
X-rays are required if fracture is suspected. Clinical examination is

usually sufficient to diagnose cartilage injury. Arthroscopy (looking into a joint) would be very helpful.

Medications and treatment

Torn cartilages can be removed through an arthroscope, or extensive open surgery will be required. Minor conditions, such as tennis elbow, may respond to injections of local anaesthetic and corticosteroids. Less serious injuries will respond to analgesics, analgesic creams and sprays, and non-steroidal anti-inflammatory drugs including: Algesal, Brufen, Feldene, Feldene Gel, Froben, Indocid, Intralgin, Mobiflex, Naprosyn, Nurofen, Orudis, Ponstan, Proflex, Relifex, Rheumox, Stugam, Traxam, Voltarol. Carpal tunnel syndrome may require surgical intervention but occasionally responds to diuretic treatment to reduce pressure on the joint.

Further advice

Make certain that you warm up and train properly to help prevent sports injuries. Trying to exercise through an injury to improve it rarely works, and rest, physiotherapy, and treatment with ice are invaluable in the treatment of all sports injuries. Occasionally steroid injections are helpful but they should not be overused.

Ankylosing spondylitis

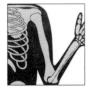 Ankylosing spondylitis, sometimes known as 'poker back', is an inflammatory condition affecting the sacro-iliac joints of the spine, and occasionally the hip and other joints. Its cause is not known but may be associated with genetic factors. It is perhaps ten times more common in men than in women and the first symptoms usually appear in people in their mid-twenties. While the females in affected families may not suffer from the symptoms, it seems that they may be carriers of the condition from one generation to the next.

Symptoms

Persistent backache with stiffness. The pain is worse after long periods of rest, so early morning pain and stiffness are common features of the condition. Occasionally, there may be associated symptoms such as iritis (redness of the eyes) or colitis (inflammation of the bowels). Other joints may become involved later, causing hip or ankle pain. Occasionally skin rashes may occur.

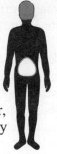

Action

If you suffer from persistent backache, you should seek medical advice.

Tests

Blood tests to check for inflammatory arthritis should be done, including full blood count, sedimentation rate, and latex tests for rheumatoid arthritis. HLAB27 tests should be carried to check for genetic factors associated with ankylosing spondylitis.

Medications and treatment

Non-steroidal anti-inflammatory medication and painkillers are used to control this condition. Physiotherapy is important to maintain mobility, and severe ankylosing spondylitis may require more radical therapy.

Further advice

If you suffer from ankylosing spondylitis, you should try to keep fit, exercise regularly, and maintain good general health.

Associated conditions

Reiter's disease is a condition that may begin as a venereal disease and may progress to a condition similar to ankylosing spondylitis.

Rheumatoid arthritis ♥♥

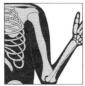 Rheumatoid arthritis is an inflammatory joint condition which is more common in women than men, particularly young women. Its cause is unknown.

Symptoms

Pain, stiffness, and swelling of joints, particularly the small joints of the hands and feet. In the morning after rest, the stiffness in the joints may be particularly noticeable. Other joints may also become involved, including the neck, shoulders, elbows, wrists, knees, and ankles. Rheumatoid arthritis may even affect the jaw joint. In some cases, the disease progresses to a severe condition with involvement of other organs such as the heart, lungs, and eyes. In others, it burns itself out but leaves some disability, particularly in the hands.

Action

If you suffer from persistent pain and stiffness in the hands or feet, you should seek medical advice.

Tests

Blood tests including rheumatoid factors, full blood counts, sedimentation rate, and tests of heart and lung function are included in the investigation of rheumatoid arthritis. X-rays will show characteristic erosion of bone and joint.

Medications and treatment

Steroids probably have little place in the management of this condition. Non-steroidal anti-inflammatory drugs, including aspirin, Distamine, Myocrisin, and Nivaquine, are often helpful, and severe cases may need more radical treatment such as gold or penicillamine. Occasionally cytotoxic chemotherapy may be used to treat rheumatoid arthritis.

Further advice

Many patients claim that they benefit from a vegetarian diet, and a diet high in essential fatty acids and oils. You should try to exercise and maintain a good standard of general health.

Associated conditions

Bornholm disease is an arthritis caused by a virus that affects the ribs. It may appear as chest pain.

Osteoarthritis and osteoporosis ♥

 Osteoporosis is loss of calcium from the bones which occurs in older people. Osteoarthritis is loss of cartilage tissue from the joints. It is a degenerative condition and also occurs in the older age groups.

Symptoms

Osteoporosis may appear with fractures, pain, and backache (*see* below). Osteoarthritis presents with pain, bony swelling in the joints, and stiffness. It can be distinguished from rheumatoid arthritis because of its occurrence in the older age groups and from the presence of Heberden's nodes (swelling of the last joint) on the fingers. Typically, the hip and the knee are the joints affected, so that difficulty in walking is a main symptom. Osteoarthritis may also affect the hands. There may be an inherited component in the female line of families. Osteoarthritis of the hip may cause pain in the groin. Osteoarthritis of the neck may cause a stiff neck

Action

The symptoms may well respond to rest, improved climate, and to simple painkillers, but persistent symptoms require medical attention.

Tests

X-rays of joints, blood tests to distinguish the condition from rheumatoid arthritis, and measurements of calcium in bone should be carried out to diagnose these conditions.

Medications and treatment

Simple painkillers, such as ibuprofen, or more powerful nonsteroidal anti-inflammatory drugs or analgesics may be required. Fractures caused by osteoporosis may need treatment with drugs, such as etidronate, and by hormone replacement to try to improve the calcium retention in bone.

Further advice

A healthy diet, high in vitamins and calcium, and light regular exercise are important in preventing bones and joints deteriorating.

Associated conditions

Backache and its associated conditions (*see* below) are clearly related to conditions such as osteoporosis and osteoarthritis.

Backache, including lumbago, sciatica, slipped disc, and spondylitis

 Backache is a very common symptom and can range from mild and temporary to permanent and disabling. The commonest cause is degeneration of the vertebrae in the spine due to osteoarthritis and osteoporosis, and leading to pressure on the nerve roots. Bulging of the discs between the vertebrae is known as a slipped disc: it can cause severe sciatica. Spondylitis is inflammation of the small joints of the spine, and lumbago is a general term used to describe low back pain probably due to muscle spasm.

Symptoms

The symptoms may occur from the neck (cervical spondylosis) to the lumbar spine, the latter being more common. Sciatica occurs where a nerve root is under pressure, and the pain goes down the back of the leg. Acute slipped disc may occur in young healthy people usually from straining or lifting; there is a sudden onset of severe back pain radiating down the back of the leg. Occasionally, bowel and bladder function may be affected. Minor degrees of backache may come and go.

Action

For severe slipped disc, the patient should be asked to lie down on his or her back on a firm board or mattress, and medical advice should be sought. Less severe conditions may respond to bed rest, physiotherapy, and simple analgesics, but if they are persistent, symptoms should be investigated.

Tests

Clinical examination followed by X-rays and, where necessary, MRI scans to look for pressure on nerve roots. Blood tests should be carried out to exclude other causes including the rare possibility of an unusual malignancy pressing on the nerves in the back (spinal meningioma)

Medications and treatment

Bed rest usually resolves the symptoms of a slipped disc in two to three weeks. If persistent, microdisc surgery may be required or even a laminectomy with removal of parts of the bone in the spine to relieve pressure. These conditions will usually respond to simple analgesics, such as ibuprofen, and to rest, heat treatment, gentle physiotherapy, and eventually muscle-building exercises to protect the spine.

Further advice

Attention to diet and maintenance of a high calcium and vitamin content may help prevent degeneration of the spine. Hormone replacement therapy might also be helpful in preventing or arresting deterioration of this condition.

Serious bone disease including cancer and infection ♥♥♥♥♥

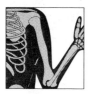

Bone sarcomas or tumours are rare. Infection of bone (osteomyelitis) may occur following a fracture.

Symptoms
These include pain and swelling of the bone. Bone pain is usually worse at night. Osteomyelitis may be accompanied by symptoms of infection such as fever.

Action
If you suspect either of these conditions, you should seek medical advice urgently.

Tests
X-ray of bone and excision biopsy may be required to diagnose this condition. Routine blood tests may detect the spread of tumour or infection to other parts of the body.

Medications and treatment
Primarily, these conditions are treated by surgery, together with anti-tumour or anti-infective therapy where appropriate.

Associated conditions
Other organs can produce sarcomas; for example, muscle may produce myosarcomas, fibrous tissues will produce fibrosarcomas, and, rarely, heart muscle will produce rhabdomyosarcomas. Joints may become infected in the same way as bones and this can cause a form of septic arthritis.

Polymyalgia rheumatica, and temporal arteritis ♥♥

These conditions are related but their cause is not known.

Symptoms

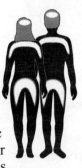

The symptoms of polymyalgia rheumatica are pain and weakness in the muscles, particularly the shoulders and around the pelvis. Temporal arteritis presents with pain and swelling in an artery on the head and may cause severe headache. The conditions often exist together, or one may lead to the other. A classic symptom of polymyalgia is inability to comb the hair because of weakness in the arm muscles. The muscles may be extremely painful.

Action

Where this condition is suspected, medical advice should be sought immediately.

Tests

A raised sedimentation rate occurs in these conditions, so that blood tests to check for this, for anaemia, and for other possible causes, including muscle enzymes, should be carried out. X-rays may be required. A biopsy of the temporal artery may be needed to make the diagnosis for temporal arteritis.

Medications and treatment

This condition usually responds to steroids. You may need to take the steroids for a prolonged period, occasionally in quite high doses.

Further advice

You should undergo gentle physiotherapy to encourage the use of your muscles.

Myasthenia gravis

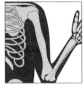

Myasthenia gravis is a disease of the neuromuscular junction. The cause of this condition is not known.

Symptoms

Severe weakness of muscles, particularly affecting the upper limbs, but also the eyes and eyelids. The muscles exhaust very quickly, so that there may be some muscle function after rest but this runs out after a short period of time.

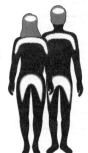

Action

Where this condition is suspected, medical advice should be sought immediately.

Tests

Diagnosis can be made by muscle biopsy and tests using drugs such as edrophonium.

Medications and treatment

Myasthenia gravis is treated with anticholinesterase drugs such as Mestinon or Prostigimin.

Associated conditions

Muscular dystrophies can be similar to myasthenia gravis. These are usually inherited. *See also* motor neurone disease, Chapter 5.

Myalgic encephalomyelitis ♥♥
(ME, yuppie flu, Royal Free disease, post-viral fatigue syndrome)

 This condition affects the nerves and the muscles, and usually occurs after a severe virus infection of the glandular fever or Epstein-Barr type.

Symptoms
Classically, fatigue and muscle ache, weakness and depression. True clinical depression may co-exist and make diagnosis difficult. Patients feel permanently exhausted and unable to work or exercise. This sets up a vicious circle from which it may be difficult to escape.

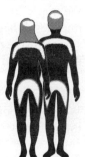

Action
Simple remedies should be tried at first but, if symptoms are persistent, you should seek medical advice.

Tests
There are no diagnostic tests for this condition which adds to the difficulty in treating and managing patients who suffer.

Medications and treatment
High doses of vitamins, sometimes given intravenously, and minerals, such as magnesium, have been tried with some success for this condition. Counselling and psychotherapy may also be of value.

Further advice
Maintaining a healthy diet and regular exercise pattern, as well as a positive attitude may prevent this condition and help recovery from it. You should begin a programme of gentle exercises.

Associated conditions
See infectious mononucleosis, Chapter 15.

Gout

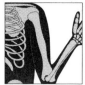 Gout is a condition caused by excess uric acid level in the blood. It may be genetic or it may be related to alcohol intake.

Symptoms
Classically, the presence of a severely painful joint, particularly in the first joint of the large toe. Gout can affect any joint, and deposits of uric acid may be found in the ear and elsewhere. Uric acid crystals may produce symptoms of renal colic (*see* above).

Action
If you are suffering from an attack of gout, you should rest, take painkillers if necessary, and drink plenty of non-alcoholic fluids. You should avoid aspirin because, even in low doses, it increases uric acid levels.

Tests
Blood tests to check the uric acid level as well as X-rays of the joint and joint aspiration may help in making a diagnosis. Urine tests will be helpful. Occasionally, uric acid levels can be secondary to other conditions, particularly blood disorders, and these should be checked.

Medications and treatment
The acute pain of gout usually responds to drugs such as colchicine or indomethacin. Long-term prevention is achieved by using allopurinol which lowers serum uric acid levels.

Further advice
It is helpful to avoid alcohol and to drink plenty of non-alcoholic drinks, especially in warm weather. Dietry changes may be helpful and you should reduce your consumption of spinach, strawberries, offal, meat extracts, asparagus, salmon, herrings, anchovies, duck and goose meat.

Associated conditions

Pseudo-gout is a condition which is similar to gout; it usually affects the knees. A number of other conditions may also produce arthritis, including psoriasis and systemic lupus erythematosus.

Prescription Medicines

Algesal

A cream used as an analgesic rub to treat rheumatic conditions.

Side effects:
Caution: in pregnant women.
Not to be used for: children under 6 years.
Caution needed with:

Brufen

A magenta-coloured, oval tablet supplied at strengths of 200 mg, 400 mg, 600 mg and used as a non-steroid anti-inflammatory drug to treat pain, rheumatoid arthritis, ankylosing spondylitis, osteoarthritis, sero-negative arthritis, peri-articular disorders, soft tissue injuries.

Side effects: dyspepsia, stomach bleeding, rash, rarely low blood platelet levels.
Caution: in pregnant women, the elderly, and in patients suffering from asthma or allergy to aspirin or anti-inflammatory drugs, or liver, kidney, or heart disease.
Not to be used for: patients suffering from peptic ulcer.
Caution needed with:

Distamine

A white tablet or a white, scored tablet according to strengths

of 50 mg, 125 mg, 250 mg and used as an anti-arthritic drug and binding agent to treat severe active rheumatoid arthritis, cystinuria, Wilson's disease (inherited disorders), heavy metal poisoning, liver disease.

Side effects: nausea, anorexia, fever, rash, loss of taste, blood changes, blood or protein in the urine, kidney changes, muscle disease.

Caution: in nursing mothers and in patients suffering from kidney disease, sensitivity to penicillin. Your doctor may advise that your blood and urine should be checked regularly.

Not to be used for: pregnant women or for patients suffering from lupus erythematosus, agranulocytosis, thrombocytopenia (rare blood and multi-system disorders).

Caution needed with: gold salts, anti-malaria or cytotoxic drugs, phenylbutazone.

Feldene

A maroon/blue capsule or a maroon capsule according to strengths of 10 mg, 20 mg and used as a non-steroid anti-inflammatory drug to treat rheumatoid arthritis, osteoarthritis, ankylosing spondylitis, acute muscle or bone problems, acute gout, juvenile chronic arthritis.

Side effects: stomach disturbances, swelling, brain disturbances, feeling of being unwell, tinnitus, skin reactions.

Caution: in pregnant women, nursing mothers, and in patients suffering from kidney or liver disease.

Not to be used for: patients suffering from anti-inflammatory- or aspirin-induced allergy, stomach ulcer, history of recurring ulcers, recent anal inflammation.

Caution needed with: anticoagulants, other non-steroid anti-inflammatory drugs, antidiabetics, lithium.

Froben

A yellow tablet supplied at strengths of 50 mg, 100 mg and

**used as a non-steroid anti-inflammatory drug to treat rheu-
matoid disease, osteoarthritis, ankylosing spondylitis.**

Side effects: stomach intolerance, rash, rarely jaundice, blood
changes, fluid retention.
Caution: in the elderly, pregnant women, nursing mothers, and in
patients suffering from asthma, kidney, liver, or heart disease,
allergy to aspirin or anti-inflammatory drugs.
Not to be used for: children or for patients suffering from stomach ulcer or stomach bleeding.
Caution needed with: frusemide, anticoagulants.

Indocid

**An ivory capsule supplied at strengths of 25 mg, 50 mg and
used as a non-steroid anti-inflammatory drug to treat rheumatoid arthritis, osteoarthritis, degenerative disease of the
hip joint, ankylosing spondylitis, acute gout, lumbago, acute
joint disorders, orthopaedic procedures, period pain.**

Side effects: gastro-intestinal bleeding, headache, corneal deposits, disturbances of the retina, gastro-intestinal intolerance, dizziness, brain disturbances, blood changes.
Caution: in the elderly, and in patients suffering from kidney or
liver disease, brain disorders.
Not to be used for: children, pregnant women, nursing mothers,
or for patients suffering from stomach ulcer, history of stomach
lesions, aspirin/anti-inflammatory drug allergy, recent proctitis,
severe allergic swelling.
Caution needed with: anticoagulants, lithium, diuretics, ß-
blockers, probenecid, aminoglycoside antibiotics, methotrexate,
steroids, some analgesics.

Intralgin

A gel used as an analgesic rub to treat muscle strains, sprains.

Side effects: may be irritant.
Caution:

Not to be used for: areas near the eyes or on broken or inflamed skin or on membranes (such as the mouth).
Caution needed with:

Mestinon

A white tablet tablet supplied at a strength of 60 mg and used as a nerve conduction enhancer to treat paralytic ileus, myasthenia gravis (muscular disorders).

Side effects: nausea, salivation, diarrhoea, colic.
Caution: in patients suffering from bronchial asthma, heart disease, epilepsy, Parkinson's disease.
Not to be used for: patients with bowel or urinary obstruction.
Caution needed with: some drugs used in anaesthesia.

Mobiflex

A brown, five-sided tablet supplied at a strength of 20 mg and used as a non-steroid anti-inflammatory drug to treat osteoarthritis, rheumatoid arthritis.

Side effects: stomach disturbances, swelling, headache, rash, blood changes, liver changes, disturbances of the eyesight.
Caution: in the elderly or in patients suffering from liver or kidney disease, heart failure.
Not to be used for: children, pregnant women, patients with a history of or suffering from stomach ulcer, gastro-intestinal bleeding, gastritis, allergy to ASPIRIN or anti-inflammatory drugs.
Caution needed with: anticoagulants, antidiabetics taken by mouth, other non-steroid anti-inflammatory drugs, lithium.

Naprosyn

A yellow, scored tablet or a yellow, oblong, scored tablet according to strengths of 250 mg, 500 mg and used as a non-steroid anti-inflammatory drug to treat rheumatoid arthritis,

osteoarthritis, ankylosing spondylitis, acute gout.

Side effects: rash, stomach intolerance, headache, tinnitus, vertigo, blood changes.
Caution: in the elderly, pregnant women, nursing mothers, and in patients suffering from kidney or liver disease, heart failure, asthma, or a history of gastro-intestinal lesions.
Not to be used for: children under 5 years, or for patients suffering from stomach ulcer or allergy to aspirin or non-steroid anti-inflammatory drugs.
Caution needed with: anticoagulants, hydantoins, some antidiabetics, lithium, ß-blockers, methotrexate, probenecid, frusemide.

Nivaquine

A yellow tablet supplied at a strength of 200 mg and used as an antimalarial drug for the prevention and treatment of malaria, and to treat rheumatoid arthritis.

Side effects: headache, stomach upset, skin eruptions, hair loss, eye disorders, blood disorders, loss of pigment, allergy.
Caution: in pregnant women, nursing mothers, or in patients suffering from porphyria (a rare blood disorder), kidney or liver disease, severe gastro-intestinal, nervous, or blood disorder, psoriasis or history of epilepsy. The eyes should be tested before and during prolonged treatment.
Not to be used for:
Caution needed with:

Orudis

A green/purple capsule or a pink capsule according to strengths of 50 mg, 100 mg and used as a non-steroid anti-inflammatory drug to treat rheumatoid arthritis, osteoarthritis, ankylosing spondylitis, acute articular and joint disorders, painful periods.

Side effects: stomach intolerance, rash.
Caution: in the elderly, pregnant women and in patients suffering from kidney, heart, or liver disease.
Not to be used for: children or for patients suffering from severe kidney disease, stomach ulcer or a history of recurring ulcer, asthma, allergy to aspirin/non-steroid anti-inflammatory drugs, inflammation of the anus or rectum.
Caution needed with: anticoagulants, sulphonamide antibiotics, hydantoins, methotrexate.

Ponstan Forte

A yellow tablet supplied at a strength of 500 mg and used as a non-steroid anti-inflammatory drug to relieve pain in rheumatoid arthritis including Still's disease, osteoarthritis, and to treat headache, period pain, excessively heavy periods.

Side effects: diarrhoea, rash, kidney damage, low platelet levels.
Caution: in the elderly, in pregnant women, and in patients suffering from bronchial asthma, allergy, heart failure.
Not to be used for: patients suffering from kidney or liver disease, gastro-intestinal ulceration, inflammatory bowel disease.
Caution needed with: anticoagulants, antidiabetics, anticonvulsants.

Proflex Cream

A cream used as a non-steroid anti-inflammatory to treat rheumatic and muscular pain, sprains, strains.

Side effects: reddening of skin.
Caution: in pregnant women, nursing mothers. Avoid broken skin, lips, and eyes.
Not to be used for: children, or for patients suffering from allergy to aspirin or anti-inflammatories.
Caution needed with:

Prostigimin

A white, scored tablet supplied at a strength of 15 mg and used as an anti-cholinesterase to treat urinary retention following surgery, bowel paralysis, myasthenia gravis (a muscle disorder).

Side effects: nausea, diarrhoea, colic, salivation, vomiting.
Caution: in patients suffering from bronchial asthma, heart disease, epilepsy, Parkinson's disease.
Not to be used for: patients suffering from intestinal or urinary obstruction.
Caution needed with: some drugs used in anaesthesia.

Relifex

A red tablet supplied at a strength of 500 mg and used as a non-steroid anti-inflammatory drug to treat rheumatoid arthritis, osteoarthritis.

Side effects: diarrhoea, dyspepsia, nausea, constipation, stomach pain, wind, headache, dizziness, rash, sedation.
Caution: in the elderly and in patients suffering from kidney or liver disease or with a history of stomach ulcer, allergy to aspirin or anti-inflammatories.
Not to be used for: pregnant women, nursing mothers, children, or for patients suffering from stomach ulcer, severe liver disease.
Caution needed with: anticoagulants taken by mouth, hydantoins, anticonvulsants, antidiabetics.

Rheumox

A light/dark orange capsule supplied at a strength of 300 mg and used as a non-steroid anti-inflammatory drug to treat rheumatoid arthritis, osteoarthritis, ankylosing spondylitis, acute gout.

Side effects: sensitivity to light, fluid retention, stomach bleeding, inflammation of the lungs, interference with some blood tests.

Caution: in pregnant women and in patients with a history of stomach ulcer, or suffering from liver disease or heart failure. Patients on long-term treatment should be checked regularly.

Not to be used for: children or for patients suffering from stomach ulcer, history of blood changes, or kidney disease.

Caution needed with: phenytoin, anticoagulants, antidiabetics, sulphonamide antibiotics.

Traxam

A clear gel used as a topical non-steroid anti-inflamatory rub to treat soft tissue injury such as strains, sprains, contusions.

Side effects: mild local redness, dermatitis, itch.

Caution: in pregnant women and nursing mothers. Use only on unbroken skin and keep out of the eyes, nose, mouth etc. It should not be used with covering dressings.

Not to be used for: children or for patients suffering from allergy to aspirin/anti-inflammatory drugs.

Caution needed with:

Voltarol

A yellow tablet or brown tablet according to strengths of 25 mg, 50 mg and used as a non-steroid anti-inflammatory drug to treat bone or muscular problems, rheumatoid arthritis, osteoarthritis, ankylosing spondylitis, acute gout, chronic juvenile arthritis.

Side effects: passing stomach pain, nausea, headache, rash, fluid retention, rarely blood changes, stomach ulcer, abnormal liver or kidney function.

Caution: in pregnant women, nursing mothers, the elderly, or patients suffering from kidney, liver, or heart weakness, blood abnormalities, history of gastro-intestinal lesions. Your doctor may advise regular check-ups.

Not to be used for: patients suffering from asthma, stomach

ulcer, or allergy to aspirin/non-steroid anti-inflammatory drugs, rectal inflammation.
Caution needed with: salicylates, methotrexate, lithium, digoxin, diuretics, cyclosporin.

Over-the-counter Medicines

Algesal

A cream used as an analgesic rub to treat rheumatic conditions.

Side effects:
Caution:
Not to be used for: children under 6 years.
Not to be used with:

Aradolene

A cream used as an analgesic rub to treat rheumatic conditions.

Side effects: may be irritant
Caution:
Not to be used for: areas such as near the eyes, on broken or inflamed skin, or on membranes (such as the mouth).
Not to be used with:

Aspellin

A liniment or a spray used as a topical analgesic to treat muscular rheumatism, sciatica, lumbago, fibrositis, chilblains.

Side effects: may be irritant.
Caution:
Not to be used for: areas near the eyes, or where the skin is broken or

inflamed, or on membranes (such as the mouth).
Not to be used with:

aspirin

A white tablet supplied at a strength of 300 mg and used as an analgesic to relieve pain and reduce fever.

Side effects: stomach upsets, allergy, asthma.
Caution: in pregnant women, the elderly, or in patients with a history of allergy to aspirin, asthma, impaired kidney or liver function, indigestion.
Not to be used for: children, nursing mothers, or for patients suffering from haemophilia or ulcers.
Not to be used with: anticoagulants (blood-thinning drugs), some antidiabetic drugs, anti-inflammatory agents, methotrexate, spironolactone, steroids, some antacids, some uric-acid lowering drugs.

Balmosa

A cream used as an analgesic rub to treat muscular rheumatism, fibrositis, lumbago, sciatica, unbroken chilblains.

Side effects: may be irritant
Caution:
Not to be used for: areas near the eyes, on broken or inflamed skin, or on membranes (such as the mouth).
Not to be used with:

Bayolin

A cream used as an analgesic rub to treat rheumatism, fibrositis, lumbago, sciatica.

Side effects: may be irritant.
Caution:
Not to be used for: areas near the eyes, broken or inflamed skin, or on

membranes (such as the mouth).
Not to be used with:

Cafadol

A yellow, scored tablet used as an analgesic to relieve pain including period pain.

Side effects:
Caution: in patients with liver or kidney disease.
Not to be used for: children under 5 years.
Not to be used with:

Caprin

A pink tablet supplied at a strength of 324 mg and used as an analgesic to treat rheumatic and associated conditions.

Side effects: stomach upsets, allergy, asthma.
Caution: in pregnant women, the elderly, and in patients with a history of allergy to aspirin, asthma, impaired kidney or liver function, indigestion.
Not to be used for: children, nursing mothers, or for patients suffering from haemophilia or ulcers.
Not to be used with: anticoagulants (blood-thinning drugs), some antidiabetic drugs, anti-inflammatory agents, methotrexate, spironolactone, steroids, some antacids, some uric-acid lowering drugs.

Co-Codamol

A tablet used as an analgesic to relieve pain.

Side effects:
Caution: in patients suffering from kidney or liver disease.
Not to be used for: children under 7 years.
Not to be used with:

Co-Codaprin Dispersible

A dispersible tablet used as an analgesic to relieve pain.

Side effects: stomach upsets, allergy, asthma.
Caution: in pregnant women, the elderly, and in patients with a history of allergy to aspirin, asthma, impaired kidney or liver function, indigestion.
Not to be used for: children, nursing mothers, or for patients suffering from haemophilia or ulcers.
Not to be used with: anticoagulants (blood-thinning drugs), some antidiabetic drugs, anti-inflammatory agents, methotrexate, spironolactone, steroids, some antacids, some uric-acid lowering drugs.

Cremalgin

A balm used as an analgesic rub to treat rheumatism, fibrositis, lumbago, sciatica.

Side effects: may be irritant.
Caution:
Not to be used for: areas near the eyes, broken or inflamed skin, or on membranes (such as the mouth).
Not to be used with:

Difflam

A cream used as an anti-inflammatory and analgesic rub to relieve muscular and skeletal pain.

Side effects: may be irritant.
Caution:
Not to be used for: areas near the eyes, broken or inflamed skin, or on membranes (such as the mouth).
Not to be used with:

Disprol Paed

A suspensions supplied at a strength of 120 mg/5 ml teaspoonful and used as an analgesic to relieve pain and fever in children.

Side effects:
Caution: in children suffering from liver or kidney disease.
Not to be used for:
Not to be used with:

Dubam

An aerosol used as a topical analgesic to relieve muscular pain.

Side effects: may be irritant.
Caution:
Not to be used for: areas near the eyes, broken or inflamed skin, or on membranes (such as the mouth).
Not to be used with:

Finalgon

An ointment supplied with an applicator and used as an analgesic rub to relieve muscular and skeletal pain.

Side effects: may be irritant.
Caution:
Not to be used for: areas near the eyes, broken or inflamed skin, or on membranes (such as the mouth).
Not to be used with:

Intralgin

A gel used as an analgesic rub to treat muscle strains, sprains.

Side effects: may be irritant.
Caution:

Not to be used for: areas near the eyes, broken or inflamed skin, or on membranes (such as the mouth).
Not to be used with:

Nurofen

A magenta-coloured, oval tablet supplied at strengths of 200 mg, 400 mg, 600 mg, and used as a non-steroid anti-inflammatory drug to treat pain, rheumatoid arthritis, ankylosing spondylitis, osteoarthritis, seronegative arthritis, peri-articular disorders, soft tissue injuries.

Side effects: dyspepsia, stomach bleeding, rash, rarely low blood platelet levels.
Caution: in pregnant women, and in patients suffering from asthma or allergy to aspirin or anti-inflammatory drugs.
Not to be used for: patients suffering from peptic ulcer.
Not to be used with:

Palaprin Forte

An orange, oval, scored tablet supplied at a strength of 600 mg and used as a non-steroid anti-inflammatory drug to treat rheumatoid arthritis, osteoarthritis, spondylitis.

Side effects: stomach upsets, allergy, asthma.
Caution: in pregnant women, the elderly, and in patients with a history of allergy to aspirin, asthma, impaired kidney or liver function, indigestion.
Not to be used for: children, nursing mothers, or for patients suffering from haemophilia or ulcers.
Not to be used with: anticoagulants (blood-thinning drugs), some antidiabetic drugs, anti-inflammatory agents, methotrexate, spironolactone, steroids, some antacids, some uric-acid lowering drugs.

paracetamol tablets

A tablet supplied at a strength of 500 mg and used as an analgesic to relieve pain and reduce fever.

Side effects:
Caution: in patients suffering from kidney or liver disease.
Not to be used for: children under 6 years.
Not to be used with:

Paracodol

A white, effervescent tablet used as an analgesic to relieve pain.

Side effects:
Caution: in patients suffering from kidney or liver disease, or who are on a limited consumption of salt.
Not to be used for: children under 6 years.
Not to be used with:

Parahypon

A pink, scored tablet used as an analgesic to relieve pain.

Side effects:
Caution: in patients suffering from kidney or liver disease.
Not to be used for: children under 6 years.
Not to be used with:

Parake

A white tablet used as an analgesic to relieve pain and reduce fever.

Side effects:
Caution: in patients suffering from kidney or liver disease.
Not to be used for: children.
Not to be used with:

Pardale

A white, scored tablet used as an analgesic to relieve head-ache, rheumatism, period pain.

Side effects:
Caution: in patients suffering from kidney or liver disease.
Not to be used for: children.
Not to be used with:

Paynocil

A white, scored tablet used as an analgesic to relieve pain, reduce fever, and to treat rheumatoid arthritis and other rheumatic conditions.

Side effects: stomach upsets, allergy, asthma.
Caution: in pregnant women, the elderly, or in patients with a history of allergy to aspirin, asthma, impaired kidney or liver function, indigestion.
Not to be used for: children, nursing mothers, or for patients suffering from haemophilia or ulcers.
Not to be used with: anticoagulants (blood-thinning drugs), some antidiabetic drugs, anti-inflammatory agents, methotrexate, spironolactone, steroids, some antacids, some uric-acid lowering drugs.

Propain

A yellow, scored tablet used as an analgesic, antihistamine treatment for headache, migraine, muscle pain, period pain.

Side effects: drowsiness.
Caution: in patients suffering from liver or kidney disease.
Not to be used for: children.
Not to be used with: alcohol, sedatives.

Salonair

An aerosol used as an analgesic rub to relieve muscular and rheumatic pain.

Side effects: may be irritant.
Caution:
Not to be used for: areas near the eyes, broken or inflamed skin, or on membranes (such as the mouth).
Not to be used with:

Salzone

A syrup supplied at a strength of 120 mg/5 ml teaspoonful and used as an analgesic to relieve pain and reduce fever.

Side effects:
Caution: in children suffering from liver or kidney disease.
Not to be used for:
Not to be used with:

Solpadeine

A white, effervescent tablet used as an analgesic to relieve rheumatic, muscle, bone pain, headache, sinusitis, influenza.

Side effects: constipation.
Caution: in patients suffering from liver or kidney disease, or who have a restricted salt consumption.
Not to be used for: children under 7 years.
Not to be used with:

Solprin

A white, soluble tablet supplied at a strength of 300 mg used as an analgesic to relieve pain and to treat rheumatic conditions.

Side effects:

Caution:
Not to be used for: children.
Not to be used with:

Syndol

A yellow, scored tablet used as an analgesic, antihistamine treatment for tension headache after dental or other surgery.

Side effects: drowsiness, constipation.
Caution: in patients suffering from liver or kidney disease.
Not to be used for: children.
Not to be used with: alcohol, sedatives.

Transvasin

A cream used as an analgesic rub for the relief of rheumatic and muscular pain.

Chapter 11

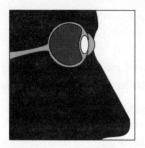

Disorders of the Eye

Please refer to 'Important Advice' on page 4 at the beginning of this book; and remember, if you are in any doubt, consult a physician.

The eye is a complex and sophisticated organ which has evolved over many millions of years to perform a vital job for humans with a very high degree of accuracy. It is reasonably well protected within the bony skull but is clearly susceptible to trauma and infection. Its need for adequate blood supply makes it vulnerable to degenerative conditions affecting the cardiovascular system.

After it passes through the conjunctiva – the outer lining of the eye – light is focused by the lens to form a sharp image on the retina at the back of the eye. The amount of light is controlled by the iris which responds like a camera shutter to changes in the available light. This movement of light takes place through fluids within the eye. The retina itself is a highly sophisticated combination of light sensors that detect colour and movement.

Treatment of eye infections in the Third World and the prevention of eye disease caused by diabetes are the major challenges of this condition.

Diseases of the retina, ♥♥♥
including detached retina, retinal artery thrombosis, retinal vein thrombosis, hypertensive and diabetic retinopathy

 The retina is a delicate membrane at the back of the eye, and is subject to a number of diseases. Detachment may occur after trauma or in someone who is very short-sighted. Hypertension and diabetes cause haemorrhages and exudates in the retina. Blockage of blood vessels to the retina can also cause damage. Rarely, tumours of the retina (retinoblastoma) may occur. These may have an hereditary factor.

Symptoms
There may be no symptoms of retinal disease until it is picked up on routine medical examination. Detachment of the retina may appear with sudden loss of vision in one eye and a film moving upwards across the field of vision. Thrombosis of the retinal artery and retinal vein may cause sudden blindness in all or part of the field of vision. Severe hypertensive diabetic retinopathy will eventually appear as loss of vision and blindness in the affected eye.

Action
Urgent specialist medical advice is required for any of these conditions.

Tests
Examination of the eye, tests for predisposing factors such as hypertension, diabetes, routine blood tests, clotting screen and search for cause of thrombosis or embolus, angiogram of the retinal vessels.

Medications and treatment
Detached retina is usually treated by bed rest and laser therapy to re-

attach the damaged retina. Hypertensive or diabetic retinopathy is treated by attention to the primary disease and by laser therapy to prevent new vessel formation and more extensive damage. Thrombosis of the retinal artery or vein may resolve spontaneously but bed rest and attention to clotting factors may be required.

Further advice
Good management of hypertension and diabetes will prevent damage to the eyes. Detached retina may indicate that you should avoid contact sports in the future.

Associated conditions
Retinoblastoma is treated by removal of the eye and treatment with drugs or radiotherapy.

Diseases of the conjunctiva and outer eye ♥

Diseases in this category include, dry eyes, Sjøgren's syndrome, styes, meibomian cysts, blepharitis, excessive tears (epiphora), subconjunctival haemorrhage, and scratched cornea through the wearing of contact lenses. Conjunctivitis is an infection of the outer eye, and, where herpes virus is concerned, this can cause an ulcer (dendritic ulcer).

Symptoms
Local symptoms, such as dry eyes or excessive tears, are usually self-explanatory. Styes and cysts can be visible and painful. Conjunctivitis usually presents with a red eye and crusts on the eyelashes. Dendritic ulcer can often be very painful but may otherwise resemble normal conjunctivitis. Subconjunctival haemorrhage may occur with spontaneous bleeding or as a result of trauma to the eye. A brick-red triangle is often visible on the white of the eye.

Action
Seek medical advice as soon as possible.

Tests
Examination of the eye and swabs from infection may be helpful.

Medications and treatment
Excision of cysts and styes may be helpful. Artificial tears, such as hypromellose, may be useful for dry eye which occurs in Sjøgren's syndrome. Conjunctivitis will respond to antibiotic eyedrops or ointment, and blepharitis may respond to treatment of associated conditions such as dandruff.

Further advice
Medications used for the eyes should be disposed of because they could become infected if kept for some time. Infections of one eye very often spread to the other eye. Conjunctivitis is highly contagious.

Associated conditions
Skin conditions such as eczema may cause disease of the eyelids or conjunctiva.

Cataract ♥♥

A cataract is a condition caused by gradual or sudden opacity of lens material.

Symptoms
Gradual lack of clarity of vision, and eventually blindness when the cataract matures. The condition is not painful.

Action
You should seek medical advice immediately if you notice any difficulty in vision.

Tests
Examination of the eye will reveal the cataract.

Medications and treatment
Cataract is usually treated by surgery to implant an artificial lens. There are no other treatments which are known to be effective.

Further advice
You should avoid ultraviolet light, and any prolonged exposure to bright sunlight, because it may precipitate cataracts. Abnormally high calcium levels in the blood may also lead to cataracts.

Iritis and uveitis

 Iritis and uveitis are auto-immune conditions whereby damage is done to the iris or the back of the eye by inflammation.

Symptoms
The symptoms of iritis are a red eye which may be painful and is particularly sensitive to light. The eye may water severely. Uveitis is a similar condition which occurs at the back of the eye. It is also painful and causes difficulty in vision.

Action
If you suspect either of these conditions, you should seek medical attention urgently.

Tests

Examination of the eye will reveal white cells as a sign of inflammation.

Medications and treatment

Steroids, given as drops, tablets, or subconjunctival injection, are used to treat these conditions.

Further advice

It is important to distinguish iritis from conjunctivitis because delay in treatment may result in impaired eyesight.

Associated conditions

Iritis and uveitis may occur as part of a generalized condition such as sarcoid or ulcerative colitis, or ankylosing spondylitis.

Glaucoma

Glaucoma is a condition caused by increased pressure in the eye which damages the nerve fibres by direct pressure.

Symptoms

There may be no symptoms of glaucoma until vision is substantially impaired in either or both eyes. Acute glaucoma may appear as a painful red eye with some sensitivity to light. Chronic glaucoma may not show symptoms other than gradually impaired vision.

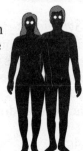

Action

Glaucoma should receive urgent medical attention.

Tests

Pressure in the eye can be measured to detect glaucoma. Precipitating causes such as diabetes should be identified and treated.

Medications and treatment

Eye drops such as Timoptol may be used. Alternatively, glaucoma can be treated by surgery.

Further advice

It is important to diagnose and treat glaucoma properly. Certain eye drops inappropriately given may make the glaucoma worse.

Prescription Medicines

Timoptol

Drops used as a ß-blocker to treat hypertension of the eye, glaucomas.

Side effects: eye irritation, systemic ß-blocker effects: slowing of the heart, low blood pressure.
Caution: in pregnant women, nursing mothers. Treatment should be withdrawn gradually.
Not to be used for: children or patients suffering from asthma, heart conduction block, heart failure, or for patients who wear soft contact lenses.
Caution needed with: verapamil, antihypertensives, adrenaline.

Over-the-counter Medicines

Brolene Eye Drops

These contain propamidine isethionate 0.1%, benzalkonium chloride 0.1%. An ointment is also available. These substances disinfect the eye and reduce redness. They may cause some local stinging and should not be used if redness of the eye persists or worsens. Allergies often in the eyes, particularly hay fever, cosmetic and dust allergies.

Eppy

Drops used as a sympathomimetic to treat glaucoma.

Side effects: pain in the eye, headache, skin reactions, melanosis, red eye, rarely systemic effects.
Caution:
Not to be used for: patients suffering from absence of the lens, narrow angle glaucoma.
Not to be used with:

Eye Dew *see* Brolene Eye Drops *and* Optrex

Fluorescein

Drops used as a dye for staining purposes to enable abrasions or foreign bodies in the eye to be found.

Hypotears

Drops used to moisten dry eyes.

Side effects:
Caution:
Not to be used for: patients who wear soft contact lenses.
Not to be used with:

Isopto Alkaline

Drops used to lubricate the eyes.

Side effects:
Caution:
Not to be used for: patients who wear soft contact lenses.
Not to be used with:

Isopto Frin

Drops used to lubricate the eyes when no infection is present.

Side effects:
Caution: in infants and in patients suffering from narrow angle glaucoma.
Not to be used for: patients who wear soft contact lenses.
Not to be used with:

Isopto Plain

Drops used to moisten dry eyes.

Side effects:
Caution:
Not to be used for: patients who wear soft contact lenses.
Not to be used with:

Lacri-Lube

An ointment used for lubricating the eyes and protecting the cornea.

Liquifilm Tears

Drops used to lubricate dry eyes.

Side effects:
Caution:
Not to be used for: patients who wear soft contact lenses.
Not to be used with:

Minims Saline

Drops used to irrigate the eyes.

Side effects:

Caution:
Not to be used for: patients who wear soft contact lenses.
Not to be used with:

Murine *see* **Brolene** *and* **Optrex**

Normasol

A solution in a sachet used for washing out eyes, burns, wounds.

Optrex eye preparations

Optrex eye preparations contain dilute solutons of witch hazel. This reduces eye reddening, and the solution acts to irrigate the eye. Some people are particularly sensitive to witch hazel and the treatment should not be continued if symptoms persist or worsen. Local sensitivity will present as stinging in or around the eye.

Opulets Saline

Drops used to irrigate the eyes.

Otrivine-Anistin

Drops used as a sympathomimetic, antihistamine treatment for allergic conjunctivitis and other eye inflammations.

Side effects: temporary smarting, headache, sleeplessness, drowsiness, rapid heart rate, congestion.
Caution: in patients suffering from high blood pressure, enlarged prostate, coronary disease, diabetes.

Not to be used for: patients suffering from glaucoma or who wear soft contact lenses.
Not to be used with: MAOIs.

Phenylephrine
Drops used as a sympathomimetic pupil dilator.
Side effects:
Caution:
Not to be used for: patients suffering from narrow angle glaucoma, high blood pressure, coronary disease, overactive thyroid.
Not to be used with: ß-blockers.

Rose Bengal
Drops used as a dye to stain the eye for finding degenerated cells in dry eye syndrome.

Side effects: severe smarting
Caution:
Not to be used for: children.
Not to be used with:

Sno Tears
Drops used to lubricate the eyes.

Side effects:
Caution:
Not to be used for: patients who wear soft contact lenses.
Not to be used with:

Tears Naturale
Drops used to lubricate dry eyes.

Side effects:
Caution:

Not to be used for: patients who wear soft contact lenses.
Not to be used with:

Topiclens

A solution in a sachet used to wash out the eyes, wounds, or burns.

Side effects:
Caution: throw away any remaining solution.
Not to be used for:
Not to be used with:

Chapter 12

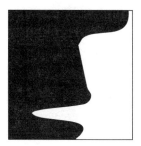

Diseases of the Mouth

Please refer to 'Important Advice' on page 4 at the beginning of this book; and remember, if you are in any doubt, consult a physician.

The mouth is the portal through which air, food, and water enter the human body. Thus, it is vulnerable to infections, but many of these are fairly visible and treatable.

Most major problems in the mouth occur in the teeth and gums, to the extent that these conditions are treated by a separate group of specialized practitioners, dentists.

The tongue contains sensors for taste and is vulnerable to benign or malignant tumours.

Dental abscess and caries ♥

 These are the main dental disorders that are referred to doctors.

Symptoms

The main symptom of dental abscess is severe pain in the mouth adjacent to a tooth. There will be associated temperature and trismus (spasm of the jaw). Dental caries (tooth decay) may lead to a variety of symptoms which are best seen by a dentist.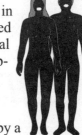

Action

Where possible, dental diseases should be treated by a dentist. Occasionally, you may need medical advice.

Tests

Dental X-rays will determine the extent of an abscess.

Medications and treatment

Antiseptic mouth washes may help resolve some of the symptoms but antibiotics are required for dental abscess. Draining an abscess is usually definitive in terms of treatment.

Further advice

The best way to prevent dental disease is to avoid eating sweet foods. Regular brushing and the use of dental floss will help prevent tooth and gum disease.

Associated conditions

Gum disease, particularly gingivitis (inflammation of the gums); aphthous ulcers are small ulcers which may appear in the mouth; and fungus infection of the mouth (thrush) may also cause pain and soreness.

Tumours of the mouth ♥♥♥♥

Tumours of the mouth are quite rare but may occur in people who are heavy smokers or who drink spirits in quantity.

Symptoms

Usually a lump or swelling on the tongue or gum. This may eventually ulcerate or bleed. There may be associated swelling of lymph nodes around the neck.

Action

Seek medical advice urgently for any lump or swelling in the mouth.

Tests

Investigations of these include biopsy to assess the degree of malignancy of the tumour.

Medications and treatment

The treatment of head and neck tumours in general is firstly surgical followed by chemotherapy and radiotherapy.

Further advice

Avoiding smoking and alcohol helps to prevent this condition and you should not smoke or drink alcohol if you are being treated for it.

Over-the-counter Medicines

AAA Spray

An aerosol used as an antibacterial and local anaesthetic to treat sore throat, minor infections of the nose and throat.

Side effects:
Caution:
Not to be used for: children under 6 years.
Not to be used with:

Anaflex

A white lozenge supplied at a strength of 30 mg and used as an antibacterial and antifungal treatment for thrush and other bacterial infections of the mouth and throat.

Side effects:
Caution:
Not to be used for: children under 6 years.
Not to be used with:

Betadine Gargle and Mouthwash

A solution used as an antiseptic to treat inflammation of the mouth and pharynx brought on by thrush and other bacterial infections.

Side effects: rarely local irritation and sensitivity.
Caution:
Not to be used for:
Not to be used with:

Bioral

A gel used as a cell-surface protector to treat mouth ulcers.

Bocasan

A sachet of white granules used as a disinfectant to treat gingivitis and mouth infections.

Side effects:

Caution:
Not to be used for: patients suffering from kidney disease.
Not to be used with:

Bonjela

Bonjela is a mouth ointment which contains choline salicylate (related to aspirin), chloride, menthol, alcohol, and glycerin. It is useful for mouth ulcers and teething problems. Small quantities should be applied every four hours because large quantities may deliver too much aspirin, especially to children.

Bradosol

A white lozenge supplied at a strength of 0.5 mg and used as a disinfectant to treat infections of the mouth and throat.

Side effects: rarely local irritation and sensitivity.
Caution:
Not to be used for:
Not to be used with:

Chloraseptic

A solution supplied with a spray and used as a disinfectant to treat sore throat, mouth ulcers, minor mouth and gum infections.

Side effects: rarely local irritation and sensitivity.
Caution:
Not to be used for: children under 6 years.
Not to be used with:

Corsodyl

A solution used as an antibacterial treatment for gingivitis,

mouth ulcers, thrush, and for mouth hygiene.

Side effects: local irritation, stained tongue or teeth, may affect taste.
Caution:
Not to be used for:
Not to be used with:

Difflam Oral Rinse

A solution used as an analgesic and anti-inflammatory treatment for painful inflammations of the throat and mouth.

Side effects: numb mouth.
Caution:
Not to be used for: children.
Not to be used with:

Eludril

A solution used as an antibacterial treatment for throat and mouth infections, gingivitis, ulcers.

Side effects:
Caution:
Not to be used for: children under 6 years.
Not to be used with:

Glandosane

An aerosol used to provide artificial saliva for dry mouth and throat.

Labosept

A red hexagonal-shaped pastille supplied at a strength of 0.25 mg and used as an antiseptic treatment for mouth and throat

infections.

Medilave

A gel used as an antiseptic and local anaesthetic to treat abrasions or ulcers in the mouth, teething.

Side effects:
Caution:
Not to be used for: infants under 6 months.
Not to be used with:

Merocaine

A green lozenge supplied at a strength of 1.4 mg and used as an antiseptic and local anaesthetic to treat painful infections of the throat and mouth, and as an additional treatment for tonsillitis and pharyngitis.

Side effects:
Caution:
Not to be used for: children.
Not to be used with:

Merocet

A solution used as an antiseptic to treat infections of the throat and mouth.

Side effects:
Caution:
Not to be used for: children under 6 years.
Not to be used with:

Naxogin 500

A white scored tablet supplied at a strength of 500 mg and

used as an antiprotozoal treatment for acute ulcerative gingivitis.

Side effects: stomach upset.
Caution: in pregnant women.
Not to be used for: children, nursing mothers, or for patients suffering from kidney weakness or brain disease.
Not to be used with: alcohol.

Orabase

An ointment used as a mucoprotectant to protect lesions in the mouth.

Oralcer

A green pellet used as an antibacterial, antifungal treatment for mouth ulcers.

Side effects: local irritation.
Caution: do not use for extended periods.
Not to be used for: patients suffering from kidney or liver disease, overactive thyroid, intolerance to iodine.
Not to be used with:

Chapter 13

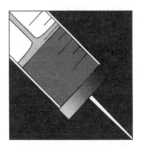

Addictions

Please refer to 'Important Advice' on page 4 at the beginning of this book; and remember, if you are in any doubt, consult a physician.

One of the failings of the complex human organism is that its nervous system has elaborated a series of psychological behaviour patterns which are not necessarily logical. These behaviour patterns can be modified by human beings themselves, and one of the things which distinguishes humans from other species is the desire to take medicines or other mind-controlling substances such as alcohol.

Alcohol has been established for many thousands of years as a drug of abuse. It is essentially a toxin and poisons all cells of the body, but particularly those of the nervous system and the liver.

More powerful toxins have been developed in the form of prescription drugs, such as tranquillizers, and illegal drugs of abuse. The danger with these compounds is in their addictive potential. Better control of alcohol, nicotine, and drug abuse would save many lives.

Addiction to alcohol (alcoholism) ♥♥♥

 Alcoholism, or addiction to alcohol, is the most common addictive disease. Sufferers may progress from social drinking to either regular heavy bout drinking or to continuous daily intake of alcohol. Spirits, in particular, are dangerous because of the damage they may cause to the body.

Symptoms
These include regular intake of alcohol either daily or several times weekly in severe bouts (bout drinking). This is followed by a deterioration of family and personal life, breakup of marriage, loss of job, loss of driving licence due to drink/driving offences, neglect of personal and social arrangements (failure to open the post is a common symptom of alcohol addiction), loss of friends, loss of trust by friends, deteriorating memory, blackouts, persistent vomiting, poor diet, malnutrition, eventually leading to brain and liver damage, alcoholic cirrhosis, and irreversible brain disorders such as encephalopathy and psychosis, suicide. Damage to family members is another significant factor that this condition causes.

Action
Early intervention is recommended to prevent the steady deterioration to the further stages of alcoholism.

Tests
Routine liver function tests will denote the degree of liver damage. Other organs that may be affected include the heart and the brain, and the appropriate tests are needed. Full blood count can assess any degree of anaemia caused by poor diet. Damage to the pancreas gland may result in diabetes. Damage to reproductive function may impair fertility in men and women.

Medications and treatment
A structured programme of peer group support (Alcoholics Anony-

mous), psychotherapy, the use of tranquillizers and ß-blockers, including Antabuse, Librium, and propanolol, to maintain withdrawal from alcohol, antidepressants, and sleeping pills all form part of the management of this difficult condition.

Further advice
Alcoholism should be regarded as an illness and taken seriously. Active management is recommended.

Associated conditions
Drinking methylated spirits or other adulterated alcohol products may cause severe damage, including blindness.

Addiction to illegal drugs including ♥♥♥♥ marijuanha, cocaine, heroin, ecstasy

 These drugs are listed together because the illegal supply of one often brings users into contact with the other drugs. Marijuanha is the most benign but prolonged use can have both psychological and physical effects including loss of immune function. Cocaine and its derivatives, including crack, produce an elevation of mood with profound withdrawal symptoms. Heroin may be taken by inhalation or by injection, the latter carrying risk of transmission of virus diseases such as hepatitis B and HIV, as well as profound serious addiction. Ecstasy is an amphetamine derivative which also produces mood elevation but profound withdrawal symptoms. Addiction occurs because of a need to overcome the withdrawal and because of other personality factors.

Symptoms
Regular drug use becomes a problem when it interferes with normal

social functioning. The expenditure of large amounts of money may lead users to commit petty crime or even more serious crime. Loss of social contacts, friends, and jobs may also occur as part of the addiction, similar to that described for alcohol addiction (*see* above). Regular use of these drugs often coexists with regular alcohol abuse. Cocaine may cause damage to the nose from repeated inhalation. Marijuanha may affect the immune system and fertility. Ecstasy occasionally causes rapid heart rate and has been known to be associated with sudden death. Deliberate or accidental overdose of these drugs is often fatal.

Tests
Blood and urine tests can determine whether drugs have been taken recently. Routine tests to determine any end organ damage can also be carried out.

Medications and treatment
The treatment of addiction to these drugs involves multidisciplinary support groups, peer groups, psychotherapy, and counselling, together with drugs such as methadone to aid the withdrawal from addictive drugs.

Further advice
As with alcohol addiction, early intervention is recommended for all these addictions.

Associated conditions
Nicotine addiction can possibly be included with this group, and the effects of regular cigarette smoking on the lungs and on the cardiovascular system are described in the relevant chapters above. Solvent abuse (eg aerosols, glue) can be fatal and often occurs in teenagers.

Addiction to prescription drugs ♥♥

 The most common prescription drugs which have caused problems with addiction are tranquillizers and sleeping pills, particularly the benzodiazepines, laxatives, and slimming pills.

Symptoms

Unlike alcoholism, this condition is more common in women than in men. Regular prescribing of these products without patient consultation colludes with the addiction. Laxative abuse and slimming pill abuse may co-exist with the anorexia/bulimia syndrome (*see* below). Addiction to sleeping pills and tranquillizers is very difficult to treat because sudden withdrawal provokes a paranoid psychosis-type syndrome, and gradual withdrawal under supervision is usually necessary.

Action

Where addiction to these medications is suspected, the patient or a family friend should discuss it with the prescribing doctor.

Tests

Psychometric testing to test brain function may be appropriate. Examination by a psychiatrist or clinical psychologist is also of value.

Medications and treatment

Gradual withdrawal under supervision is necessary, in association with psychotherapy and support groups. Attention to any underlying condition which has precipitated the addiction is also necessary.

Further advice

Prescription drugs should always be used in small quantities and under the advice of the prescriber. Repeat prescriptions should not be issued unless it is perfectly clear that the condition is a chronic one requiring long-term treatment.

Prescription Medicines

Antabuse

A white, scored tablet supplied at a strength of 200 mg and used as an enzyme inhibitor, additional treatment for alcoholism.

Side effects: drowsiness, tiredness, nausea, bad breath, reduced sex drive, rarely mental disturbances.
Caution: in patients suffering from liver, kidney, or breathing diseases, diabetes, epilepsy, drug addiction.
Not to be used for: children, pregnant women, or patients suffering from heart failure, coronary artery disease, mental disorders.
Caution needed with: alcohol, barbiturates, paraldehyde, sedatives.

Librium

A yellow-green, light blue-green, or dark blue-green tablet according to strengths of 5 mg, 10, mg, 25 mg and used as a tranquillizer to treat anxiety, symptoms of acute alcohol withdrawal, short-term treatment of sleeplessness where sedation during the day does not cause difficulty.

Side effects: drowsiness, confusion, unsteadiness, low blood pressure, rash, changes in vision, changes in libido, retention of urine. Risk of addiction increases with dose and length of treatment. May impair judgement.
Caution: in the elderly, pregnant women, nursing mothers, in women during labour, and in patients suffering from lung disorders, kidney or liver disorders. Avoid long-term use and withdraw gradually.
Not to be used for: children or for patients suffering from acute lung diseases, some chronic lung diseases, some obsessional and psychotic diseases.
Caution needed with: alcohol and other tranquillizers and anticonvulsants.

Chapter 14

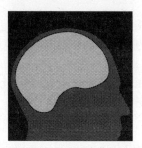

Psychological Disorders

Please refer to 'Important Advice' on page 4 at the beginning of this book; and remember, if you are in any doubt, consult a physician.

The complexity of the nervous system carries with it the need to have a sophisticated command structure for the human body. This includes the need for developing feelings which help humans in their creative quest. These feelings may be entirely positive – hope, creativity, excitement, and ambition – but inevitably such a complex system must be liable to malfunction and break-down. Depression, phobias, compulsive disorders, schizophrenia, and anorexia are merely a few of a wide range of psychiatric disorders which afflict human beings. These conditions are to be judged with equal seriousness when compared with disorders of the rest of the body, and psychological illness should not be regarded as being of less importance.

A great deal of research has been carried out in an effort to understand the human psyche and to develop better methods of treatment. Much psychological illness may relate to addiction, e.g. to alcohol. A better understanding of psychological disease, with earlier diagnosis and intervention, and wider use of counselling and support services would probably reduce the impact of psychological diseases.

Depression

 Depression is probably the most common psychiatric disease. It exists in a range of forms from mild through to very severe. Depression can sometimes be divided into two types, endogenous depression with no outside precipitating factor, or reactive depression. Many patients do not fall simply into either of these two categories, however.

Symptoms

These include a feeling of slowness, sadness, inability to make decisions, poor sleep particularly with early morning waking, lack of self-esteem, lack of self-worth, sometimes excessive sleeping, slow metabolism, constipation, poor appetite, changes in the sense of taste, sometimes excessive comfort eating with weight gain, loss of libido (impotence), hypochondriasis, addiction to alcohol or prescription drugs, suicide.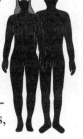

Action

Depressed patients are sometimes too depressed to motivate themselves to seek medical advice. A friend or relative, however, should encourage depressed patients to see their depression as an illness rather than as personal failure, and to seek medical advice.

Tests

Clinical examination and psychometric tests may be useful. There are recognized depression rating scales which help to diagnose the condition. Medical examination should try to exclude organic causes for depression such as brain tumour, heart and lung disease, hormonal disturbances such as underactive thyroid, or associated causes such as alcoholism or drug addiction.

Medications and treatment

The treatment consists of attacking the underlying organic cause, dealing with any associated drug addiction or alcoholism, counselling and psychotherapy, antidepressant medication, and ECT (electro-convulsive therapy). Anafranil, Asendis, Aventyl, Bolvidon, Faverin, Fluanxol, Gamanil, Lentizol, Liskonum, Lustral, Marplan, Molipaxin, Motival, Nardil, Norval, Parnate. Parstelin, Priadel, Prothiaden, Prozac, Seroxat, Surmontil, Tofranil, Triptafen

Further advice
Depression often lifts spontaneously even without the use of medication. Depression may be worse in the winter (seasonal affective disorder) or may clearly be associated with a sudden loss or bereavement.

Associated conditions
Bipolar depression (manic depressive psychosis) is where the patient swings from a low mood to a high mood. Agitated depression is depression mixed with anxiety (*see* below). Anxiety states probably exist on their own and are usually best treated with anxiolytic drugs for short periods only. Persistently elevated mood such as occurs in mania or hypomania usually responds to treatment with lithium. Anxiety states or mania may appear as phobias or obsessive compulsive disorders (*see* below). Severe hypochondriasis in depression may result in a hysterical conversion syndrome whereby severe organic symptoms are presented to mask an underlying depression.

Phobias and obsessive compulsive disorders

Phobias, such as claustrophobia (fear of closed spaces) or agoraphobia (fear of open spaces or of going out), are irrational fears. Obsessive compulsive disorders may be similar in that they are irrational, and very often the patient is compelled to undertake repetitive actions for fear that something bad will happen to them.

Symptoms

Specific phobias, such as fear of spiders or fear of birds, usually do not trouble the sufferer unless they are placed in the particular situation of stress. Claustrophobia will mean that patients will avoid travelling by air or by underground, and fear of flying may be a specific phobia in itself. Agoraphobia usually presents as a gradual withdrawal from social life and going out. In general terms, the phobias may represent some underlying trauma, anxiety, or depressive state. Obsessive compulsive disorders usually appear as a need to carry out repetitive actions such as hand washing (which may be more than 100 times a day), or checking that lights are switched off, or the gas switched off, or that doors are locked. Some patients have a series of set rituals which they must follow before they can go out. The eventual climax is that they are unable to go out, i.e. they are agoraphobic, because the ritual takes them all day. Some people need to dress and wash in exactly the same pattern each day and become disturbed if they cannot follow this procedure. Like the phobias, the obsessive compulsive disorders mask an underlying anxiety, trauma, or depression. The possibility of sexual abuse at some stage of the patient's life might also be considered.

Action

Where these conditions are disturbing the patient's normal life in terms of working or socializing, then professional help is required.

Tests

Psychometric testing and evaluation by a clinical psychologist and psychiatrist are necessary to evaluate these conditions. As in all psychiatric conditions, clinical examination should exclude the possibility of some underlying organic condition, such as a brain tumour which may appear with psychological features.

Medications and treatment

Psychotherapy combined with certain antidepressant drugs (*see* above), such as clomipramine, may be helpful in the management of these conditions.

Further advice

These conditions may be chronic and patients may relapse under stress.

Associated conditions

Certain types of manic disorder such as kleptomania or nymphomania may be a variant of an obsessive compulsive disorder rather than part of true mania.

Eating disorders including anorexia ♥♥♥ nervosa, bulimia, and obesity

 Eating disorders are commonly known as slimming diseases but their roots are to be found in the patient's disturbed emotional integrity rather than purely in an obsession with food and slimming. Like the phobias and obsessive compulsive disorders described above, these eating disorders may represent some underlying anxiety, trauma (such as sexual abuse in childhood), or depression.

Symptoms

The symptoms of anorexia nervosa are persistent weight loss, deceptive fiddling with food, laxative abuse (*see* above), loss of secondary sexual characteristics (i.e. reduction in breast size), and eventually amenorrhoea in females (anorexia nervosa occurs rarely in men). The patients are typically manipulative about food and hide food or vomit food after it has been eaten. Anorexia nervosa may end in the death of the sufferer. Bulimia is a similar condition where starvation may be followed by bouts of bingeing, often associated with the vomiting of food. Patients may be of any weight depending on how much food is retained and how the cycle of bingeing and vomiting varies. Thus, unlike the anorexia patients, the bulimics may be of normal weight or even overweight. Patients with anorexia or bulimia will also show other signs of disturbed personality function including attention-seeking and manipulative behaviour.

Action
Where these conditions are suspected, immediate medical advice should be sought.

Tests
Patients with weight loss should be evaluated for organic causes including cancers, diabetes, and overactive thyroid gland. Similarly, patients suffering from repeated vomiting should be evaluated for gastro-intestinal or liver disorders which may cause vomiting.

Medications and treatment
The treatment of these conditions involves a complex interplay of counselling support with psychotherapy, and the use of appropriate antidepressant and sedative medication.

Further advice
These conditions are chronic and recurrent. It has been said that once you suffer from bulimia you will always suffer from it in some shape or form, and the condition may relapse under moments of stress.

Associated conditions
Compulsive eating and severe obesity may be variants of these conditions which may overlap with the obsessive compulsive disorders described above.

Schizophrenia

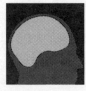 Schizophrenia is disturbed mental function and is not the split personality that many believe it to be. The disturbance of mental function may be severe enough to cause a schizophrenic psychosis or it may be mild. Schizophrenia may have a

genetic or biochemical basis for its origin.

Symptoms

These range from a mild delusion with paranoia which may include hallucinations, particularly auditory hallucinations. Patients may hear voices which may be critical voices. These voices may be scolding the patient or instructing the patient to carry out certain activities or functions. The voices are often described as coming from an electrical source such as a radio or television; schizophrenic patients may become obsessed with electricity and the thought that they are somehow wired up and are being listened to. The paranoia may increase or the patient may develop a frozen or catatonic state. Holding conversations with these unheard voices may be part of the deterioration into full schizophrenic psychosis which may appear to the layman as frank madness. Milder forms of schizophrenia may be difficult to detect and may appear as a depressive disorder. Here the patient simply cannot carry out normal working tasks and withdraws.

Action

Professional medical help is necessary as soon as this condition is suspected.

Tests

Full evaluation by psychiatrists and clinical psychologists are necessary to help detect this condition. As with all psychiatric disorders, organic conditions, such as brain tumour, should be excluded as a cause for bizarre presenting symptoms.

Medications and treatment

Neuroleptic drugs, such as Largactil, are valuable in the management of this condition. Medication should be accompanied by supportive psychotherapy. Surgical and electrical treatments are rarely used for the management of this condition nowadays. Anquil, Clopixol, Clozaril, Depixol, Dolmatil, Dozic, Fentazin, Heminevrin, Largactil, Melleril, Moditen, Nozinan, Orap, Serenace, Stelazine, Sulpitil.

Prescription Medicines

Anafranil

A yellow/caramel capsule, orange/caramel capsule, or blue/ caramel capsule according to strengths of 10 mg, 25 mg, 50 mg and used as a tricyclic antidepressant to treat depression, obsessions, phobias.

Side effects: dry mouth, constipation, urine retention, blurred vision, palpitations, drowsiness, sleeplessness, dizziness, low blood pressure, weight change, skin reactions, jaundice or blood changes, loss of libido may occur.

Caution: in nursing mothers or in patients suffering from heart disease, liver disease, thyroid disease, adrenal tumour, glaucoma, urine retention, epilepsy, diabetes, some other psychiatric conditions. Your doctor may advise regular blood tests.

Not to be used for: children, pregnant women, or for patients suffering from heart attacks, liver disease, heart block.

Caution needed with: alcohol, anticholinergics, adrenaline, barbiturates, MAOIs, other antidepressants, antihypertensives, cimetidine, oestrogens, some local anaesthetics.

Anquil

A white tablet supplied at a strength of 0.25 mg and used as an antipsychotic drug for controlling unacceptable sexual behaviour.

Side effects: muscle spasms, restlessness, hands shaking, dry mouth, urine retention, palpitations, low blood pressure, weight gain, changes in libido, low body temperature, breast swelling, menstrual changes, jaundice, blood and skin changes, stomach upset, drowsiness, rarely fits.

Caution: in nursing mothers, and in patients suffering from liver or kidney disease, epilepsy, or Parkinson's disease. Your doctor may advise regular blood and liver tests.

Not to be used for: children or for pregnant women.

Caution needed with: alcohol, tranquillizers, pain killers,

antihypertensives, antidepressants, anticonvulsants, antidiabetic drugs, levodopa.

Asendis

A white, orange, blue, or white, hexagonal tablet according to strengths of 25 mg, 50 mg, 100 mg, 150 mg and used as a tricyclic antidepressant to treat depression.

Side effects: anticholinergic effects, drowsiness, impotence, nausea, vomiting, breast enlargement, convulsions at high doses.
Caution: in the elderly, and in patients who are a suicide risk, or who are suffering from epilepsy, glaucoma, urine retention, confusion, agitation.
Not to be used for: pregnant women, nursing mothers, or for patients suffering from recent heart attack, heart block, heart rhythm disturbances, severe liver disease, mania.
Caution needed with: MAOIs, sympathomimetics, barbiturates, alcohol, antihypertensives, anaesthetics.

Aventyl

A white/yellow capsule supplied at a strength of 10 mg, 25 mg and used as a tricyclic antidepressant to treat depression, bed wetting in children.

Side effects: dry mouth, constipation, urine retention, blurred vision, palpitations, drowsiness, sleeplessness, dizziness, hands shaking, low blood presure, weight change, skin reactions, jaundice or blood changes, loss of libido may occur.
Caution: in nursing mothers or in patients suffering from heart disease, thyroid disease, epilepsy, diabetes, some other psychiatric conditions. Your doctor may advise regular blood tests.
Not to be used for: children under 6 years, pregnant women, or for patients suffering from heart attacks, liver disease, heart block.
Caution needed with: alcohol, anticholinergics, adrenaline, MAOIs, barbiturates, other antidepressants, antihypertensives,

cimetidine, oestrogens, some local anaestetics.

Bolvidon

A white tablet supplied at a strength of 10 mg, 20 mg, and 30 mg and used as tetracyclic antidepressant to treat depression.

Side effects: drowsiness, bone marrow depression, possibility of jaudice, hypomania or convulsions when the drug should be withdrawn.
Caution: in pregnant women, the elderly, and in patients suffering from epilepsy, enlarged prostate, or heart attacks. Your doctor may advise regular blood tests.
Not to be used for: children, nursing mothers, or for patients suffering from mania or severe liver disease.
Caution needed with: MAOIs, alcohol, anticoagulants.

Clopixol

A pink tablet, light-brown tablet, or brown tablet according to strengths of 2 mg, 10 mg, 25 mg and used as a tranquillizer to treat mental disorders especially schizophrenia.

Side effects: muscle spasms, restlessness, hands shaking, dry mouth, urine retention, palpitations, low blood pressure, weight gain, changes in libido, low body temperature, breast swelling, menstrual changes, jaundice, blood and skin changes, drowsiness, rarely fits.
Caution: in pregnant women, nursing mothers, in the elderly who should take smaller dosage, and in patients suffering from Parkinson's disease, kidney, liver, or heart disease, or breathing disorders.
Not to be used for: children or for patients suffering from acute opiate, alcohol, or barbiturate poisoning, advanced kidney, liver, or heart disease, senility, apathy, or withdrawal, Parkinson's disease, severe arteriosclerosis, or for anyone who is intolerant of these drugs taken by mouth.
Caution needed with:

Clozaril

A yellow, scored tablet supplied at strengths of 25 mg, 100 mg, and used as a sedative to treat schizophrenia.

Side effects: blood changes, drowsiness, watering of the mouth, rapid heart beat, tiredness, dizziness, headache, difficulty in passing urine, stomach upset, change in electrical activity of the brain and heart, temporary upset of automatic body functions.
Caution: in the elderly, and in patients with a history of epilepsy or suffering from enlarged prostate, glaucoma, liver disease,.or intestinal abnormality. Patients should report any symptoms of infection. Your doctor may advise regular blood tests.
Not to be used for: children, pregnant women, nursing mothers, or for patients suffering from severe kidney or liver disease, alcoholism, drug intoxication, drowsiness or reduced reactions, or for those in a coma or having a history of drug-induced blood disorder.
Caution needed with: other drugs which cause blood disorder, some sedatives, alcohol, MAOIs, anticholinergics, drugs which lower blood pressure.

Depixol

A yellow tablet supplied at a strength of 3 mg and used as a sedative to treat schizophrenia and other mental disorders, especially withdrawal or apathy.

Side effects: muscle spasms, restlessness, hands shaking, dry mouth, urine retention, palpitations, low blood pressure, weight gain, changes in libido, low body temperature, breast swelling, menstrual changes, jaundice, blood and skin changes, drowsiness, rarely fits.
Caution: in pregnant women, the elderly, and in patients suffering from kidney, liver, heart, or lung disease, Parkinson's disease, or anyone who is intolerant of those drugs taken by mouth.
Not to be used for: children, or for very excitable or overactive patients.
Caution needed with: alcohol, tranquillizers, pain killers,

antihypertensives, antidepressants, anticonvulsants, antidiabetic drugs, levodopa.

Dolmatil

A white, scored tablet supplied at a strength of 200 mg and used as a sedative to treat schizophrenia.

Side effects: muscle spasms, restlessness, hands shaking, dry mouth, urine retention, palpitations, low blood pressure, weight gain, changes in libido, low body temperature, breast swelling, menstrual changes, jaundice, blood and skin changes, drowsiness, rarely fits.
Caution: in pregnant women or for patients suffering from hypomania, kidney disease, or epilepsy.
Not to be used for: for children under 14 years or for patients suffering from phaeochromocytoma (a disease of the adrenal glands).
Caution needed with: alcohol, tranquillizers, pain killers, antihypertensives, antidepressants, anticoagulants, antidiabetic drugs, levodopa, antacids, sucralfate.

Dozic

A liquid used as a sedative to treat schizophrenia, mania, hypomania, organic psychoses, alcohol withdrawal symptoms, delirium tremens, behaviour problems among children.

Side effects: muscle spasms, restlessness, hands shaking, dry mouth, urine retention, palpitations, low blood pressure, weight gain, changes in libido, low body temperature, breast swelling, menstrual changes, jaundice, blood and skin changes, drowsiness, rarely fits.
Caution: in pregnant women or in patients suffering from liver or kidney disease, epilepsy, severe cardiovascular disease, Parkinson's disease, or overactive thyroid gland.
Not to be used for: unconscious patients.
Caution needed with: alcohol, tranquillizers, pain killers,

antihypertensives, antidepressants, anticonvulsants, antidiabetic drugs, levodopa, rifampicin, lithium.

Faverin

A yellow tablet supplied at a strength of 50 mg and used as an antidepressant to treat depression.

Side effects: nausea, vomiting, sleepiness, diarrhoea, agitation, anorexia, tremor, convulsions
Caution: in patients suffering from liver or kidney disease.
Not to be used for: children, pregnant women, nursing mothers, or for patients with a history of epilepsy.
Caution needed with: propanolol, theophylline, phenytoin, warfarin, MAOIs, alcohol, lithium, tryptophan.

Fentazin

A white tablet supplied at strengths of 2 mg, 4 mg and used as a sedative to treat anxiety, tension, chronic mental disorders, schizophrenia, vomiting, nausea, and other psychiatric problems.

Side effects: muscle spasms, restlessness, hands shaking, blurred vision, dry mouth, urine retention, palpitations, low blood pressure, weight gain, changes in libido, low body temperature, breast swelling, menstrual changes, jaundice, blood and skin changes, drowsiness, rarely fits.
Caution: in pregnant women, nursing mothers, and in patients suffering from Parkinson's disease, liver disease, cardiovascular disease, kidney failure, epilepsy, glaucoma, myaesthenia gravis, adrenal tumour, enlarged prostate.
Not to be used for: children, unconscious patients, or those suffering from bone marrow depression.
Caution needed with: alcohol, tranquillizers, pain killers, antihypertensives, antidepressants, anticonvulsants, antidiabetic drugs, levodopa.

Fluanxol

A red tablet supplied at strengths of 0.5 mg, 1 mg and used as a sedative for the short-term treatment of depression and anxiety.

Side effects: muscle spasms, restlessness, hands shaking, blurred vision, dry mouth, urine retention, palpitations, low blood pressure, weight gain, changes in libido, low body temperature, breast swelling, menstrual changes, jaundice, blood and skin changes, drowsiness, rarely fits.

Caution: in pregnant women, and in patients suffering from Parkinson's disease, severe hardening of the arteries, confusion in the elderly, severe kidney, liver, or heart disease.

Not to be used for: children or for excitable, overactive, or severely clinically depressed patients.

Caution needed with: alcohol, tranquillizers, pain killers, antihypertensives, antidepressants, anticonvulsants, antidiabetic drugs, levodopa.

Gamanil

A maroon, scored tablet supplied at a strength of 70 mg and used as an antidepressant to treat depression.

Side effects: dry mouth, constipation, urine retention, blurred vision, palpitations, drowsiness, sleeplessness, dizziness, hands shaking, low blood presure, weight change, skin reactions, jaundice or blood changes, loss of libido may occur.

Caution: in nursing mothers or in patients suffering from heart disease, thyroid disease, epilepsy, diabetes, glaucoma, adrenal tumour, urinary retention, some other psychiatric conditions. Your doctor may advise regular blood tests.

Not to be used for: children, pregnant women, or for patients suffering from heart attacks, heart block, liver disease.

Caution needed with: alcohol, anticholinergics, adrenaline, MAOIs, barbiturates, other antidepressants, antihypertensives, oestrogens, cimetidine.

Heminevrin

A syrup used as a sedative for the short-term treatment of sleeplessness in the elderly, agitated states, tension and anxiety, daytime sedation in senile mental disorder, confusion, alcohol withdrawal symptoms, pre-eclamptic toxaemia, severe epilepsy.

Side effects: blocked and irritating nose, irritating eyes, stomach disturbances, severe allergy, sedation, excitement, confusion.
Caution: in patients suffering from long-term lung weakness, kidney or liver disease. Patients should be warned of impaired ability.
Not to be used for: children, nursing mothers, or patients suffering from acute lung weakness.
Caution needed with: alcohol and sedatives.

Largactil

A white tablet supplied at strengths of 10 mg, 25 mg, 50 mg, 100 mg and used as a sedative to treat brain disturbances needing sedation, premedication, inducing hypothermia, nausea, vomiting, schizophrenia, mood change.

Side effects: muscle spasms, restlessness, hands shaking, dry mouth, urine retention, palpitations, low blood pressure, weight gain, blurred vision, changes in libido, low body temperature, breast swelling, menstrual changes, jaundice, blood and skin changes, drowsiness, rarely fits.
Caution: in pregnant women and nursing mothers.
Not to be used for: unconscious patients, the elderly, or for patients suffering from bone marrow depression, liver or kidney disease, heart failure, epilepsy, parkinsonism, underactive thyroid, enlarged prostate, glaucoma.
Caution needed with: alcohol, tranquillizers, pain killers, antihypertensives, antidepressants, anticonvulsants, antidiabetic drugs, levodopa.

Lentizol

A pink capsule or pink/red capsule according to strengths of 25 mg, 50 mg and used as a tricyclic antidepressant to treat depression especially where sedation is needed.

Side effects: dry mouth, constipation, urine retention, blurred vision, palpitations, drowsiness, sleeplessness, dizziness, hands shaking, low blood presure, weight change, skin reactions, jaundice or blood changes, loss of libido may occur.
Caution: in nursing mothers or in patients suffering from heart disease, thyroid disease, epilepsy, diabetes, glaucoma, adrenal tumour, urinary retention, some other psychiatric conditions. Your doctor may advise regular blood tests.
Not to be used for: children, pregnant women, or for patients suffering from heart attacks, liver disease, heart block.
Caution needed with: alcohol, anticholinergics, adrenaline, MAOIs, barbiturates, other antidepressants, cimetedine, oestrogens, antihypertensives.

Liskonum

A white, scored, oblong tablet supplied at a strength of 450 mg and used as a sedative to treat mania, hypomania, manic depression.

Side effects: nausea, diarrhoea, hand tremor, muscular weakness, brain and heart disturbances, weight gain, fluid retention, underactive or over active thyroid gland, thirst and frequent urination, kidney changes, skin reactions, intoxication.
Caution: treatment should be started in hospital and a careful check on the functioning of the kidneys and thyroid should be made, as well as ensuring that there is an adequate consumption of salt and fluid. Your doctor may advise blood tests to gauge dose.
Not to be used for: children, for pregnant women, nursing mothers, or for patients suffering from disturbed sodium balance, Addison's disease, kidney or heart disease, or underactive thyroid.

Caution needed with: diuretics, non-steroid anti-inflammatory drugs, carbamazepine, phenytoin, haloperidol, flupenthixol, methyldopa, phenytoin, fluoxamine.

Lustral

White, capsule-shaped tablets supplied at strengths of 50 mg, 100 mg, and used to treat the symptoms of depression, and to prevent relapse and further depressive episodes.

Side effects: dry mouth, nausea, diarrhoea, shaking, sweating, stomach discomfort, sexual disturbances.
Caution: in pregnant women, nursing mothers, patients undergoing electroconvulsive therapy, or suffering from unstable epilepsy.
Not to be used for: children, or for patients suffering from kidney or liver disorder.
Caution needed with: MAOIs, lithium, tryptophan.

Melleril

A white tablet supplied at strengths of 10 mg, 25 mg, 50 mg, 100 mg and used as a sedative to treat schizophrenia, manic mental disorders, senile confusion, behavioural disorders, epilepsy in children.

Side effects: muscle spasms, restlessness, blurred vision, hands shaking, constipation, dry mouth, urine retention, palpitations, low blood pressure, weight gain, changes in libido, low body temperature, breast swelling, menstrual changes, jaundice, blood and skin changes, drowsiness, rarely fits.
Caution: in patients suffering from liver disease, kidney disease, cardiovascular disease, epilepsy, glaucoma, myaesthenia gravis, enlarged prostate, severe lung disease, parkinsonism, adrenal tumour.
Not to be used for: pregnant women, nursing mothers, severely depressed or unconscious patients or for patients suffering from blood disorders, severe heart disease.

Caution needed with: alcohol, tranquillizers, pain killers, antihypertensives, antidepressants, anticonvulsants, antidiabetic drugs, levodopa.

Moditen

A pink tablet, yellow tablet, or white tablet according to strengths of 1 mg, 2.5 mg, 5 mg and used as a sedative to treat schizophrenia, behavioural problems, anxiety, tension, senile disorders.

Side effects: muscle spasms, restlessness, constipation, blurred vision, hands shaking, dry mouth, urine retention, palpitations, low blood pressure, weight gain, changes in libido, low body temperature, breast swelling, menstrual changes, jaundice, blood and skin changes, drowsiness, rarely fits.
Caution: in the elderly, pregnant women, nursing mothers, and in patients suffering from tremor or rigidity, liver, lung, or heart disorder, thyroid disorder, epilepsy, glaucoma, myaesthenia gravis, or enlarged prostate.
Not to be used for: children or for patients suffering from phaeochromocytoma, kidney or liver failure, poor brain circulation, severe heart weakness, severe depression or coma.
Caution needed with: alcohol, tranquillizers, pain killers, antihypertensives, antidepressants, anticonvulsants, antidiabetic drugs, levodopa.

Molipaxin

A pink, scored tablet supplied at a strength of 150 mg and used as a sedative to treat depression and anxiety.

Availability: NHS and private prescription.
Side effects: drowsiness, dizziness, headache, penile erection.
Caution: in patients suffering from epilepsy, severe kidney or liver disease.
Not to be used for: children.
Caution needed with: muscle relaxants, anaesthetics, alcohol,

sedatives, MAOIs, clonidine.

Motival

A triangular, pink tablet used as a sedative to treat anxiety/depression

Side effects: muscle spasms, restlessness, sleeplessness, dizziness, hands shaking, dry mouth, constipation, blurred vision, urine retention, palpitations, low blood pressure, weight change, changes in libido, low body temperature, breast swelling, menstrual changes, jaundice, blood and skin changes, drowsiness, rarely fits.

Caution: in patients with a history of epilepsy or brain damage, nursing mothers, and in patients suffering from heart disease, urinary retention, adrenal tumour, glaucoma, thyroid disease, epilepsy, diabetes, some other psychiatric conditions. Your doctor may advise regular blood and liver tests.

Not to be used for: children, pregnant women or for patients suffering from Parkinson's disease, heart attacks, liver disease, heart block.

Caution needed with: alcohol, anticholinergics, adrenaline, MAOIs, barbiturates, cimetidine, tranquillizers, pain killers, antihypertensives, antidepressants, anticonvulsants, antidiabetic drugs, levodopa.

Nardil

An orange tablet supplied at a strength of 15 mg and used as an MAOI to treat depression, phobias.

Side effects: severe high blood pressure reactions with certain foods, sleeplessness, low blood pressure, dizziness, drowsiness, weakness, dry mouth, constipation, stomach upset, blurred vision, urinary difficulties, ankle swelling, rash, jaundice, weight gain, confusion, sexual desire changes.

Caution: in the elderly and in patients suffering from epilepsy.

Not to be used for: children, or for patients suffering from liver

disease, blood changes, heart disease, phaeochromocytoma, overactive thyroid, brain artery disease.
Caution needed with: amphetamines or similar sympathomimetic drugs, tricyclic antidepressants, pethidine and other similar analgesics, some cough mixtures and appetite supressants containing sympathomimetics. barbiturates, sedatives, alcohol, and antidiabetics may be enhanced. anticholinergic side effects are increased. Cheese, Bovril, Oxo, meat extracts, broad beans, banana, Marmite, yeast extracts, wine, beer, other alcohol, pickled herrings, vegetable proteins. (Up to 14 days after cessation.)

Norval

An orange tablet supplied at strengths of 10 mg, 20 mg, 30 mg and used as a tetracyclic anti-depressant to treat depression.

Side effects: drowsiness, bone marrow depression, possible jaundice, hypomania, or convulsions.
Caution: in pregnant women, the elderly or patients suffering from epilepsy, glaucoma, enlarged prostate, heart attack; discontinue if jaundice, hypomania, or convulsions happen. Your doctor may advise that blood tests should be taken once a month for the first 3 months.
Not to be used for: children, nursing mothers, or for patients suffering from mania or severe liver disease.
Caution needed with: MAOIs, alcohol, anticoagulants.

Nozinan

A white, scored tablet supplied at a strength of 25 mg, and used as a sedative to treat schizophrenia and other mental disorders, and to treat severe pain accompanied by restlessness, distress, or vomiting.

Side effects: muscle spasms, restlessness, hands shaking, constipation, blurred vision, dry mouth, urine retention, palpitations, low blood pressure, weight gain, changes in libido, low body temperature, breast swelling, menstrual changes, jaundice, blood and skin changes, drowsiness, fits.

Caution: in pregnant women, nursing mothers, and in patients suffering from cardiovascular disease, liver damage, Parkinson's disease, or epilepsy.

Not to be used for: children, or for patients with bone marrow disorder, or who are in a coma.

Caution needed with: alcohol, tranquillizers, pain killers, antihypertensives, antidepressants, anticonvulsants, antidiabetics, levodopa.

Orap

A white, scored tablet or a green, scored tablet according to strengths of 2 mg, 4 mg, 10 mg and used as a sedative to treat schizophrenia.

Side effects: muscle spasms, restlessness, hands shaking, blurred vision, constipation, dry mouth, urine retention, palpitations, low blood pressure, weight gain, abnormal heart rhythm, changes in libido, low body temperature, breast swelling, menstrual changes, jaundice, blood and skin changes, drowsiness, rarely fits.

Caution: in pregnant women and in patients suffering from endogenous depression, Parkinson's disease, epilepsy, kidney or liver damage, electrolyte disturbance.

Not to be used for: children or for patients suffering from some heart disorders.

Caution needed with: alcohol, tranquillizers, pain killers, antihypertensives, antidepressants, anticonvulsants, antidiabetic drugs, levodopa, some heart drugs, some tranquillizers.

Parnate

A red tablet used as an MAOI antidepressant to treat depression.

Side effects: severe high blood pressure reactions with certain

foods, sleeplessness, low blood pressure, dizziness, drowsiness, weakness, dry mouth, constipation, stomach upset, blurred vision, urinary difficulties, ankle swelling, rash, jaundice, weight gain, confusion, sexual desire changes.
Caution: in the elderly and in patients suffering from epilepsy.
Not to be used for: children, or for patients suffering from liver disease, blood changes, heart disease, phaeochromocytoma, overactive thyroid, brain artery disease.
Caution needed with: amphetamines or similar sympathomimetic drugs, tricyclic antidepressants, pethidine and other similar analgesics, some cough mixtures and appetite supressants containing sympathomimetics. barbiturates, sedatives, alcohol, and antidiabetics may be enhanced. anticholinergic side effects are increased. Cheese, Bovril, Oxo, meat extracts, broad beans, banana, Marmite, yeast extracts, wine, beer, other alcohol, pickled herrings, vegetable proteins. (Up to 14 days after cessation.)

Parstelin

A green tablet used as an MAOI to treat depression with anxiety.

Side effects: severe high blood pressure reactions with certain foods, low blood pressure, muscle spasms, restlessness, low body temperature, breast swelling, menstrual changes, sleeplessness, low blood pressure, dizziness, drowsiness, weakness, dry mouth, constipation, stomach upset, blurred vision, urinary difficulties, ankle swelling, rash, blood and skin changes, jaundice, weight gain, confusion, sexual desire changes.
Caution: in the elderly, pregnant women, nursing mothers, and in patients suffering from epilepsy. Your doctor may advise regular blood and liver checks.
Not to be used for: children, or for patients suffering from liver disease, blood changes, heart disease, phaeochromocytoma, overactive thyroid, brain artery disease, Parkinson's disease.
Caution needed with: amphetamines or similar sympathomimetic drugs, tricyclic antidepressants, tranquillizers,

levodopa, pethidine and other similar analgesics, some cough mixtures and appetite supressants containing sympathomimetics. barbiturates, sedatives, alcohol, and antidiabetics may be enhanced. anticholinergic side effects are increased. Cheese, Bovril, Oxo, meat extracts, broad beans, banana, Marmite, yeast extracts, wine, beer, other alcohol, pickled herrings, vegetable proteins. (Up to 14 days after cessation.)

Priadel

A white, scored tablet supplied at strengths of 200 mg, 400 mg and used as a lithium salt to treat mania, manic depression, recurring depression, agression, and self-injuring behaviour.

Side effects: nausea, diarrhoea, hand tremor, muscular weakness, brain and heart disturbances, weight gain, fluid retention, under- or overactive thyroid, thirst and excessive urination, skin reactions. Your doctor may advise blood tests to gauge dose.
Caution: treatment should start in hospital. Kidney, heart, and thyroid function should be checked regularly. Salt and fluid consumption should be maintained.
Not to be used for: children, pregnant women, nursing mothers, or for patients suffering from Addison's disease, weak kidneys or heart, underactive thyroid, disturbed sodium balance.
Caution needed with: diuretics, non-steroid anti-inflammatory drugs, phenytoin, carbamazepine, flupenthixol, haloperidol, diazepam, methyldopa, tetracyclines.

Prothiaden

A red/brown capsule supplied at a strength of 25 mg and used as a tricyclic antidepressant to treat depression, anxiety.

Side effects: dry mouth, constipation, urine retention, blurred vision, palpitations, drowsiness, sleeplessness, dizziness, hands shaking, low blood presure, weight change, skin reactions, jaundice or blood changes, loss of libido may occur, weakness,

lack of co-ordination, convulsions, stomach upset, heart irregu-
larities.
Caution: in nursing mothers or in patients suffering from heart
disease, thyroid disease, epilepsy, diabetes, retention of urine,
liver disorder, adrenal tumour, some other psychiatric conditions.
Your doctor may advise regular blood tests.
Not to be used for: children, pregnant women, or for patients
suffering from heart attacks, liver disease, heart block.
Caution needed with: alcohol, anticholinergics, adrenaline,
MAOIs, barbiturates, other antidepressants, antihypertensives,
cimetidine, oestrogens.

Prozac

**A green/off-white capsule supplied at a strength of 20 mg and
used as an antidepressant to treat depression, bulimia nervosa (an eating disorder).**

Side effects: nausea, headache, anxiety, sleeplessness, dizziness,
rash, weakness, reduced judgement and abilities; rarely convulsions, hypomania, mania.
Caution: in pregnant women and in patients suffering from
unstable epilepsy, liver failure, moderate kidney failure, heart
disease, diabetes.
Not to be used for: children, nursing mothers, or for patients
suffering from severe kidney failure or allergy to fluoxetine.
Caution needed with: MAOIs, tryptophan (this is in many health
foods), lithium.

Serenace

**A green/pale-green capsule supplied at a strength of 0.5 mg
and used as a sedative for an additional treatment in the
short-term management of anxiety. (Serenace Tablets and
Liquid used to treat schizophrenia and behavioural disorders.)**

Side effects: muscle spasms, restlessness, hands shaking, constipation, blurred vision, dry mouth, urine retention, palpitations, low blood pressure, weight gain, changes in libido, low body temperature, breast swelling, menstrual changes, jaundice, blood and skin changes, drowsiness, rarely fits.

Caution: in pregnant women or in patients suffering from hyperthyroidism, liver or kidney failure, severe cardiovascular disease, tardive dyskinesia (a movement disorder), epilepsy.

Not to be used for: nursing mothers, unconscious patients, or for patients suffering from Parkinson's disease.

Caution needed with: alcohol, tranquillizers, pain killers, antihypertensives, antidepressants, anticonvulsants, antidiabetic drugs, levodopa.

Seroxat

A white, oval, scored tablet or a blue, oval, scored tablet according to strengths of 20 mg, 30 mg, and used as an antidepressant to treat depression and anxiety.

Side effects: nausea, sleepiness, sweating, tremor, tingling, dry mouth, insomnia, sexual disturbance.

Caution: in pregnant women, nursing mothers, and in patients suffering from severe kidney or liver damage, cardiovascular disease, epilepsy, or a history of mental disturbance.

Not to be used for: children.

Caution needed with: MAOIs, tryptophan, lithium, phenytoin, anticonvulsants, drugs affecting liver enzymes (eg barbiturates, carbamazepine, primidone, rifampicin, allopurinol, ciprofloxacin, cimetidine, erythromycin).

Stelazine

A blue tablet supplied at strengths of 1 mg, 5 mg and used as a sedative to treat anxiety, depression, agitation, schizophrenia, mental disorders, severe agitation, dangerous impulsive behaviour, nausea, vomiting.

Side effects: brain disturbances, dry mouth, blurred vision, ECG and hormone changes, allergies, impaired judgement and ability, rarely extrapyramidal symptoms (shaking and rigidity).

Caution: in the elderly, pregnant women, nursing mothers, and in patients suffering from undiagnosed vomiting, epilepsy, cardiovascular disease or Parkinson's disease. Your doctor may advise you to watch for loss of dexterity.

Not to be used for: patients in an unconscious state or patients suffering from liver disease, bone marrow depression.

Caution needed with: sedatives, alcohol, analgesics, antihypertensives.

Sulpitil

A white, scored tablet supplied at a strength of 200 mg and used as a sedative to treat schizophrenia.

Side effects: muscle spasms, restlessness, hands shaking, constipation, blurred vision, dry mouth, urine retention, palpitations, low blood pressure, weight gain, changes in libido, low body temperature, breast swelling, menstrual changes, jaundice, blood and skin changes, drowsiness, rarely fits.

Caution: in pregnant women and in patients suffering from hypertension, kidney disease, hypomania, or epilepsy

Not to be used for: children under 14 years or for patients suffering from phaeochromocytoma (a disease of the adrenal glands).

Caution needed with: alcohol, tranquillizers, pain killers, antihypertensives, antidepressants, anticonvulsants, antidiabetic drugs, levodopa.

Surmontil

A white tablet supplied at strengths of 10 mg, 25 mg and used as a tricyclic antidepressant to treat depression, anxiety, sleep disturbance, agitation.

Side effects: dry mouth, constipation, urine retention, blurred vision, palpitations, drowsiness, sleeplessness, dizziness, hands shaking, low blood presure, weight change, skin reactions, unsteadiness, convulsions, jaundice or blood changes. Loss of sexual desire may occur.

Caution: in nursing mothers or in patients suffering from adrenal tumour, heart or liver disease, thyroid disease, epilepsy, diabetes, some other psychiatric conditions. Your doctor may advise regular blood tests.

Not to be used for: children, pregnant women, or for patients suffering from heart attacks, liver disease, heart block.

Caution needed with: alcohol, anticholinergics, adrenaline, MAOIs, barbiturates, other antidepressants, antihypertensives, cimetidine, oestrogens.

Tofranil

A red-brown, triangular tablet or red-brown, round tablet according to strengths of 10 mg, 25 mg and used as a tricyclic antidepressant to treat depression, night-time bed wetting in children

Side effects: dry mouth, constipation, urine retention, blurred vision, palpitations, drowsiness, sleeplessness, dizziness, hands shaking, low blood presure, weight change, skin reactions, jaundice or blood changes. Loss of sexual desire may occur.

Caution: in nursing mothers or in patients suffering from heart disease, thyroid disease, epilepsy, diabetes, glaucoma, urine retention, some other psychiatric conditions. Your doctor may advise regular blood tests.

Not to be used for: children under 6 years, pregnant women, or for patients suffering from heart attacks, liver disease, heart block.

Caution needed with: alcohol, anticholinergics, adrenaline, MAOIs, barbiturates, other antidepressants, antihypertensives, cimetidine, oestrogens.

Triptafen

A pink tablet used as a tricyclic antidepressant to treat depression with anxiety.

Side effects: dry mouth, constipation, urine retention, blurred vision, palpitations, drowsiness, sleeplessness, dizziness, hands shaking, low blood presure, weight change, skin reactions, jaundice or blood changes. Loss of sexual desire may occur.

Caution: in nursing mothers and in patients suffering from Parkinson's disease, heart or liver disease, thyroid disorder, adrenal tumour, diabetes, glaucoma, urine retention, epilepsy.

Not to be used for: children or for patients suffering from bone marrow depression, heart attack, heart block, severe liver disease.

Caution needed with: alcohol, anticholinergics, adrenaline, MAOIs, barbiturates, other antidepressants, antihypertensives, cimetidine, oestrogens.

Chapter 15

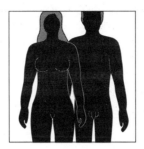

Generalized Infections

Please refer to 'Important Advice' on page 4 at the beginning of this book; and remember, if you are in any doubt, consult a physician.

Many of the infections covered in this book relate to specific organ sites but, occasionally, an infection may affect the whole body. Septicaemia is a blood-borne infection that affects the whole body, as is malaria. Many virus infections – particularly conditions such as mumps, measles, and chicken-pox – affect the entire body and we have covered these elsewhere. These conditions may all be asymptomatic, i.e. they may be carried by a person who does not have symptoms but who may still be able to pass on the infection to others. Within this chapter we will also cover virus diseases such as glandular fever which are blood-borne viruses affecting many parts of the body.

Malaria

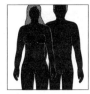 Malaria is an infection caused by a protozoan carried by insects, namely the mosquito. Infection is commonly contracted in tropical areas where there is poor sanitation, but the symptoms can appear at any time thereafter.

Symptoms
The symptoms are similar to those of severe influenza, and the diagnosis can often be missed. Fever, shaking, headache, pains in the limbs, abdominal pain, weakness, depression, tiredness, are all symptoms of malaria. Malaria may be mild and recurrent or it may progress to a severe state with haemorrhage, kidney failure, brain haemorrhage, and death.

Action
If you suspect malaria, you should seek immediate medical advice by a specialist in tropical medicine.

Tests
Blood tests to look for malaria parasites can make the diagnosis. Other tests for severe infections might be helpful.

Medications and treatment
Antimalarial drugs, such as pymethamine or chloroquine, are used in the management of the acute case. These and other drugs are also used as preventative measures taken before travelling to potential malaria areas. Avloclor, Daraprim, Fansidar, Halfan, Lariam, Maloprim, Nivaquine, Paludrine.

Further advice
Malaria is normally prevented by taking antimalarial medication prior to, and for four weeks after, a visit to a malaria area. The type of medication taken depends on the area, and updated reports of required medication can be obtained from tropical medicine institutes.

Associated conditions

Tropical diseases include a number of insect-borne infections, such as lyme disease, rocky mountain spotted fever, and a number of other protozoal diseases and infections caused by bathing in or drinking infected water. Any infection in someone who has returned from a tropical country should be investigated for full tropical screen.

Septicaemia

 Septicaemia is a condition of generalized infection. Theoretically, any bacterium or fungus can affect the blood stream, usually in unwell or immuno-compromised patients. Toxic shock can occur in patients who have infection with certain types of gram-negative bacteria. These can occasionally be caused by infected tampons.

Symptoms

The symptoms for septicaemia are similar to those of influenza with fever, headache, shaking, chills, weakness, collapse, and death.

Action

Where septicaemia is suspected, urgent medical attention is required.

Tests

Blood cultures can help to diagnose the infecting agent and help with instituting appropriate treatment.

Medications and treatment

Antibacterial, antifungal medication should be given, usually by intravenous infusion. Monoclonal antibodies are available for treatment of gram-negative toxic shock.

Further advice
Septicaemia can be prevented in hospitals by adequate aseptic techniques and by awareness of the likelihood of diagnosis so that early treatment can be instituted.

Associated conditions
Bacterial endocarditis may be associated with septicaemia.

HIV infection and AIDS

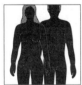 The human immuno-deficiency virus is normally a blood-borne virus which, after many years of infection, causes acquired immune deficiency syndrome (AIDS). The virus can be transmitted by unprotected (particularly rectal) intercourse, by blood products, and by infected needles. It is found in all ages and groups of patients (including newborn children who catch it from their infected mothers), but the nature of transmission makes it common in haemophiliacs, needle-sharing drug addicts, and male homosexual patients.

Symptoms
There are almost certainly no symptoms of acquiring HIV infection, although some patients have reported the presence of a rash after accidental needlestick injuries carrying the HIV virus. The period of asymptomatic presentation may persist for many years and varies from patient to patient, but the symptoms of AIDS include weakness, fatigue, muscle loss, weight loss, opportunistic infections particularly with fungi such as oral thrush, oesophageal thrush, pneumocystis infections in the lung, septicaemia, endocarditis, and central nervous system effects including dementia, with a gradual progression to death.

Action

Specialist medical advice should be sought where HIV or AIDS is suspected.

Tests

HIV antibody tests on blood can be reported within a few hours. Tests for AIDS would include checking for opportunistic infections and for the presence of activity of T-lymphocytes.

Medications and treatment

Opportunistic infections need to be treated with appropriate antiviral, antifungal, or antibacterial medications. Retrovir is an antiviral drug which has been used in HIV-infected patients to delay progression to AIDS although this is still under research. A number of other interesting antiviral drugs are under development.

Further advice

Prevention of HIV transmission is important, and advice on the use of condoms, safe sex, use of clean needles, and testing of blood products is important.

Associated conditions

There are almost certainly at least two types of HIV virus. Patients presenting with HIV infections may also have other venereal diseases or other blood-borne viruses such as hepatitis.

Other virus infections ♥♥
including Epstein-Barr virus and infectious
mononucleosis (glandular fever)

Virus infections, such as measles and chickenpox, have been covered in the section on skin disorders. Glandular fever and Epstein-Barr viruses are common causes of minor virus infections. But they are most commonly associated with a severe post-viral syndrome, sometimes known as myalgic encephalomyelitis (ME) or yuppie flu (*see* above).

Symptoms

The symptoms of glandular fever include swollen glands, sore throat, vomiting, severe headache, general debility, occasionally skin rash particularly where an ampicillin has been used, and occasionally swelling of the liver and spleen with jaundice and intolerance of alcohol. Epstein-Barr virus is similar but the symptoms are often not as severe. The symptoms of ME include profound lethargy, weakness, depression, with aches in the muscles.

Tests

There are specific blood tests to look for Epstein-Barr and glandular fever (infectious mononucleosis) viruses. A Paul Burnell test is specific for glandular fever. Clinical examination will reveal enlargement of glands and occasionally liver and spleen. Liver function tests may be carried out. A similar picture can be obtained with the Epstein-Barr virus. ME is difficult to diagnose on specific testing, and the diagnosis is often made by clinical history.

Action

These conditions will often resolve without specific medication, and supportive therapy can include non-alcoholic fluids and analgesics, such as aspirin and paracetamol. If symptoms persist or are severe, you should seek medical advice.

Medications and treatment

Apart from general supportive treatment, antidepressant medication may be helpful in ME. High doses of vitamins and minerals such as magnesium may be helpful in the treatment of prolonged post-viral symptoms.

Further advice

These viruses may be transmitted by oral contact, such as kissing and probably through infected saliva transmitted by sneezing. There are no vaccines available to prevent their spread.

Associated conditions

There is a number of other virus conditions which may appear with similar symptoms but, in general, these conditions are self-limiting and improve after seven to ten days.

Prescription Medicines

Avloclor

A white, scored tablet supplied at a strength of 250 mg and used as an antimalarial, amoebicide preparation for the prevention of malaria, and the treatment of hepatitis, amoebiasis.

Side effects: headache, stomach upset, skin eruptions, hair loss, blurred vision, eye damage, blood disorders, loss of pigments.
Caution: in pregnant women, nursing mothers, and in patients suffering from porphyria (a rare blood disorder), kidney or liver disease, or psoriasis. Your doctor may advise regular eye tests before and during treatment.
Not to be used for:
Caution needed with:

Daraprim

A white, scored tablet supplied at a strength of 25 mg and used as an antimalarial drug for the prevention of malaria.

Side effects: rash, anaemia.
Caution: in pregnant women, nursing mothers, and in patients suffering from liver or kidney disease.
Not to be used for: children under 5 years.
Caution needed with: co-trimoxazole, lorazepam.

Fansidar

A white, quarter-scored tablet used as a sulphonamide for the prevention and treatment of malaria.

Side effects: rash, inflammation of the pharynx, itch, stomach upset, rare skin and blood changes.
Caution: patients should keep out of the sun. Your doctor may advise regular blood tests if the treatment is prolonged.
Not to be used for: new-born infants, pregnant women, nursing mothers or for patients suffering from severe kidney or liver disease, or sensitivity to sulphonamides.
Caution needed with: trimethoprim.

Halfan

A white, scored, capsule-shaped tablet used to treat malaria.

Side effects: stomach upset, abdominal pain, blood changes.
Caution: in women of child-bearing age, and in patients suffering from complicated malarial conditions, or malaria involving the brain.
Not to be used for: children under 37 kg body weight, pregnant women, nursing mothers, or for preventing malaria.
Caution needed with:

Lariam

A white, quarter-scored tablet supplied at a strength of 250 mg, and used to treat and prevent malaria.

Side effects: dizziness, nausea, vomiting, stomach upset, loss of appetite, headache, slow pulse rate, skin changes, psychological changes.
Caution: in patients suffering from heart conduction disorders. Women must use reliable contraception during treatment and for 3 months afterwards.
Not to be used for: pregnant women, nursing mothers, or for patients suffering from liver or kidney damage, or history of

psychiatric disorder or convulsions.
Caution needed with: quinine, sodium valproate, typhoid vaccination.

Maloprim

A white, scored tablet used as a sulphone preparation for the prevention of malaria.

Side effects: blood disorders, sensitive skin.
Caution: in pregnant women, nursing mothers, and in patients suffering from liver or kidney disease.
Not to be used for:
Caution needed with: trimethoprim.

Nivaquine

A yellow tablet supplied at a strength of 200 mg and used as an antimalarial drug for the prevention and treatment of malaria, and to treat rheumatoid arthritis.

Side effects: headache, stomach upset, skin eruptions, hair loss, eye disorders, blood disorders, loss of pigment, allergy.
Caution: in pregnant women, nursing mothers, or in patients suffering from porphyria (a rare blood disorder), kidney or liver disease, severe gastro-intestinal, nervous, or blood disorder, psoriasis or history of epilepsy. The eyes should be tested before and during prolonged treatment.
Not to be used for:
Caution needed with:

Paludrine

A white, scored tablet supplied at a strength of 100 mg and used as an antimalarial drug for the prevention of malaria.

Side effects: stomach upset, skin reactions, hair loss, mouth ulcers.

Caution: in patients suffering from severe kidney failure.
Not to be used for:
Caution needed with:

Chapter 16

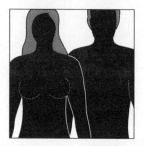

Endocrine Disorders

Please refer to 'Important Advice' on page 4 at the beginning of this book; and remember, if you are in any doubt, consult a physician.

Careful control of many functions of the body relies on a number of powerful peptides called hormones. These are released by endocrine glands which appear in various sites of the body. The pancreas is an endocrine gland that secretes insulin and other hormones such as glucagon. The pituitary gland controls other endocrine glands and, on its own, secretes hormones such as oxytocin and vasopresin. The thyroid gland in the neck secretes thyroid hormone, and the nearby parathyroid glands secrete a substance that controls calcium level in the body. The adrenal glands, next to the kidney, produce cortisone, adrenalin, and other related hormones.

The main problem with these endocrine glands is that they can overproduce or underproduce. Classically, diabetes mellitus results when there is an underproduction of insulin, and a similar pattern exists for most of the other endocrine glands. The most common overproduction of hormones seen clinically is thyrotoxicosis where there is overproduction of thyroxin from the thyroid gland. In general terms, the management of these conditions is relatively straightforward with replacement hormones being given for underactivity, but they have such profound metabolic effects that they often appear with complex and difficult medical problems.

Diabetes mellitus   ♥♥

 Diabetes mellitus is a condition caused by inter-
action of genetic, viral, and possibly dietary
components resulting in failure of the pancreas
gland to produce enough insulin. Type 1 diabetes
occurs usually in young adults who require insulin, whereas type 2 diabetes occurs in the older age group who
may be maintained on diet and tablets alone.

Symptoms

These include weight loss, thirst, passing a lot of urine,
infections especially of the urine and genitalia and
particularly with thrush or other fungi, weakness,
tiredness, loss of concentration, poor performance at
work or school, loss of libido, impotence, infertility.
Diabetes may be symptomless and may be detected
on routine blood or urine examination. Progressive
deterioration of diabetes, with elevation of blood sugar
and ketones in the blood (ketoacidosis), may eventually
lead to hyperglycaemic coma and death. Hypoglycaemia (low blood
sugar) may occur when the treatment of diabetes with excess insulin
or tablets results in a low blood sugar, and this too may appear with
unconsciousness or coma.

Action

Where diabetes is suspected, urgent medical attention is required,
particularly for diabetic coma states. Appropriate first aid depends
on whether the blood sugar is high or low. If in doubt, assume the
blood sugar is low and treat patients with glucose tablets or an oral
solution of sweet tea to elevate blood sugar. Glucagon injections
may be given.

Tests

The tests for diabetes include measurement of blood and urine sugar.
Urine tests can also be carried out to look for protein and ketones.
Blood tests can look for the presence of acidosis and other factors

contributing to a deterioration and state of dehydration. Glycosylated haemoglobin tests can check the control of diabetes.

Medications and treatment

The treatment of hypoglycaemia includes the administration of glucose or glucagon as indicated above. The treatment of diabetes involves the use of diet, tablets such as metformin or glibenclamide, and insulin preparations. Diabenese, Diamicron, Daonil, Glibenese, Glucophage, Glurenorm, Rastinon.

Further advice

The management of diabetes involves specialist advice, particularly from dietitians. The pattern of insulin, food, and exercise needs to be adjusted. Self-monitoring of blood sugar and urine is important in maintaining the condition and making appropriate adjustments in treatment.

Associated conditions

Diabetes insipidus is a rare condition where brain damage destroys the production of vasopressin from the pituitary gland in the brain. The symptoms are thirst and the passing of a great deal of urine, but blood and urine tests do not show elevated sugar. Treatment is by the administration of synthetic vasopressin analogues. Hypercalcaemia may also appear with thirst and passing a lot of urine. This is usually associated with disease of the parathyroid glands. Similarly, diseases of the parathyroid may appear with hypocalcaemia where the patients may develop muscular spasms due to a lack of calcium in the circulation.

Disorders of the pituitary gland

 The pituitary gland is situated just below the brain. It controls many hormonal functions in the body including the thyroid growth hormones, sex hormones, and the hormones of the posterior pituitary gland (*see* diabetes insipidus above)

The pituitary gland can be damaged or destroyed by trauma or by tumour. Tumours of the pituitary gland may produce excess hormone or may destroy the controls of the other hormonal systems.

Symptoms

The symptoms of pituitary disease include a lack of pituitary function where the tumour has destroyed the pituitary gland. Thus, patients will develop symptoms of underactive thyroid gland (*see* below), failure of ovulation with infertility, amenorrhoea, and impotence (due to lack of sex hormones), and collapse and wasting similar to Addison's disease (*see* below) due to lack of cortisone in the blood. Occasionally, excess hormone is produced by the pituitary gland, the most common of which is excess growth hormone resulting in a condition known as gigantism or acromegaly with overgrowth of the bones and jaw. Destruction of the posterior pituitary gland not only causes diabetes insipidus (*see* above) but also failure of lactation.

Action

Where pituitary failure or hyperactivity is suspected medical advice should be sought as soon as possible.

Tests

Pituitary function tests include routine blood tests for levels of hormones such as thyroid, oestrogen, testosterone, growth hormone, and insulin stress test for the ability of the pituitary gland to produce growth hormone in response to stress.

Medications and treatment

Excess growth hormone or prolactin production may respond to drugs such as bromocriptine, but often surgery is needed to remove tumours of the pituitary gland, thereby treating gigantism or acromegaly. Underactive pituitary glands necessitate treatment of the cause as well as replacement of hormones, particularly cortisone and thyroxine. Children will also need growth hormone supplements. Additional hormones will be required for the treatment of impotence and infertility.

Further advice

Insulin stress tests need to be carried out with caution. Overactive pituitary glands may also cause diabetes.

Disorders of the adrenal glands

 The adrenal gland is an endocrine gland which is located above the kidney. Its function is controlled partially by the pituitary hormones. Overactivity of the adrenal gland can result in Cushing's syndrome, phaeochromocytoma, or Conn's syndrome. Underactivity of the pituitary gland results in Addison's disease.

Symptoms

The symptoms of Addison's disease include weakness, weight loss, lethargy, pigmentation of the skin, drop in blood pressure, and eventually collapse and death. It is caused by an absence of cortisone due to failure of the adrenal glands. The cause of this adrenal failure may be tumour or tuberculosis of the adrenal gland, or occasionally wasting of the adrenal gland due to overuse of steroids. Addison's disease may appear as a separate entity in itself with possibly an auto-immune destructive element of the adrenal gland. Cushing's and Conn's syndrome are due to excess corticoid drugs. Cushing's syndrome presents with obesity, stretch marks, diabetes, high blood pressure, and cataracts, and is due to excess cortisone. Conn's syndrome presents with elevated blood pressure and potassium and is due to excess mineralocorticoids. Phaeochromocytoma, due to excess adrenaline, presents with hypertension which may be spasmodic. It is worth noting that the weakness in Addison's disease may be due to a low blood potassium (hypokalaemia).

Action
Where adrenal disorders are suspected, urgent medical attention is required.

Tests
Blood tests include measurements of potassium and sodium, adrenaline, and urine tests for hormones and their breakdown products. Clinical examination will reveal typical features of the condition concerned. X-rays of the pituitary and adrenal glands may help make the diagnosis, and adrenal function tests, such as using ACTH, will determine whether there is functioning adrenal capacity present.

Medications and treatment
Surgical treatment may be required for conditions such as phaeochromocytoma, Cushing's, or Conn's disease. Underactive adrenal glands in Addison's disease can be treated by the administration of replacement hormones usually by mouth.

Further advice
Continued monitoring is required to establish that adequate replacement therapy has been given. Where oral steroids are being used in high doses for other conditions, the possibility of shrinkage of the adrenal glands should always be borne in mind.

Diseases of the thyroid gland

 The thyroid gland controls the rate of metabolism of the body, and an underactive thyroid gland (myxoedema or hypothyroidism) produces a slow, sluggish metabolism whereas an overactive thyroid gland (thyrotoxicosis or hyperthyroidism) will produce a fast metabolism.

Symptoms
The symptoms of an underactive thyroid gland are coldness, tiredness, weight gain, depression, sleepiness, loss of hair particularly

from the eyebrows, dry skin, elevated cholesterol, heart disease, carpal tunnel syndrome, anaemia, and infertility. The symptoms of an overactive thyroid gland are anxiety, hypertension, weight loss, excessive appetite, sweating, rapid pulse, and insomnia.

Action
Either of these conditions may come on insidiously without being noticed by the patient's friends or relatives. Where suspected, medical attention should be sought as soon as possible.

Tests
Thyroid function tests and other routine blood tests including full blood count will make the diagnosis. Examination of the thyroid gland itself to look for goitres, cysts, or tumours, is important, using clinical examination and other means such as ultrasound. Pituitary function might also need to be investigated.

Medications and treatment
Myxoedema is easily treated with thyroid replacement Tertroxin or Eltroxin. An overactive thyroid may respond to a single dose of radioactive thyroxine, or surgery may be necessary, particularly where a cyst or tumour needs to be removed. Carbimazole may also be used to treat an overactive thyroid.

Further advice
Continuous assessment may be required to establish the correct dose of treatment. An overactive thyroid gland may often swing to be underactive during or after treatment.

Disorders of lipid metabolism

There are rare lipid storage diseases, such as Gaucher's disease, which normally affect children. In adults, the most common problems are elevation of cholesterol and triglycerides, usually as part of an inherited disorder but sometimes due to outside factors, such as alcohol or poor diet.

Symptoms

Usually none, but it may appear with heart disease such as angina or heart attack. Deposits of lipid around the eyes or joints may be noticeable. Furring up of peripheral arteries may appear with intermittent claudication (limping).

Action

A low-fat diet is important but, where a serious lipid disorder is suspected, medical advice should be sought.

Tests

Heart and blood tests for HDL and LDL cholesterol, as well as triglycerides, are important. Other conditions, such as an underactive thyroid gland, may produce elevation of lipids and these should also be checked.

Medications and treatment

Apart from weight loss and diet, there is a number of medications, particularly the more recently developed drugs, such as Zocor, which lower cholesterol levels. Atromid-S, Bezalip-Mono, Bradilan, Colestid, Lipantil, Lipostat, Lopid, Lurselle, Maxepa, Modalim, Olbetam, Questran-A, Zocor.

Further advice

It is important to drink less alcohol to control elevated lipids. Relatives of patients with elevated lipids should be screened to be checked for familial problems.

Prescription Medicines

Atromid-S

A red capsule supplied at a strength of 500 mg and used as a lipid-lowering agent to treat elevated cholesterol.

Caution: in patients with low serum proteins. Your doctor may advise diet and other changes in lifestyle as well as regular blood tests.
Not to be used for: children, pregnant women, or for patients with a history of gall bladder problems or kidney or liver disease.
Caution needed with: anticoagulants, antidiabetic drugs, phenytoin.

Bezalip-Mono

A white tablet supplied at a strength of 400 mg and used as a lipid-lowering drug to treat high blood lipids.

Side effects: stomach upset, muscle aches, rash.
Caution: in patients with kidney disease. Your doctor may advise change in diet or lifestyle.
Not to be used for: children, pregnant women, nursing mothers, or for patients suffering from severe kidney or liver disease.
Caution needed with: anticoagulants, antidiabetics, MAOIs.

Bradilan

A white tablet supplied at a strength of 250 mg and used as a vasodilator to treat peripheral vascular problems including intermittent difficulty walking, night cramps, chilblains, Raynaud's phenomenon (spasm of the arteries), some brain disorders. Also used to control high blood lipids.

Side effects: flushes.
Caution:
Not to be used for: children.
Caution needed with:

Colestid

Granules in sachets containing 5 g used as a lipid-lowering agent to reduce lipids.

Side effects: constipation.
Caution: in pregnant women, nursing mothers. Vitamin A, D, and K supplements should be taken.
Not to be used for: patients suffering from complete biliary blockage.
Caution needed with: digoxin, antibiotics, diuretics. Take any other drugs 1 hour before or 4 hours after Colestid.

Daonil

A white, oblong, scored tablet supplied at a strength of 5 mg and used as an antidiabetic drug to treat diabetes.

Side effects: allergy including skin rash.
Caution: in the elderly and in patients suffering from kidney failure.
Not to be used for: children, pregnant women, nursing mothers, during surgery, or for patients suffering from juvenile diabetes, liver or kidney impairment, hormone disorders, stress, infections.
Caution needed with: ß-blockers, MAOIs, steroids, diuretics, alcohol, the contraceptive pill, anticoagulants, lipid-lowering agents, aspirin, antibiotics (rifampicin, sulphonamides antibiotics, chloramphenicol), glucagon, cyclophosphamide.

Diabinese

A white, scored tablet supplied at strengths of 100 mg, 250 mg and used as an antidiabetic treatment for diabetes.

Side effects: allergy, including skin rash.
Caution: in the elderly and in patients suffering from kidney failure.
Not to be used for: children, pregnant women, nursing mothers, during surgery, or for patients suffering from juvenile diabetes,

liver or kidney disorders, stress, infections.
Caution needed with: ß-blockers, MAOIs, steroids, diuretics, alcohol, anticoagulants, lipid-lowering agents, aspirin, some antibiotics (rifampicin, sulphonamides, chloramphenicol), glucagon, cyclophosphamide, the contraceptive pill.

Diamicron

A white, scored tablet supplied at a strength of 80 mg and used as an anti-diabetic treatment for diabetes.

Side effects: allergy, including skin rash.
Caution: in the elderly and in patients suffering from kidney failure.
Not to be used for: children, pregnant women, nursing mothers, during surgery, or for patients suffering from juvenile diabetes, liver or kidney disorders, stress, infections.
Caution needed with: ß-blockers, MAOIs, steroids, diuretics, alcohol, anticoagulants, lipid-lowering agents, aspirin, some antibiotics (rifampicin, sulphonamides, chloramphenicol), glucagon, cyclophosphamide, the contraceptive pill.

Glibenese

A white, oblong, scored tablet supplied at a strength of 5 mg and used as a sulphonylurea to treat diabetes.

Side effects: allergy including skin rash.
Caution: in the elderly and in patients suffering from kidney failure.
Not to be used for: children, pregnant women, nursing mothers, during surgery, or for patients suffering from juvenile diabetes, liver or kidney impairment, hormone disorders, stress, infections.
Caution needed with: ß-blockers, MAOIs, steroids, diuretics, alcohol, anticoagulants, lipid-lowering agents, aspirin, some antibiotics (rifampicin, sulphonamides, chloramphenicol), glucagon, cyclophosphamide, the contraceptive pill.

Glucophage

A white tablet supplied at strengths of 500 mg, 850 mg and used as an antidiabetic to treat diabetes.

Side effects: allergy including skin rash, rarely acidosis (a metabolic disorder).
Caution: in the elderly and in patients suffering from kidney failure.
Not to be used for: children, pregnant women, nursing mothers, during pregnancy, or for patients suffering from juvenile diabetes, liver or kidney impairment, hormone disorders, stress, infections.
Caution needed with: ß-blockers, MAOIs, steroids, diuretics, alcohol, anticoagulants, lipid-lowering agents, aspirin, some antibiotics (rifampicin, sulphonamides, chloramphenicol), glucagon, cyclophosphamide, the contraceptive pill.

Glurenorm

A white, scored tablet supplied at a strength of 30 mg and used as an antidiabetic to treat diabetes.

Side effects: allergy including skin rash.
Caution: in the elderly and in patients suffering from kidney failure.
Not to be used for: children, pregnant women, nursing mothers, during surgery, or for patients suffering from juvenile diabetes, liver or kidney impairment, hormone disorders, stress, infections.
Caution needed with: ß-blockers, MAOIs, steroids, diuretics, alcohol, anticoagulants, lipid-lowering agents, aspirin, some antibiotics (rifampicin, sulphonamides, chloramphenicol), glucagon, cyclophosphamide, the contraceptive pill.

Lipantil

A white capsule supplied at a strength of 100 mg and used as a lipid-lowering agent to lower cholesterol or triglycerides.

Side effects: stomach upset, dizziness, headache, tiredness, rashes.
Caution: in patients suffering from kidney impairment.
Not to be used for: pregnant women, nursing mothers, or for patients suffering from severe kidney or liver problems, gall bladder disease.
Caution needed with: anticoagulants, phenylbutazone, antidiabetic drugs taken by mouth.

Lipostat

A pink, oblong tablet supplied at a strength of 10 mg, 20 mg, and used as a lipid-lowering agent to treat raised cholesterol.

Side effects: rash, muscle pain, headache, chest pain, nausea, vomiting, diarrhoea, tiredness.
Caution: in patients with a history of liver disease. Your doctor may advise regular tests during treatment.
Not to be used for: children, pregnant women, nursing mothers, or for patients suffering from liver disease.
Caution needed with: cholestyramine, colestipol.

Lopid

A white/maroon capsule and white oval tablet supplied at strengths of 300 mg, 600 mg and used as a lipid-lowering agent to treat raised lipid levels.

Side effects: stomach upset, rashes, impotence, headache, dizziness, painful extremities, muscle aches, blurred vision.
Caution: your doctor may advise a lipid check; blood count, and liver function should be checked before treatment; eyes, blood, and serum should be checked regularly.
Not to be used for: pregnant women, nursing mothers, alcoholics, or patients suffering from gallstones or liver disease.
Caution needed with: anticoagulants.

Lurselle

A white, scored tablet supplied at a strength of 250 mg and used as a lipid-lowering agent to treat elevated lipids.

Side effects: diarrhoea, stomach upset.
Caution: in patients suffering from heart disorders. Cease treatment 6 months before a planned pregnancy.
Not to be used for: children, pregnant women, or nursing mothers.
Caution needed with:

Maxepa

A clear, soft capsule used as a lipid-lowering agent to treat elevated lipids.

Side effects: nausea, belching
Caution: in patients suffering from bleeding disorders.
Not to be used for: children.
Caution needed with: anticoagulants.

Modalim

A white, capsule-shaped tablet supplied at a strength of 100 mg and used to treat high blood lipid levels which cannot be controlled by diet alone.

Side effects: headache, vertigo, rash, stomach upset, muscle pain, impotence, hair loss, dizziness, drowsiness.
Caution: in patients suffering from liver or kidney disease.
Not to be used for: children, pregnant women, nursing mothers, or for patients suffering from severe liver or kidney disease.
Caution needed with: anticoagulants, antidiabetics, the contraceptive pill.

Olbetam

A red-brown/dark-pink capsule supplied at a strength of 250

mg and used as a lipid-lowering agent to treat elevated lipids.

Side effects: flushes, rash, redness, stomach upset, headache, general feeling of being unwell.
Caution:
Not to be used for: children, pregnant women, nursing mothers, or for patients suffering from stomach ulcer.
Caution needed with:

Questran

A powder in a sachet used as a lipid-lowering agent to treat elevated lipids, and to relieve some cases of diarrhoea and itching.

Side effects: constipation, vitamin K deficiency.
Caution: in pregnant women, nursing mothers, and patients on long-term treatment should take Vitamin A, D, K supplements.
Not to be used for: children under 6 years or for patients suffering from complete biliary blockage.
Caution needed with: digoxin, antibiotics, diuretics; allow 1 hour between treatment and any other drugs.

Rastinon

A white, scored tablet supplied at a strength of 500 mg and used as an antidiabetic treatment for diabetes.

Side effects: allergy including skin rash.
Caution: in the elderly and in patients suffering from kidney failure.
Not to be used for: children, pregnant women, nursing mothers, during surgery, or for patients suffering from juvenile diabetes, liver or kidney disorders, stress, infections, endocrine disorder.
Caution needed with: ß-blockers, MAOIs, steroids, diuretics, alcohol, anticoagulants, lipid-lowering agents, aspirin, some antibiotics (rifampicin, sulphonamides, chloramphenicol), glucagon, cyclophosphamide, the contraceptive pill.

Zocor

A peach-coloured, oval tablet or a tan, oval tablet according to strengths of 10 mg, 20 mg and used as a lipid-lowering agent to treat raised cholesterol.

Side effects: headache, indigestion, diarrhoea, tiredness, rash, constipation, wind, nausea, muscle weakness.
Caution: in patients suffering from liver disease. Your doctor may advise liver and eye checks.
Not to be used for: pregnant women, nursing mothers, or for patients suffering from liver disease.
Caution needed with: digoxin, some anticoagulants, cyclosporin, gemifibrozil, nicotinic acid.

Chapter 17

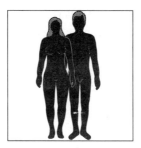

General Conditions

Please refer to 'Important Advice' on page 4 at the beginning of this book; and remember, if you are in any doubt, consult a physician.

Allergies are very common and are a product of our need to protect ourselves against the outside world. Thus, our defence mechanism, designed to protect against invasion, occasionally reacts against non-harmful substances, e.g. grass pollen, producing the common allergy known as hay fever. Very occasionally, profound and severe allergy to substances that enter the body when, for example, a bee stings, may occur with the result that the patient collapses in anaphylactic shock. It is clear from the complex nature of our environment, as well as the pollutants that occur in it, that allergies are becoming more common and, therefore, a greater clinical challenge.

This defence mechanism occasionally turns in on itself resulting in auto-immune disorders, where the body destroys its own tissues using its own antibodies. These often appear with complex and dangerous clinical conditions that are difficult to identify and even harder to treat.

Anaphylactic shock and allergy

The cause of allergy is not known but the body does produce antibodies as a protective mechanism. Sometimes, these cause harm by provoking an allergy. Severe allergy may cause anaphylactic shock.

Symptoms

The symptoms of anaphylactic shock are collapse with swelling of the lips and tongue, difficulty in breathing, and generalized oedema. This may occur in response to a sudden allergy, particularly to a wasp or bee sting. Other allergies, such as hay fever, appear with a runny nose, whereas penicillin and drug allergies often appear with skin rashes. Itchy skin and swelling of any part of the body may also be part of the presentation of allergic disorders.

Action

Severe anaphylactic shock requires emergency medical treatment. Many patients carry emergency medications for this purpose. Medical advice should be sought as soon as possible. Other allergies may respond to self-medication with antihistamines.

Tests

Skin tests and blood tests may be carried out to determine the cause of the allergy and an exact profile of what the patient is allergic to. Allergies run in families and many people are allergic to a large number of extraneous substances.

Medications and treatment

The emergency treatment of anaphylactic shock includes the use of steroids, adrenaline, antihistamines, and other measures for resuscitation if cardiac arrest occurs. Allergies usually respond to antihistamines, and occasionally steroids may be required.

Further advice

Try to avoid those factors to which you are allergic. If you suffer from severe allergies and you are prone to anaphylactic shock you should equip yourself with a self-medication kit.

Auto-immune disorders

There is a number of auto-immune disorders which have been referred to above. Thyroid disease, adrenal disease, and diabetes may all be caused by the destruction of the body by itself. There is a number of conditions which are also classified as auto-immune that are, in effect, multisystem disorders affecting many parts of the body. These include scleroderma, systemic lupus erythematosus (SLE), and polyarteritis nodosa. SLE is related to arthritis; it is an auto-immune disorder that destroys tissues in the skin, joints, lungs, and heart.

Symptoms

The symptoms of systemic lupus erythematosus include skin rash, particularly across the bridge of the nose and the cheeks, and arthritis. The condition may also cause fibrosis of the lungs, damage to the kidneys, and the heart valves. Like scleroderma it may also cause an arthritis, particularly of the small joints of the hand. Scleroderma is similar and usually presents with tight skin, particularly around the mouth and joints. Polyarteritis nodosa is a condition where painful nodules appear, particularly in the legs and especially in men. It may affect the testes and may result in testicular failure.

Action

Minor degrees of arthritis will respond to self-medication, but, where suspected, these conditions need to be investigated and diagnosed.

Tests

Biopsies may be necessary to make the diagnosis definitively. Blood tests include looking at the sedimentation rate and other measures of auto-immune function.

Medications and treatment
These conditions respond to anti-inflammatory drugs and to steroids.

Associated conditions
Raynaud's syndrome may be a precursor of conditions such as SLE or scleroderma. It presents with severe chilblains of the hand brought about by spasm of the arteries.

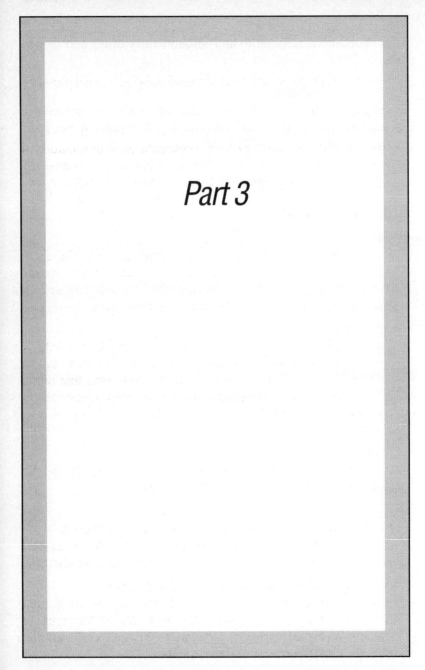

Part 3

Glossary

Words in SMALL CAPITAL letters are defined elsewhere in the glossary.

abortion
> loss of foetus, where a foetus is an unborn child of up to 28 weeks of pregnancy. Abortion may be therapeutic as in termination of pregnancy or spontaneous (often described as a miscarriage). After 28 weeks of pregnancy, loss of a child is considered to be a stillbirth. Example: spontaneous abortion may occur if the foetus is abnormal.

abscess
> collection of infection and PUS. The abscess may often be under pressure and the infection has usually arrived from an external source. Abscesses generally need to be drained. Example: a perinephric abscess is an infection near the KIDNEY.

ACE inhibitor
> an ACE inhibitor is an Angiotension-Converting ENZYME inhibitor. An angiotension-converting ENZYME is a PROTEIN in the KIDNEY which enables the production of a HORMONE that raises blood pressure. By inhibiting this enzyme it can reduce blood pressure. Example: blood pressure may be reduced by captopril, an ACE inhibitor.

ACTH
> Adreno-CorticoTrophic Hormone. a substance secreted by the pituitary GLAND to control the adrenal CORTEX.

acute
> of short duration. It does not mean severe, although acute illnesses may also be severe, hence the confusion. Example: acute bronchitis usually resolves in a few days. *See also* **chronic**.

AIDS (Acquired Immune Deficiency Syndrome)
> this is a collection of symptoms and signs caused by human immuno-deficiency VIRUS HIV. The virus attacks the immune system and leaves patients open to infections. Example: candida infections often occur in AIDS patients.

anaemia

inadequate blood. Low HAEMOGLOBIN, the iron-containing pigment which carries oxygen in the RED BLOOD CELLS, is a sign of anaemia. Example: poor diet may lead to iron-deficiency anaemia.

anaesthetic

a drug which relieves pain. An anaesthetic may be applied locally or generally when the patient is put to sleep during an operation. Example: lignocaine is a local anaesthetic.

analgesic

a painkiller. A number of medications have pain-killing properties as well as other effects, such as being ANTI-INFLAMMATORIES. Example: aspirin has analgesic properties.

aneurysm

blood vessel swelling. Weakness of the blood vessel wall can result in a swelling or dilation. This can occur in the blood vessels in the brain or in the large vessels near the heart, such as the AORTA. Example: an aortic aneurysm may burst and simulate a heart attack.

angiogram

see **arteriography**

angioplasty

unblocking an ARTERY in the heart. During X-RAY of the arteries around the heart, a balloon can be inserted to push open any blockage in the coronary arteries. Example: angioplasty is one of the treatments for angina.

antibiotic

a drug which kills BACTERIA. Some antibiotics are very specific (narrow-spectrum) while others kill a wide range of bacteria and are considered to be broad-spectrum antibiotics. Antibiotics are of no value in the treatment of VIRUS infections such as the common cold or influenza. Example: tetracycline is a broad-spectrum antibiotic.

antibody

an antibody is a PROTEIN, produced by the body, that is specific for certain infections or toxic substances. Example; a second infection of measles is uncommon because there are circulating antibodies produced in response to the first infection.

anticoagulant

a blood-thinning agent. Anticoagulants are used where there is a clotting tendency as in PULMONARY EMBOLUS or after surgery. Example: warfarin is an anticoagulant.

anticholinesterase

an ENZYME that prevents the breakdown of chemical transmitters and encourages muscle contraction. Example: anticholinesterases are useful in myasthenia gravis.

antidepressant

a drug used to treat depression. These drugs work by changing the concentrations of various chemicals in the brain. Antidepressants take several days to have their full effect.

antihistamine

a preparation that blocks the histamine response in the body which occurs during an allergic reaction. Antihistamines are used to treat all types of allergy (skin rashes, hay fever, etc). Example: chlorpheniramine is an antihistamine.

anti-inflammatory

a drug that reduces inflammation. Many medications not only function as painkillers but actively reduce swelling and inflammation, particularly in joints. Example: ibuprofen is an anti-inflammatory drug.

aorta

the main ARTERY that leads away from the heart.

arrhythmia

an unusual heart rhythm. Heart rhythm disturbances can occur where there is underlying heart disease. These rhythms may arise in the upper part of the heart, the atria, or lower part of the heart, the VENTRICLES. Example: atrial FIBRILLATION is a cardiac arrhythmia.

arteriography

dye testing of an ARTERY. This investigation is done to see

whether there is any blockage or narrowing of an artery. Example: RENAL arteriography may show a KIDNEY TUMOUR.

artery

a blood vessel that takes blood away from the heart. Arteries carry blood with oxygen and supply the major organs. Example: the RENAL artery supplies the KIDNEY.

arthritis

joint inflammation. There are various types of arthritis ranging from RHEUMATOID arthritis, which is an inflammatory condition, to simple wear and tear as may occur in sports injuries. Example: rheumatoid arthritis is common in young women.

arthroscopy

telescope into a joint. Under local ANAESTHETIC, a small telescope can be inserted into a joint, and the joint can be both visualized and cleaned out. In addition, BIOPSIES may be taken.

ascites

fluid in the abdomen. The cavity around the gut or peritoneum may contain fluid. Example: MALIGNANT ascites can occur with BOWEL CANCER.

atherosclerosis

hardening of the ARTERIES, i.e. they become less elastic. Example: heart disease may be caused by atherosclerosis because there is insufficient oxygen delivery to the heart muscle. *Also* arteriosclerosis.

atopic

allergic, whereby the patient has a reaction to certain materials, such as grass pollen or food. Atopy can be detected by the use of PATCH TESTS. Example: an atopic reaction to fish in a patch test denotes allergy to fish.

bacterium

a microscopic agent which may cause infection. Some bacteria are not harmful but, occasionally, serious infections may be caused by bacteria. Example: cystitis is usually caused by bacteria.

benign

not CANCEROUS. CYSTS and other swellings in various parts of the body are considered TUMOURS but, if they are benign, they will not spread to other parts of the body. Example: benign prostatic hypertrophy is enlargement of the prostate.

bilirubin

a bile pigment made from the breakdown of RED BLOOD CELLS.

biopsy

sample of living tissue. The sample is obtained usually through a needle inserted through the skin. Example: KIDNEY biopsy is valuable in diagnosing kidney disease.

bladder

a sac in the pelvis which can stretch and which collects urine from the KIDNEYS. Under voluntary control, it expels the urine through the URETHRA. Example: cystitis is infection of the bladder.

blood cells, red

cells carrying haemoglobin, an iron-containing pigment which binds to oxygen. Example: inadequate red blood cells occur in ANAEMIA. *See also* blood cell, white.

blood cells, white

cells whose main activity is to protect against infection and therefore provide immunity. Example: excess white blood cells may be found in leukaemia and may take over the bone marrow causing a very severe anaemia. This can be fatal.

bone scan

a type of X-ray of bones which determines how much calcium is present and whether there are any other deposits in the bones. Example: a bone scan may be used to check for CANCER deposits.

bowel

the large and small intestines that transfer food from the stomach and also absorb nutrients,

bronchitis

inflammation of the lining of the bronchial tubes, or BRONCHI. Example: CHRONIC bronchitis is caused by cigarette smoking.

bronchodilator

a drug which relaxes muscle in the bronchial tubes, or BRONCHI, and opens them up enabling air to be inhaled and exhaled more easily. Example: Ventolin is a bronchodilator.

bronchoscopy

investigation whereby a telescope is passed into the lungs and BRONCHUS. Samples for BIOPSIES may be taken and the bronchial tree can be visualized. Example: coughing blood should be investigated with a bronchoscopy.

bronchus

a tube supplying air to the lungs which connects up to the TRACHEA. There are two bronchi. Inflammation of the bronchi results in BRONCHITIS. Example: CANCER of the bronchus is the commonest cancer.

bypass graft

replacing heart ARTERIES with another artery such as the internal mammary artery or VEINS from the leg. Example: bypass grafting is one of the treatments available after a heart attack.

calcium antagonist

a drug that blocks calcium uptake into heart muscle and therefore reduces the oxygen demand of the heart muscle, thus improving conditions such as angina and high blood pressure. Example: verapamil is a calcium antagonist.

cancer

a disease which appears as a growth or TUMOUR that is made of body cells that are multiplying abnormally. The cancer may penetrate the tissues in which it has formed and spread further. It is therefore described as malignant and may recur even if the initial growth is removed surgically, for example. If it is not treated, cancer may lead to the death of the patient as normal cells are invaded. Example: blood in the urine may be a symptom of kidney cancer.

carcinoma

a MALIGNANT growth or CANCER that forms in surface tissues of the body, such as the skin, or the linings of the internal ORGANS or GLANDS. Carcinoma is the commonest form of cancer.

catatonic

describing a state in which the patient is frozen into inactivity. Example: catatonic schizophrenia may result in the patient lying absolutely still for days on end.

CEA

Carcino-Embryonic Antigen. An ENZYME which is elevated in patients suffering from colon CANCER. Example: a reduction in CEA may occur during the treatment of colon cancer.

cerebellum

part of the rear of the brain, separate from the main part of the brain which is known as the CORTEX. Example: the cerebellum controls co-ordination.

chemotherapy

treatment of disease, especially CANCER, using chemicals that destroy cancerous cells or invading BACTERIA or VIRUSES. Example: chemotherapy is used to treat leukaemia.

cholangiography

see **cholecystography/cholangiography**

cholecystography/cholangiography

these are both methods of X-RAY used to detect the presence of stones or obstructions in the bile duct. Example: during surgery, an operative cholangiogram may be perfomed to check that the bile duct is free from stones.

cholesterol

a fat circulating in the blood. It is derived from food stuffs and also manufactured by the body. Example: raised cholesterol is a risk factor for a heart attack.

chronic

of long duration. Chronic illnesses are not usually as severe as acute illnesses and are not immediately life threatening, but they still may be very debilitating. Example: chronic bronchitis may persist for many years. *See also* **acute**.

claudication

limping. Pain in the leg on walking is diagnosed as claudication. Example: intermittent claudication may be caused by blockage of an ARTERY in the leg.

coagulation

clotting of the blood. This clotting is brought about by a number of clotting factors which circulate within the blood. Example: impaired coagulation occurs in haemophilia.

colic

painful internal spasms of the BOWEL, WOMB, or KIDNEY tubes. Example: kidney stones cause RENAL colic.

colitis

inflammation of the colon, or large BOWEL. Example: ulcerative colitis is a cause of bloody diarrhoea.

colonoscopy

see **sigmoidoscopy/colonoscopy**

congenital disorders

are not necessarily hereditary but they are simply present at the time of birth. Example: congenital heart disease often requires surgery in young babies.

cortex

the part of the brain that controls the main higher functions of the body.

counselling

support service for emotional problems. Counselling usually takes the form of encouraging the patients to express their own feelings under the guidance of a trained counsellor. Example: bereavement counselling is of value after the death of a relative.

CT Computerized Tomography. An X-RAY system which uses computers to take repeated slices of X-rays and then combine them to produce an overall picture. Example: brain TUMOURS may be seen on computerized tomography.

culture

incubation of bacterial sample to determine the type of BACTERIA growing and its sensitivity to ANTIBIOTICS. Example: culture of urine will determine the cause of infection.

cyst

> collection of fluid in a sac. Cysts can occur anywhere under the skin within an organ such as the LIVER or breast. Example: cyst in the breast may feel like a lump.

cystoscopy

> telescope introduced under a local or general ANAESTHETIC to investigate the BLADDER and to take **biopsy** samples. Example: blood in the urine should be investigated with a cystoscopy.

cytology

> the study of cells to determine disease in the body. Example: cervical cytology studies cells from the cervix to check for CANCER.

cytotoxic

> cell killing, in order to remove infectious or CANCEROUS cells from the body. Example: cytotoxic drugs are used to treat cancer.

D & C

> dilation and curettage of the WOMB (i.e. stretching of the cervix and scraping of the lining of the womb). Example: menstrual abnormalities may improve after a D & C.

DC shock

> Direct Current shock applied to the chest wall to restart a heart that has gone into an abnormal rhythm. Example: VENTRICULAR FIBRILLATION is an abnormal rhythm of the heart muscle which would be fatal if not treated because blood is not being circulated. DC shock can change ventricular fibrillation into a normal heartbeat.

dementia

> worsening mental function, usually detected by loss of recent memory and memory for names.

dialysis

> purification through a membrane. Dialysis clears toxins from the body and can use blood circulation in haemodialysis or tubes into the stomach in peritoneal dialysis. Example: peritoneal dialysis is used in KIDNEY failure.

dopamine/dopaminergic

certain brain cells have a high content of the substance dopamine (related to adrenaline). Damage to these brain cells may cause Parkinson's disease. Example: dopaminergic nerve fibres may become depleted of dopamine after an attack of ENCEPHALITIS.

Doppler ultrasound

investigation of moving parts using sound waves to build up a picture of blood flow. Example: Doppler ultrasound can measure blood flow in ARTERIES and VEINS.

DVT

Deep-Vein Thrombosis. Thrombosis is the presence of a clot in a VEIN which may cause further blockage or may detach and travel elsewhere in the body as an EMBOLUS. Example: blood clots may form in the legs or after surgery causing DVT.

ECG

ElectroCardioGram. This picks up electrical impulses from the heart and displays them so that various regions of the heart can be investigated for abnormalities. Electrodes are applied to the chest wall using a conductive jelly. Example: one test for a suspected heart attack is an electrocardiogram.

ECT

ElectroConvulsive Therapy. Electrical impulses are applied to the brain to treat certain conditions. The patients are given muscle relaxants to prevent muscle spasm during ECT. Example: ECT may be used to treat depression.

ectopic

not in its normal place. Example: ectopic pregnancy takes place in the FALLOPIAN TUBE instead of the WOMB.

EEG

Electro-EncephaloGraph. Brain wave patterns are recorded using electrodes attached to the scalp with jelly. Example: the investigation of epilepsy includes performing an EEG.

electrolytes

sodium, potassium, etc, that are measured in the blood. They are important because they reflect the fluid balance as controlled by the KIDNEYS, and serious deviations in the electrolyte balance can be potentially fatal. Example: dehydration and vomiting will lead to a change in electrolytes.

embolus

a clot (or, rarely, air or other substance) that travels in the blood stream. An embolus may detach from a THROMBUS in a blood vessel. Example: a PULMONARY embolus is a cause of severe lung disease.

encephalitis

inflammation of the brain usually caused by VIRUSES. Example: encephalitis may be a late complication of measles.

endoscopy

internal investigation with a telescope. The telescope or endoscope is introduced under gentle anaesthesia, and biopsies or samples may be taken of the stomach or duodenum. Example: ULCERS need to be investigated with an endoscopy.

enzymes

enzymes are PROTEINS which the body uses to help carry out its metabolic function. The enzymes function as catalysts, that is, they take part in and speed up chemical reactions without being changed by those reactions. Certain enzymes can be measured in blood tests to detect abnormalities. Example cardiac enzymes are elevated after a heart attack.

erythropoietin

a PROTEIN produced by the KIDNEY which regulates blood production. It is now available as a medication. Example: erythropoietin injections may treat the ANAEMIA of kidney failure.

ESR

Erythrocyte Sedimentation Rate. An erythrocyte is a RED BLOOD CELL, and a high sedimentation rate is caused by excess PROTEIN and viscosity in the blood as a sign of MALIGNANCY or other disease.

faeces

see **stool**

fallopian tube

the tube that conducts eggs from the OVARY to the WOMB.

fibrillation

abnormal muscle contraction. This type of contraction may be seen in heart muscle or in other muscle such as the muscles of the legs.

fibrinogen

a blood PROTEIN which is involved in the process of clotting. Fibrinogen depletion in wasting diseases may cause a tendency to bleed. Example: bleeding disorders may need to be investigated by measuring fibrinogen levels.

fistula

a connection between two membranes. Example: CANCER of the BLADDER may cause a fistula into the BOWEL.

frequency of urination

repeated BLADDER emptying. Example: frequency of urination is a symptom of prostate disease.

gall bladder

an organ near the LIVER which stores bile. Bile is a mixture of ENZYMES and thinning agents which help to digest the fat that we eat. Example: gallstones may be found in the gall bladder.

gangrene

death of tissue, usually caused by loss of oxygen supply with superadded infection. Example: diabetes may result in gangrene of the toes.

gland

an organ with specific activity. This may apply to endocrine glands, which secrete HORMONES, or other glands in the body. Example: lymph glands drain infected sites.

gonorrhoea

a sexually transmitted or venereal disease caused by a BACTERIUM. Example: a discharge from the URETHRA may indicate gonorrhoea.

gram negative

negative staining of bacteria under a microscope. Thick-walled bacteria that have certain properties do not take up the stain and are known as gram negative bacteria. Thin-walled bacteria take up the gram stain and are thus gram positive. Example: kidney infections are often caused by gram negative bacteria.

granuloma

internal ABSCESS or collection of material of poorly defined nature. Example: sarcoid is a granulomatous disease.

gynaecological

referring to female disorders. Example: CANCER of the uterus or WOMB is a gynaecological disorder.

haematuria

blood in the urine, sometimes visible to the naked eye, somtimes visible only under a microscope. Example: haematuria may be a symptom of kidney stones.

haemoglobin

the iron-containing pigment that carries oxygen in the RED BLOOD CELLS or erythrocites. Example: low haemoglobin may be found in ANAEMIA.

haemorrhage

bleeding caused by a ruptured blood vessel. Example: a STROKE may be caused by haemorrhage in the ARTERIES supplying the brain.

heart valves

heart valves, such as the mitral and tricuspid valves, work to regulate the blood flow in the heart and to prevent back flow of blood during the heart beat. Example: rheumatic fever may affect the mitral and tricuspid valves.

hepatic

relating to the LIVER. The liver is the largest organ in the body and its function is to store and metabolize materials. Example: the ARTERY to the liver is the hepatic artery.

HIV

Human Immuno-deficiency Virus, a VIRUS that replicates in the lymph GLANDS and eventually causes a decrease in immunity. Example: HIV infection may be transmitted by contaminated blood transfusion.

hormone

chemical messenger secreted by a GLAND which travels in the blood stream to have a specific effect elsewhere. Example: insulin is a hormone.

hypertension

high blood pressure which throws additional strain on the heart and may lead to heart attacks. Example: hypertension may be caused by cigarette smoking.

hypnotic

a drug which works as a sleeping pill. Example: addiction to hypnotics occurs if they are used for too long.

hypotension

low blood pressure caused by a loss of blood volume or blood vessel tone, as in SHOCK. Example: hypotension is common after a heavy loss of blood.

immune system

parts of the body used to protect against infection. They work by producing ANTIBODIES and by blocking harmful substances, toxins. Example: lymph nodes are part of the immune system.

infection

invasion by disease caused by bacteria or viruses. These infectious agents may be transmitted by any method, but usually they are passed on in food or they are inhaled. Example: MENINGITIS is infection of the lining of the brain.

inotropic

heart stimulating causing increased heart rate. Example: digoxin is an inotropic drug.

interferon

a drug which inhibits VIRUSES and CANCERS by blocking their effect on cells. Example: interferon is used in the treatment of some warts.

-itis

suffix used to indicate inflammation or infection. Example: appendicitis is infection of the appendix.

IUCD

Interuterine Contraceptive Device. It usually consists of a plastic coil inserted through the cervix leaving threads which may be detected on vaginal examination. Example: the coil or IUCD may cause ECTOPIC pregnancy.

IVF

In-Vitro Fertilization. The bringing together of the sperm and ovum outside the body in order to assist conception. Example: IVF is used to treat infertility.

IVP

IntraVenous Pyelogram. A dye test of the KIDNEY whereby an injection into the arm releases a dye that is concentrated in the kidney allowing the kidney obstructions to be visualized. Example: kidney CANCER may be investigated with an IVP.

jaundice

yellow pigment in the skin caused by elevation of BILIRUBIN. Example: LIVER disease may cause jaundice.

kidney

one of a pair of organs that filter the blood and secrete urine.

kidney function tests

blood tests of KIDNEY function which detect whether the kidneys are working normally or not. Example: testing for and finding raised blood urea indicates possible kidney failure.

Kveim test

a test for sarcoidosis whereby an injection of animal PROTEINS causes allergic reaction to confirm the diagnosis. Example: a positive Kveim test may take six weeks to appear.

lactation

milk production by the breasts. Example: lactation after child-birth is maintained by hormones secreted by the pituitary GLAND at the base of the brain.

laparoscopy

telescope investigation into the stomach. A telescope, or laparoscope, is inserted under local anaesthesia into the abdominal cavity. Example: laparoscopy can diagnose appendicitis.

LFT

Liver Function Tests. Measurements of ENZYMES and BILIRUBIN to assess LIVER function. Example LFTs may give altered results in hepatitis.

libido

sex drive. Example: antihistamine drugs may cause loss of libido.

lipid

a fat secreted by the LIVER and also produced by the conversion of fat that we eat. Lipids are found in the blood. Example: CHOLESTEROL is a lipid.

liver

the organ which stores and breaks down materials.

lumbar puncture

the taking of a sample of the fluids surrounding the brain and the spine. Example: lumbar puncture should be performed in cases of suspected MENINGITIS and will show BACTERIA in the spinal fluid if meningitis is present.

lung perfusion scan

investigation of lungs using radioactive isotopes. Example: one test for PULMONARY EMBOLUS is a lung perfusion scan.

lymphatic

relating to the lymph and IMMUNE SYSTEMS which are there to protect the body against infections. Example: infection causes swelling of the lymphatic GLANDS.

malignant

see **cancer** Example: CARCINOMA of the BRONCHUS is a malignant disease.

mania

irrational desire or mood elevation. Example: kleptomania is a desire to steal.

melaena

altered blood (black tar) in the STOOLS. Example: melaena is a symptom of bleeding duodenal ULCER.

meningitis

inflammation of the lining of the brain. Example: bacterial meningitis causes stiff neck.

mitral valve

see **heart valves**

monoclonal

single clone, that is, describing a single 'breed' of ANTIBODIES used to treat infections with certain agents. Example: monoclonal antibodies may be used to treat certain types of shock.

MRI

Magnetic Resonance Imaging. Using magnetic fields to obtain pictures of internal organs. Example: pressure on the spine may be seen by MRI.

nerve, parasympathetic

part of the NERVOUS SYSTEM that is not under conscious control. The nervous system consists of the voluntary nervous system and the autonomic nervous system of which the parasympathetic and SYMPATHETIC NERVOUS systems are part. Example: the heart is slowed by parasympathetic nerves.

nerve, sympathetic

part of the NERVOUS SYSTEM that is not under conscious control. Example the heart is speeded up by sympathetic nerves.

nervous system

the electrical 'wiring' system that controls the functions of the body. Example: the movement of a limb is brought about by the voluntary nervous system, the message moving from the brain to the limb muscle.

neuropathy

NERVE damage which is manifested by loss of sensation and pins and needles, and caused by a variety of factors including vitamin deficiency. Example: diabetes may cause neuropathy in the feet.

NSAID

Non-Steroidal Anti-Inflammatory Drug. NSAIDs comprise a class of drugs which are used to treat inflammation but they are not related to the STEROIDS that may have damaging side effects. Example: indomethacin is an NSAID used to treat ARTHRITIS.

osteoporosis

thinning of bones caused by gradual loss of calcium. Example: osteoporosis occurs in women after the menopause.

ovary

the female organ in which eggs and female HORMONES are produced.

papilloma

wart. Example: multiple papillomata can be transmitted sexually.

paralysis

loss of movement. Example: NERVE damage in the spine may cause paralysis of the lower limbs.

paranoia

a psychological state characterized by feelings of persecution. Example: paranoid schizophrenia may cause sufferers to think that their thoughts are being monitored.

parotid gland

salivary GLAND. Example: the parotid gland is enlarged in mumps infection.

patch test

a skin test where a potentially harmful material is put on to a patch and applied to the skin. A red reaction indicates a positive allergy to the material. Example: hay fever sufferers will show a positive patch test response to pollen.

pericardium

membrane around the heart. Example: the pericardium may be affected by a VIRUS infection causing pericarditis which may give chest pains similar to a heart attack.

peritonitis

inflammation of the lining of the intestines. Example: appendicitis may lead to peritonitis.

pessary

medicine inserted into the vagina. Example: thrush responds to Canesten pessaries.

phlebitis

inflamed VEIN. Example: a painful foot can be caused by phlebitis.

phobia

irrational fear. Example: dysmorphophobia is fear of one's own appearance.

physiotherapy

training in joint and muscle use. Example: clearing the chest may be aided by physiotherapy.

pleuritic pain

pain on breathing caused by irritation of the pleura or lining of the lungs. Example: PULMONARY EMBOLUS may cause pleuritic chest pain.

pneumonia

lung infection or inflammation which causes difficulty with breathing. Example: AIDS patients may develop pneumocystis pneumonia.

prostration

collapse with fatigue or illness. Example: patients with SEPTICAEMIA may have fever and prostration.

prostate gland

a GLAND in men that secretes fluids into the genital tract.

protein

any of the building blocks of many organic substances. We derive protein from food such as meat.

psychiatric

relating to an abnormal mental process that requires medical intervention. Example: schizophrenia is a psychiatric disorder.

psychiatrist

a doctor who specializes in psychological disorders, that is, disorders of the mind and thoughts. Example: antidepressants may be prescribed by a psychiatrist.

psychometric

psychometric testing uses questionnaires and interview to determine certain aspects of behaviour such as how depressed a person is. Example: DEMENTIA can be measured using psychometric testing.

psychotherapy

interpretation and COUNSELLING technique which analyses the patient's past and present experiences and tries to relate them to the treatment of their condition. Example: depression can be treated by psychotherapy.

pulmonary

relating to the lungs. Example: a blood clot in the lungs is a pulmonary EMBOLUS.

pus

a mixture of BACTERIA, blood, and inflammtory cells.

pyelography

see **IVP**

pyloric stenosis

pyloric stenosis is caused by ulceration narrowing (stenosis) the exit valve (pyloris) of the stomach. Example: pyloric stenosis may also rarely occur as a disease in newborn children.

radiotherapy

high dose of X-RAYS and other radioactive materials used to treat CANCER by killing off rapidly dividing cancer cells. Example: radiotherapy is useful in treating lung cancer.

renal

relating to the KIDNEY. Example: renal failure may be caused by infection.

retina

membrane at the back of the eye which detects light and converts it into images for the brain. Example: detached retina needs to be treated with laser and rest.

retinopathy

damage to the RETINA or membrane at the back of the eye.

rheumatoid

resembling rheumatism. Example: the early symptoms of rheumatoid ARTHRITIS may resemble rheumatism.

sarcoma

CANCER. Unlike CARCINOMAS, sarcomas involve bone, muscle, and fibrous tissue. Examples: fibrosarcomas, myosarcomas. and rhabdosarcomas are all TUMOURS.

scan

investigation. *See* **MRI** and **CTscans**.

septicaemia

blood infection. Example: toxic shock is a HYPOTENSION caused by a BACTERIA infection presenting as SEPTICAEMIA.

sialogram

an X-RAY of the PAROTID GLAND to detect stone or other obstruction, eg, a stone results in a shadow seen on the sialogram.

sigmoidoscopy/colonoscopy

ENDOSCOPY involving the large bowel (colon). Example: polyps (small growths) may be removed during sigmoidoscopy.

smear

cells taken from the beck of the WOMB. Example: abnormal smear is a test for early detection of CANCER by the visualization of abnormal cells in the cervical smear.

sputum

phlegm. Example: MALIGNANT cells in sputum may indicate lung CANCER.

steroid

anti-inflammatory drug (corticosteroid) or body-building drug (anabolic steroid). Example: steroids are used to treat polymyalgia rheumatica.

stool

faeces or excrement. Example: parasites may be found on examination of the stools.

stroke

a blockage of one of the ARTERIES to the brain. Example: a stroke may result in loss of speech. *Also* **cerebrovascular accident**, **CVA**.

suppository

medicine inserted into the rectum. Example: Predsol suppositories are used in the treatment of proctitis.

syndrome

a pattern of symptoms and signs occurring together in a disease. Example: AIDS is a syndrome which includes multiple infections.

syphilis

a sexually transmitted or venereal disease caused by a BACTERIUM. Example: the spread of HIV may be worsened by the presence of syphilis.

thallium scan

a radioactive scan of the heart using the radioactive element thallium. Its distribution in the heart can be detected on exercise. Example: exercise testing with thallium is one of the tests for angina.

thrombus

a clot in a blood vessel or elsewhere. Example: after an operation, a thrombus may form in the leg.

thrush

fungus infection. Example: vaginal thrush responds to antifungal pessaries.

TIA

Transitory Ischaemic Attack. A brief episode of lack of oxygen supplying the brain. Example: minor STROKES: can cause TIAs with brief loss of speech or power.

tinnitus
buzzing in the ears. Example: tinnitus is a symptom of Ménière's disease.

T lymphocyte
a certain 'breed' of LYMPHATIC cells.

tourniquet
a tight bandage anywhere around the body, usually used when a blood sample is being taken. Example: a bleeding ARTERY can be treated by applying a tourniquet but this should only be carried out under expert supervision.

tranquillizer
sedative drug. Example: anxiety may be treated with tranquillizers.

trachea
the tube that carries air from the exterior into the lungs.

trauma
injury. Example: unconsciousness may be caused by trauma to the head.

tricuspid valve
see **heart valves**

triglyceride
a blood fat produced from the LIVER or from the fat that is taken in in food. Example: diabetes causes raised triglycerides.

tumour
an abnormal swelling in any part of the body.

ulcer
a crater in a membrane where the normal surface is replaced by an inflamed pit that may eventually lead to complications. Example: gastric ulcer is a cause of stomach pain.

urethra
a tube which connects the BLADDER to the exterior.

vaccination
injection with materials to protect against infection by causing

the production of ANTIBODIES. Example: vaccines are now available against some types of MENINGITIS.

vein

blood vessel returning blood to the heart. Example: the RENAL vein drains the KIDNEYS.

ventricle

the main chamber of the heart.

virus

a small infectious agent. Example: AIDS is caused by the human immuno-deficiency VIRUS.

womb

the uterus, the organ in which the foetus develops.

X-ray

internal view of the chest, for example, by the use of radioactive films that can detect abnormalities. Example: one test for a suspected lung CANCER is a chest X-ray

Part 4
Alphabetical listing and index

Each of the conditions described in Part 2 of the book under the relevant body system is included here in alphabetical order so that you can turn quickly to any one of them, such as Angina pectoris. This is followed by a comprehensive Index of Part 2.

Addiction to alcohol (alcoholism) ♥♥♥

Alcoholism, or addiction to alcohol, is the most common addictive disease. Sufferers may progress from social drinking to either regular heavy bout drinking or to continuous daily intake of alcohol. Spirits, in particular, are dangerous because of the damage they may cause to the body.

Symptoms

These include regular intake of alcohol either daily or several times weekly in severe bouts (bout drinking). This is followed by a deterioration of family and personal life, breakup of marriage, loss of job, loss of driving licence due to drink/driving offences, neglect of personal and social arrangements (failure to open the post is a common symptom of alcohol addiction), loss of friends, loss of trust by friends, deteriorating memory,

blackouts, persistent vomiting, poor diet, malnutrition, eventually leading to brain and liver damage, alcoholic cirrhosis, and irreversible brain disorders such as encephalopathy and psychosis, suicide. Damage to family members is another significant factor that this condition causes.

Action

Early intervention is recommended to prevent the steady deterioration to the further stages of alcoholism.

Tests

Routine liver function tests will denote the degree of liver damage. Other organs that may be affected include the heart and the brain, and the appropriate tests are needed. Full blood count can assess any degree of anaemia caused by poor diet. Damage to the pancreas gland may result in diabetes. Damage to reproductive function may impair fertility in men and women.

Medications and treatment

A structured programme of peer group support (Alcoholics Anonymous), psychotherapy, the use of tranquillizers and ß-blockers, including Antabuse, Librium, and propanolol, to maintain withdrawal from alcohol, antidepressants, and sleeping pills all form part of the management of this difficult condition.

Further advice
Alcoholism should be regarded as an illness and taken seriously. Active management is recommended.

Associated conditions
Drinking methylated spirits or other adulterated alcohol products may cause severe damage, including blindness.

Addiction to illegal drugs including ♥♥♥♥ marijuanha, cocaine, heroin, ecstasy

 These drugs are listed together because the illegal supply of one often brings users into contact with the other drugs. Marijuanha is the most benign but prolonged use can have both psychological and physical effects including loss of immune function. Cocaine and its derivatives, including crack, produce an elevation of mood with profound withdrawal symptoms. Heroin may be taken by inhalation or by injection, the latter carrying risk of transmission of virus diseases such as hepatitis B and HIV, as well as profound serious addiction. Ecstasy is an amphetamine derivative which also produces mood elevation but profound withdrawal symptoms. Addiction occurs because of a need to overcome the withdrawal and because of other personality factors.

Symptoms
Regular drug use becomes a problem when it interferes with normal social functioning. The expenditure of large amounts of money may lead users to commit petty crime or even more serious crime. Loss of social contacts, friends, and jobs may also occur as part of the addiction, similar to

that described for alcohol addiction. Regular use of these drugs often coexists with regular alcohol abuse. Cocaine may cause damage to the nose from repeated inhalation. Marijuanha may affect the immune system and fertility. Ecstasy occasionally causes rapid heart rate and has been known to be associated with sudden death. Deliberate or accidental overdose of these drugs is often fatal.

Tests
Blood and urine tests can determine whether drugs have been taken recently. Routine tests to determine any end organ damage can also be carried out.

Medications and treatment
The treatment of addiction to these drugs involves multidisciplinary support groups, peer groups, psychotherapy, and counselling, together with drugs such as methadone to aid the withdrawal from addictive drugs.

Further advice
As with alcohol addiction, early intervention is recommended for all these addictions.

Associated conditions
Nicotine addiction can possibly be included with this group, and the effects of regular cigarette smoking on the lungs and on the cardiovascular system are described in the relevant chapters above. Solvent abuse (eg aerosols, glue) can be fatal and often occurs in teenagers.

Addiction to prescription drugs

 The most common prescription drugs which have caused problems with addiction are tranquillizers and sleeping pills, particularly the benzodiazepines, laxatives, and slimming pills.

Symptoms

Unlike alcoholism, this condition is more common in women than in men. Regular prescribing of these products without patient consultation colludes with the addiction. Laxative abuse and slimming pill abuse may co-exist with the anorexia/bulimia syndrome. Addiction to sleeping pills and tranquillizers is very difficult to treat because sudden withdrawal provokes a paranoid psychosis-type syndrome, and gradual withdrawal under supervision is usually necessary.

Action

Where addiction to these medications is suspected, the patient or a family friend should discuss it with the prescribing doctor.

Tests

Psychometric testing to test brain function may be appropriate. Examination by a psychiatrist or clinical psychologist is also of value.

Medications and treatment

Gradual withdrawal under supervision is necessary, in association with psychotherapy and support groups. Attention to any underlying condition which has precipitated the addiction is also necessary.

Further advice

Prescription drugs should always be used in small quantities and under the advice of the prescriber. Repeat prescriptions should not be issued unless it is perfectly clear that the condition is a chronic one requiring long-term treatment.

Adrenal glands, disorders of

The adrenal gland is an endocrine gland which is located above the kidney. Its function is controlled partially by the pituitary hormones. Overactivity of the adrenal gland can result in Cushing's syndrome, phaeochromocytoma, or

Conn's syndrome. Underactivity of the pituitary gland results in Addison's disease.

Symptoms

The symptoms of Addison's disease include weakness, weight loss, lethargy, pigmentation of the skin, drop in blood pressure, and eventually collapse and death. It is caused by an absence of cortisone due to failure of the adrenal glands. The cause of this adrenal failure may be tumour or tuberculosis of the adrenal gland, or occasionally wasting of the adrenal gland due to overuse of steroids. Addison's disease may appear as a separate entity in itself with possibly an auto-immune destructive element of the adrenal gland. Cushing's and Conn's syndrome are due to excess corticoid drugs. Cushing's syndrome presents with obesity, stretch marks, diabetes, high blood pressure, and cataracts, and is due to excess cortisone. Conn's syndrome presents with elevated blood pressure and potassium and is due to excess mineralocorticoids. Phaeochromocytoma, due to excess adrenaline, presents with hypertension which may be spasmodic. It is worth noting that the weakness in Addison's disease may be due to a low blood potassium (hypokalaemia).

Action

Where adrenal disorders are suspected, urgent medical attention is required.

Tests

Blood tests include measurements of potassium and sodium, adrenaline, and urine tests for hormones and their breakdown products. Clinical examination will reveal typical features of the condition concerned. X-rays of the pituitary and adrenal glands may help make the diagnosis, and adrenal function tests, such as using ACTH, will determine whether there is functioning adrenal capacity present.

Medications and treatment

Surgical treatment may be required for conditions such as phaeochromocytoma, Cushing's, or Conn's disease. Underactive adrenal glands in Addison's disease can be treated by the administration of replacement hormones usually by mouth.

Further advice
Continued monitoring is required to establish that adequate replacement therapy has been given. Where oral steroids are being used in high doses for other conditions, the possibility of shrinkage of the adrenal glands should always be borne in mind.

AIDS

see **HIV infection and AIDS**

Alcoholism

see **Addiction to alcohol**

Allergy

see **Anaphylactic shock and allergy**

Alopecia

see **Hair loss**

Alzheimer's disease

see **Dementia**

Amyotrophic lateral sclerosis

see **Multiple sclerosis**

Anaemia

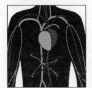

Anaemia is a condition caused by a deficiency of iron in the red blood cells (iron-deficiency anaemia). There are other types of anaemia caused by lack of vitamin B_{12} or folic acid, low thyroxine level, or anaemia may be caused by loss of blood through excessive bleeding. In addition, any chronic disorder may cause anaemia by affecting general health and bone marrow production of red blood cells. Any illness that invades the bone marrow, e.g. leukaemia can cause anaemia. Rarely the body will destroy its own red blood cells (auto-immune haemolytic anaemia).

Symptoms
Tiredness with associated pallor and some general weakness. Anaemia may be completely symptomless and picked up only on routine blood tests. Breathlessness on exercise and angina may also be symptoms of anaemia. There may be symptoms of the causes of anaemia, such as underactive thyroid gland, or excessive bleeding.

Action
Simple, mild anaemia may respond to self-medication but, where symptoms are severe, medical investigation is required.

Tests
Blood tests for haemoglobin red-cell count, iron level, iron binding capacity, vitamin B_{12}, folic acid, thyroxine, and other routine blood tests, such as kidney function (because kidney failure is another cause of anaemia due to lack of erythropoietin).

Medications and treatment
Medications, including iron and vitamins, are included at the end of this chapter. Thyroxine may be required in underactive thyroid patients, and erythropoietin in those with kidney failure. Blood transfusion may be required in severe cases of anaemia.

Further advice
Strict vegetarians may suffer from vitamin deficiency, particularly vitamin B_{12} deficiency. Iron deficiency may also occur when the diet is poor in meat. Dietary supplements may be required in children, the elderly, during pregnancy, and in vegetarians.

Associated conditions
Sickle-cell anaemia and thalassemia are conditions where changes in the haemoglobin cause anaemia or an anaemia-like syndrome. Iron should not be given to patients with thalassemia.

Anaphylactic shock and allergy
see also Shock

 The cause of allergy is not known but the body does produce antibodies as a protective mechanism. Sometimes, these cause harm by provoking an allergy. Severe allergy may cause anaphylactic shock.

Symptoms
The symptoms of anaphylactic shock are collapse with swelling of the lips and tongue, difficulty in breathing, and generalized oedema. This may occur in response to a sudden allergy, particularly to a wasp or bee sting. Other allergies, such as hay fever, appear with a runny nose, whereas penicillin and drug allergies often appear with skin rashes. Itchy skin and swelling of any part of the body may also be part of the presentation of allergic disorders.

Action
Severe anaphylactic shock requires emergency medical treatment. Many patients carry emergency medications for this purpose. Medical advice should be sought as soon as possible. Other allergies may respond to self-medication with antihistamines.

Tests
Skin tests and blood tests may be carried out to determine the cause

of the allergy and an exact profile of what the patient is allergic to. Allergies run in families and many people are allergic to a large number of extraneous substances.

Medications and treatment
The emergency treatment of anaphylactic shock includes the use of steroids, adrenaline, antihistamines, and other measures for resuscitation if cardiac arrest occurs. Allergies usually respond to antihistamines, and occasionally steroids may be required.

Further advice
Try to avoid those factors to which you are allergic. If you suffer from severe allergies and you are prone to anaphylactic shock you should equip yourself with a self-medication kit.

Angina pectoris

 Angina pectoris is a condition where pain in the heart is caused by an inadequate blood supply to the heart muscle. The condition is similar to, and may eventually lead to, a heart attack. The factors that precipitate angina include: a family history of heart disease, smoking, obesity, a sedentary lifestyle, high blood pressure, high cholesterol, high triglycerides, cold weather.

Main symptom
Chest pain. Typically, the chest pain of angina pectoris is a central, gripping chest pain that may radiate to the left arm or jaw, and that may be worse on exercise, particularly in cold weather. The pain is relieved by rest. Any chest pain, however, that is worse on exercise and relieved by rest may be angina. Angina may sometimes come on at rest (atypical angina).

Associated symptoms
Nausea, breathlessness, collapse, dizziness, unconsciousness.

Action
Seek advice to investigate and treat angina. Pay particular attention to risk factors for heart disease and to treating these where possible.

Tests
Investigations for angina include: ECG, exercise ECG, chest X-ray, blood tests for precipitating factors, coronary angiography, thallium scanning of the heart, echocardiography.

Medications and treatment
Anti-anginal medications include ß-blockers and nitrates.

Further advice
After the treatment of the risk factors for heart disease, you may be investigated and considered for coronary artery bypass grafting (CABG) which replaces diseased arteries with fresh arteries or veins. You should lose weight, take light, regular exercise, stop smoking, and eat a low-fat diet. Angioplasty (balloon flattening of blockages) may also be used for treatment.

Ankylosing spondylitis

Ankylosing spondylitis, sometimes known as 'poker back', is an inflammatory condition affecting the sacro-iliac joints of the spine, and occasionally the hip and other joints. Its cause is not known but may be associated with genetic factors. It is perhaps ten times more common in men than in women and the first symptoms usually appear in people in their mid-twenties. While the females in affected families may not suffer from the symptoms, it seems that they may be carriers of the condition from one generation to the next.

Symptoms
Persistent backache with stiffness. The pain is worse after long periods of rest, so early morning pain and stiffness are common features of the condition. Occasionally, there may be associated

symptoms such as iritis (redness of the eyes) or colitis (inflammation of the bowels). Other joints may become involved later, causing hip or ankle pain. Occasionally skin rashes may occur.

Action
If you suffer from persistent backache, you should seek medical advice.

Tests
Blood tests to check for inflammatory arthritis should be done, including full blood count, sedimentation rate, and latex tests for rheumatoid arthritis. HLAB27 tests should be carried to check for genetic factors associated with ankylosing spondylitis.

Medications and treatment
Non-steroidal anti-inflammatory medication and painkillers are used to control this condition. Physiotherapy is important to maintain mobility, and severe ankylosing spondylitis may require more radical therapy.

Further advice
If you suffer from ankylosing spondylitis, you should try to keep fit, exercise regularly, and maintain good general health.

Associated conditions
Reiter's disease is a condition that may begin as a venereal disease and may progress to a condition similar to ankylosing spondylitis.

Anorexia nervosa

see **Eating disorders**

Aortic aneurysm

Aortic aneurysm is a swelling of the main artery leading to the

 heart. These aneurysms are most commonly found in the upper abdomen/lower chest area. The cause of aortic aneurysm is most commonly hardening of the arteries or arteriosclerosis. Occasionally aneurysms have been associated with previous syphilis infections, but these are rarely seen nowadays.

Main symptom
A swelling in the upper abdomen through which a pulse can clearly be felt. Occasionally, these aneurysms may dissect or rupture and this may appear as a medical emergency similar to a heart attack.

Action
If the patient is fit, aortic aneurysms will lend themselves to bypass surgery. The acute presentation of a ruptured or dissected aortic aneurysm should be treated as a medical emergency in the same way as a heart attack.

Tests
These involve routine tests such as abdomen and chest X-ray, ECG, coronary arteriography, and aortic angiogram.

Medications and treatment
Treatment of the acute condition includes treatment of shock with fluids, plasma, or blood, and treatment of associated conditions including kidney failure which can arise as a result of a dissecting aortic aneurysm.

Further advice
Because aortic aneurysms are related to hardening of the arteries, you should adopt similar changes to lifestyle as you would following a heart attack, i.e. you should lose weight, stop smoking, reduce alcohol intake, and take light, regular exercise.

Appendicitis

see **Intestinal obstruction**

Arrhythmias

see **Heart rhythm disturbances**

Arteritis, temporal

see **Polymyalgia rheumatica**

Asthma

 Asthma is a condition caused by spasm of the muscles in the bronchial tree (the tubes taking air from the mouth to the lungs) resulting in wheezing. Asthma may occur in adults or children and may be precipitated by allergic factors, cold, exercise, stress, or dust inhalation.

Symptoms
Typically coughing and wheezing, the cough often producing thick sputum.

Action
Severe asthma (status asthmaticus) is a medical emergency and help should be sought urgently. Less severe asthma may respond to humidification of the room, rest, and avoidance of precipitating factors.

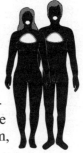

Tests
Tests for asthma include lung function tests, particularly peak flow rate, chest X-ray, allergy tests.

Medications and treatment
Asthma treatments include bronchodilators and steroids. Anti-allergy treatments are also helpful.

Further advice

Where possible, you should avoid precipitating factors, and take medications to prevent asthma attack rather than wait until it is well established.

Associated conditions

Asthma may be associated with hay fever and eczema and may run in allergic (atopic) families.

Auto-immune disorders

 There is a number of auto-immune disorders which have been referred to above. Thyroid disease, adrenal disease, and diabetes may all be caused by the destruction of the body by itself. There is a number of conditions which are also classified as auto-immune that are, in effect, multisystem disorders affecting many parts of the body. These include scleroderma, systemic lupus erythematosus (SLE), and polyarteritis nodosa. SLE is related to arthritis; it is an auto-immune disorder that destroys tissues in the skin, joints, lungs, and heart.

Symptoms

The symptoms of systemic lupus erythematosus include skin rash, particularly across the bridge of the nose and the cheeks, and arthritis. The condition may also cause fibrosis of the lungs, damage to the kidneys, and the heart valves. Like scleroderma it may also cause an arthritis, particularly of the small joints of the hand. Scleroderma is similar and usually presents with tight skin, particularly around the mouth and joints. Polyarteritis nodosa is a condition where painful nodules appear, particularly in the legs and especially in men. It may affect the testes and may result in testicular failure.

Action

Minor degrees of arthritis will respond to self-medication, but, where suspected, these conditions need to be investigated and diagnosed.

Tests
Biopsies may be necessary to make the diagnosis definitively. Blood tests include looking at the sedimentation rate and other measures of auto-immune function.

Medications and treatment
These conditions respond to anti-inflammatory drugs and to steroids.

Associated conditions
Raynaud's syndrome may be a precursor of conditions such as SLE or scleroderma. It presents with severe chilblains of the hand brought about by spasm of the arteries.

Backache, including lumbago, sciatica, slipped disc, and spondylitis ♥

 Backache is a very common symptom and can range from mild and temporary to permanent and disabling. The commonest cause is degeneration of the vertebrae in the spine due to osteoarthritis and osteoporosis, and leading to pressure on the nerve roots. Bulging of the discs between the vertebrae is known as a slipped disc: it can cause severe sciatica. Spondylitis is inflammation of the small joints of the spine, and lumbago is a general term used to describe low back pain probably due to muscle spasm.

Symptoms
The symptoms may occur from the neck (cervical spondylosis) to the lumbar spine, the latter being more common. Sciatica occurs where a nerve root is under pressure, and the pain goes down the back of the leg.

Acute slipped disc may occur in young healthy people usually from straining or lifting; there is a sudden onset of severe back pain radiating down the back of the leg. Occasionally, bowel and bladder function may be affected. Minor degrees of backache may come and go.

Action
For severe slipped disc, the patient should be asked to lie down on his or her back on a firm board or mattress, and medical advice should be sought. Less severe conditions may respond to bed rest, physiotherapy, and simple analgesics, but if they are persistent, symptoms should be investigated.

Tests
Clinical examination followed by X-rays and, where necessary, MRI scans to look for pressure on nerve roots. Blood tests should be carried out to exclude other causes including the rare possibility of an unusual malignancy pressing on the nerves in the back (spinal meningioma)

Medications and treatment
Bed rest usually resolves the symptoms of a slipped disc in two to three weeks. If persistent, microdisc surgery may be required or even a laminectomy with removal of parts of the bone in the spine to relieve pressure. These conditions will usually respond to simple analgesics, such as ibuprofen, and to rest, heat treatment, gentle physiotherapy, and eventually muscle-building exercises to protect the spine.

Further advice
Attention to diet and maintenance of a high calcium and vitamin content may help prevent degeneration of the spine. Hormone replacement therapy might also be helpful in preventing or arresting deterioration of this condition.

Bell's palsy

see **Neuropathy**

Bladder, functional disorders of the

 The bladder functions to expel urine and is under the control of the parasympathetic nervous system. Various conditions may affect bladder function, including multiple sclerosis, paralysis, or simply prolapse.

Symptoms
Stress incontinence has been dealt with above. Difficulty passing urine, a poor stream of urine, frequency of urination, passing of small volumes of urine with blood, and incontinence - particularly nocturnal incontinence.

Action
Where symptoms are distressing and persistent, they should be fully investigated.

Tests
Specialized tests involving cystometry, cystoscopy, measurement of flow rates of urine, testing for infection, and examination for prolapse are all part of the investigation of the neurogenic bladder.

Medications and treatment
A number of medications, such as Cystrin, may be helpful in this condition. Occasionally surgery may be required to improve sphincter function.

Further advice
Chronic low-grade infection may appear with symptoms similar to neurogenic bladder.

Bleeding disorders

see **Haemophilia and other bleeding disorders**

Bone disease, serious, including cancer and infection

♥♥♥♥♥

Bone sarcomas or tumours are rare. Infection of bone (osteomyelitis) may occur following a fracture.

Symptoms
These include pain and swelling of the bone. Bone pain is usually worse at night. Osteomyelitis may be accompanied by symptoms of infection such as fever.

Action
If you suspect either of these conditions, you should seek medical advice urgently.

Tests
X-ray of bone and excision biopsy may be required to diagnose this condition. Routine blood tests may detect the spread of tumour or infection to other parts of the body.

Medications and treatment
Primarily, these conditions are treated by surgery, together with anti-tumour or anti-infective therapy where appropriate.

Associated conditions
Other organs can produce sarcomas; for example, muscle may produce myosarcomas, fibrous tissues will produce fibrosarcomas, and, rarely, heart muscle will produce rhabdomyosarcomas. Joints may become infected in the same way as bones and this can cause a form of septic arthritis.

Bowel cancer
(including cancer of the rectum)

Bowel cancer is a common form of cancer and is separate from stomach cancer.

Symptoms
The symptoms of bowel cancer may be difficult to detect. Alteration in bowel habit, e.g. changing from constipation to diarrhoea or vice versa, may be the only sign. The condition may be symptomless and picked up on routine examination either by rectal examination or on fuller sigmoidoscopy or colonoscopy. Certain patients with polyps may be more prone to this condition and will need regular investigation. Passing blood, or altered blood with or without mucus may also be a sign of bowel cancer. Occasionally, the condition presents with intestinal obstruction because the tumour fills the bowel. Fatigue, anaemia, and weight loss may also be features of bowel cancer.

Action
Any persistent alteration in bowel habits should be reported to a physician for investigation.

Tests
Sigmoidoscopy, colonoscopy, barium enema, blood tests (including tests for the CEA which is specific for bowel cancer) are all part of the investigations for this condition. Biopsies should be taken.

Medications and treatment
Generally, this condition is treated surgically, and cytotoxic chemotherapy with drugs such as 5FU may be useful.

Further advice
Eating a high-roughage diet will help to prevent bowel cancer.

Associated conditions

Cancer of the rectum and anus are rare. Cancer of the small bowel is very unusual. Bowel cancer often spreads to the liver and may appear with evidence of liver enlargement or liver failure.

Bowel disorders, inflammatory: ♥♥ ulcerative colitis and Crohn's disease

 These are distinct conditions which occasionally overlap. Ulcerative colitis normally affects the colon whereas Crohn's disease normally affects the small bowel. There are mixed variants of these conditions, however. Neither disease has a known cause. They are thought to be associated with a family history and with stress.

Symptoms

Abdominal pain, passing blood or mucus from the back passage, weight loss, and diarrhoea. Ulcerative colitis may be associated with more profuse bleeding whereas Crohn's disease is often associated with abdominal pain and the formation of fistulae and abscesses including anal fistulae. Patients may become thin and anaemic.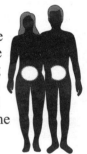

Action

Persistent bloody diarrhoea should be referred for investigation. Short-term symptoms, such as diarrhoea with or without blood, may be caused by gastro-enteritis.

Tests

Endoscopy and biopsy are often required as are barium enema or barium meal with follow-through barium to the small bowel. Blood tests for anaemia, liver-function tests, raised sedimen' raised white-cell count, and other signs of auto-immun' help in making the diagnosis.

Medications and treatment

Steroids, either in tablet form or enema (Predsol), may be useful as are drugs such as Salazopyrin or mesalazine. The objective is to control symptoms with the minimum dose of steroids. Drugs such as Salazopyrin need to be continued on a long-term basis. Surgical treatment should be avoided where possible but, occasionally, removal of part of the bowel may be necessary. Also: Anusol HC; Asacol; Colifoam; Dipentum; Salofalk; Scheriproct.

Further advice

Keeping to a low-roughage diet and low stress levels may be helpful in the management of these conditions.

Associated conditions

Diverticulitis is different from these conditions and responds to antibiotic therapy and high roughage diet. Ulcerative colitis may rarely be associated with a condition resembling ankylosing spondylitis with involvement of the joints in the back and inflammation of the eyes. Skin rashes may also occur. Fistulae in ano or anal tear may be associated with ulcerative colitis or Crohn's disease.

Bowel infections including gastro-enteritis ♥

 Bowel infections are often caused by bacterial infection, e.g. staphylococcus, salmonella, and more rarely by cholera and typhoid. They are usually caused by eating infected food or drinking infected water. Occasionally, gastro-enteritis may be caused by a virus infection.

Symptoms

Abdominal pain and diarrhoea, often associated with vomiting. Staphylococcal gastro-enteritis usually occurs within a few hours whereas salmonella may take between 12 and 24 hours to present itself. The abdominal pain may be very severe and is usually centred the umbilicus. The vomiting may continue for some time until eventually bile is being vomited.

Action
These conditions usually respond to starving and to maintaining fluid intake where possible. If patients are unable to keep fluids down for 24 hours then medical advice is usually required.

Tests
Blood tests and cultures of bowel material should be taken to check whether the patient has salmonella, cholera, or typhoid. Blood tests should also be checked to see if there is dehydration or change in electrolytes such as sodium and potassium.

Medications and treatment
Fluid replacement, possibly using intravenous fluid, may be required. Antinausea drugs, such as Stemetil or Maxolon, may be used and can be given by injection. Imodium or Lomotil can be used for diarrhoea. Antibiotics may be required.

Further advice
Gastro-enteritis may be prevented by strict hygiene, particularly when travelling abroad. Certain foods, particularly seafoods, may have grown in infected water.

Associated conditions
Tapeworm or threadworm infections may also be included in this category, and specific antiworm preparations are available for their treatment. Examples: Alcopar; Avloclor; Combantrin; Eskazole; Flagyl; Mintezol; Pripsen; Vermox; Zadstat.

Bowel, inflammatory diseases of

see **Intestinal obstruction**

Bowel syndrome, irritable ♥

Irritable bowel syndrome is caused by spasm of the small or large bowel and is often related to stress.

Symptoms
The symptoms of irritable bowel syndrome are intermittent abdominal pain with the passing of diarrhoea with or without mucus. Occasionally blood may be seen but this is not usually a feature in this condition. The patient is often tender in the abdomen close to the left hip or in the groin.

Action
Irritable bowel syndrome may respond to self-medication.

Tests
Prolonged symptoms may lead to investigation for other conditions. The investigations would include blood tests and possible endoscopy, and barium meal or barium enema.

Medications and treatment
Peppermint oils, such as Colpermin, or drugs such as Colofac may be helpful in the management of this condition.

Further advice
Reducing stress and eating a high-roughage diet may improve the symptoms of irritable bowel syndrome.

Associated conditions
This condition is also sometimes known as spastic colon.

Brain tumour ♥♥♥♥♥

 tumours may be benign or malignant. In both cases, they

cause their effects by local pressure rather than by spreading to other parts of the body. Very often, brain tumours are secondary to other cancers, such as lung cancer. Brain tumours may affect the main brain (cortex), lower brain (cerebellum), or spinal cord.

Symptoms

The symptoms of brain tumours are manifold because the tumour can mimic symptoms in any part of the body depending on where it sits in the brain or spinal column. The main symptoms of increased brain pressure are headache, nausea and vomiting, slowing of the pulse, loss of consciousness, or dementia. More specific symptoms include loss of speech, loss of vision, loss of hearing, loss of power, paralysis, loss of sensation, confusion, and disorientation. Epilepsy may also be a symptom of a brain tumour. The symptoms of brain tumours are persistent and worsening, whereas benign headache may come and go. Brain tumour symptoms seem to get worse gradually. Symptoms of raised brain pressure are worse in the morning.

Action

Where symptoms have persisted and where the patient is clearly deteriorating, medical attention is required. In the first place, you should try simple remedies for headaches, including analgesics such as aspirin or paracetamol.

Tests

The main tests for brain or spinal tumours are CT (computerized tomography) and MRI (magnetic resonance imaging) scans. Both of these scans give detailed pictures of internal organs. Tests, such as chest X-ray to look for for primary cancers, are important as are routine blood tests.

Medications and treatment

Dexamethasone is useful to reduce brain pressure. Brain tumours are treated by surgery, followed by chemo- and radiotherapy where appropriate for malignant tumours.

Further advice
Patients may suffer from post-operative epilepsy even if they did not have it before. This may require anticonvulsive medication.

Breast abscess

see **Breast, diseases of**

Breast cancer

see **Breast, diseases of**

Breast cysts

see **Breast, diseases of**

Breast, diseases of, ♥♥♥♥♥
including breast cysts, breast abscess, fibroadenosis, and breast cancer

 The breast is an organ which is highly susceptible to hormonal changes, and various conditions may appear as a lump in a breast. Most breast lumps are benign but breast cancer is one of the commonest diseases in women. Rarely, breast cancer may occur in men.

Symptoms
Usually the presence of a lump in the breast. A painful lump usually indicates breast abscess whereas a collection of painful lumps may

indicate fibroadenosis or mastitis. Mastitis or breast tenderness is usually worse before a period. Breast tenderness also occurs during pregnancy. A single painless lump may well be a cyst, but it may also be breast cancer. Breast cancer may additionally be complicated by changes to the nipple, including nipple retraction, changes to the skin above the lump giving it an orange-peel type texture. Lumps may appear elsewhere including in the armpit and other breast. Symptomatically, it may be difficult to diagnose breast cancer and further investigation may be required.

Action
If you find a new lump in a breast, then you should seek medical advice immediately.

Tests
Clinical examination and special investigations, including aspiration of cysts, aspiration biopsy, mammography, and breast ultrasound, are all part of the investigation of lumps in the breast. Full clinical examination may also include bone scans, liver scans, and brain scans. Routine blood tests, such as full blood count, ESR, alkaline phosphatase, and liver function tests may also be included.

Medications and treatment
Breast lumps are usually treated by surgery. Severe fibroadenosis and premenstrual syndromes may respond to various hormonal treatments, however. Breast abscesses need to be treated with antibiotics or by drainage. Breast cysts may be treated by aspiration.

Further advice
Regular self-monitoring of breasts for lumps is a good way to identify changes in the breast. Breast abscesses may occur during lactation when bacteria enter through a crack in the nipple. Improved nipple hygiene may prevent this occurring.

Bronchiectasis

see **Lower respiratory infections, chronic**

Bronchitis, acute

see **Lower respiratory infections, acute**

Bronchitis, chronic

see **Lower respiratory infections, chronic**

Bronchus, carcinoma of

see **Lung cancer**

Bulimia

see **Eating disorders**

Carpal tunnel syndrome

see **Neuropathy**

Cataract

 A cataract is a condition caused by gradual or sudden opacity of lens material.

Symptoms
Gradual lack of clarity of vision, and eventually blindness when the cataract matures. The condition is not painful.

Action
You should seek medical advice immediately if you notice any

difficulty in vision.

Tests
Examination of the eye will reveal the cataract.

Medications and treatment
Cataract is usually treated by surgery to implant an artificial lens. There are no other treatments which are known to be effective.

Further advice
You should avoid ultraviolet light, and any prolonged exposure to bright sunlight, because it may precipitate cataracts. Abnormally high calcium levels in the blood may also lead to cataracts.

Cerebral vascular accident ♥♥♥♥♥ (CVA, Stroke, Cerebral vascular disease, Hardening of the arteries)

CVAs and strokes are caused by thrombosis, i.e. blood clot in a vessel supplying blood and oxygen to pass to the brain, or by haemorrhage, i.e. breakdown of a major vessel which has the same ultimate effect of denying oxygen to the brain. Cerebral haemorrhage may occur as a result of trauma or rupture of a congenital aneurysm. Major catastrophic strokes may occur or the strokes may may be smaller and minor (including so-called transient ischaemic attacks - TIA - a brief and temporary loss of oxygen to the brain).

Symptoms
The symptoms of major stroke are sudden collapse with paralysis, often of one side of the body, loss of speech (if the right side of the body is involved). Patients may lapse into unconsciousness and may not recover. More commonly, gradual recovery occurs

with residual paralysis of one side of the body. Depending on the severity of the stroke, recovery may be rapid over a few days or may be more prolonged with spasticity of one half of the body, loss of bowel and bladder function, loss of speech, and loss of sensation. Although many cases resolve, some do not. This may be a cause of permanent paralysis of one side of the body (haemiparesis). The stroke may be secondary to a blood clot travelling through the body (embolus) which may arise after a heart attack. Therefore, patients suffering from a stroke may also show the symptoms of a heart attack.

Action
A stroke or CVA is a medical emergency and urgent medical attention is required. Transient ischaemic attacks, where brief loss of speech or brief tremor of the hand occurs, also need medical intervention because they could be caused by travelling blood clots.

Tests
Tests, such as ECG, chest X-ray, and blood tests for precipitating factors are important. Also tests for blood-clotting factors and for high blood pressure are valuable. Arteriography of brain circulation is helpful, particularly where there is an aneurysm which may be treatable surgically. Brain scan is also valuable in the diagnosis.

Medications and treatment
Anticoagulants are required for repeated thrombosis or embolus. Treating haemorrhagic disorders involves appropriate replacement therapy (e.g. factor 8 for haemophilia). Otherwise treatment and recovery from stroke include general supportive measures and treatment of high blood pressure or other precipitating factors.

Cerebral vascular disease

see **Cerebral vascular accident**

Cervix, diseases of

see **Uterus and cervix, diseases of**

Cholecystitis

see **Gall bladder disorders**

Claudication, intermittent

see **Peripheral arterial disease**

Coeliac disease

 Coeliac disease is caused by an allergy to gluten which is used for making bread, pasta, etc. It is probably an inherited disease.

Symptoms
The symptoms of coeliac disease usually occur in childhood but may appear in adults. These include diarrhoea, weight loss, fatty stools (steatorrhea). Malabsorption of various vitamins and minerals with associated weakness, bone thinning, and even rickets. There may be some liver enlargement.

Action
Where coeliac disease is suspected, investigation is required and the patient should go on a gluten-free diet.

Tests
Measurement of the fat content of stools, blood counts, vitamin levels in the blood, and biopsy of the intestinal mucosa are required in a full investigation of this condition.

Treatment
A gluten-free diet.

Further advice
If gluten is reintroduced into the diet, there will be a relapse.

Associated conditions

Tropical sprue and bowel infections may cause a malabsorption state. Overuse of antibiotics can produce similar results.

Collapse

see **Shock**

Conjunctiva and outer eye, diseases of the ♥

Diseases in this category include, dry eyes, Sjøgren's syndrome, styes, meibomian cysts, blepharitis, excessive tears (epiphora), subconjunctival haemorrhage, and scratched cornea through the wearing of contact lenses. Conjunctivitis is an infection of the outer eye, and, where herpes virus is concerned, this can cause an ulcer (dendritic ulcer).

Symptoms

Local symptoms, such as dry eyes or excessive tears, are usually self-explanatory. Styes and cysts can be visible and painful. Conjunctivitis usually presents with a red eye and crusts on the eyelashes. Dendritic ulcer can often be very painful but may otherwise resemble normal conjunctivitis. Subconjunctival haemorrhage may occur with spontaneous bleeding or as a result of trauma to the eye. A brick-red triangle is often visible on the white of the eye.

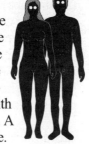

Action

Seek medical advice as soon as possible.

Tests

Examination of the eye and swabs from infection may be helpful.

Medications and treatment

Excision of cysts and styes may be helpful. Artificial tears, such as hypromellose, may be useful for dry eye which occurs in Sjøgren's syndrome. Conjunctivitis will respond to antibiotic eyedrops or ointment, and blepharitis may respond to treatment of associated conditions such as dandruff.

Further advice
Medications used for the eyes should be disposed of because they could become infected if kept for some time. Infections of one eye very often spread to the other eye. Conjunctivitis is highly contagious.

Associated conditions
Skin conditions such as eczema may cause disease of the eyelids or conjunctiva.

Coryza

see **Upper respiratory tract infections, acute**

Crohn's disease

see **Bowel disorders, inflammatory**

CVA

see **Cerebral vascular accident** *and* **Cerebrovascular accident**

Cystitis

see **Renal tract, infections of**

Deep-vein thrombosis (DVT)

Deep-vein thrombosis is a condition where there is clotting of blood in one of the deeper veins, usually in the leg or pelvis. It is caused by prolonged bed rest, some diseases which increase the clotting of the blood, and some medications, such as the contraceptive pill, which increase clotting of the blood. Deep-vein thromboses are common after surgery, particularly surgery to the abdomen or pelvis, or gynaecological surgery.

Main symptoms
These include: pain and tenderness over the vein, swelling of the leg (oedema), difficulty and pain in walking. The thrombus in the leg may detach and cause a pulmonary embolus. Deep-vein thrombosis may, therefore, lead to serious conditions including death.

Action
Deep-vein thrombosis needs to be diagnosed and treated quickly. Patients should rest with the leg elevated while medical assistance is sought.

Tests
These include: a venogram, and X-ray of the veins in the legs. In addition, routine investigations, such as chest X-ray, ECG, and blood tests, should be performed and a proper history taken to identify precipitating factors.

Medications and treatment
These include blood-thinning agents (anticoagulants) as well as general support such as elastic stockings which will support the leg. Prevention of deep-vein thrombosis is obtained in surgical patients by pre-operative administration of heparin by injection. Heparin, warfarin, and other anticoagulants may be used in treatment.

Further advice
If you have suffered from a deep-vein thrombosis, you should avoid medications, such as hormones, which may precipitate DVT. You should follow general advice about your health, such as losing weight, stopping smoking, taking light, regular exercise, and reducing alcohol intake.

Associated conditions
Superficial inflammation of the veins or phlebitis is similar but not as serious.

Dementia, including presenile dementia (Alzheimer's disease)

 Dementia is a condition where brain function deteriorates gradually. It usually occurs in older people but certain forms may appear in the younger age group. It may be caused by hardening of the arteries (athero-sclerotic dementia), but, often, the cause is not known.

Main symptoms
Progressive deterioration in mental function, including loss of memory, particularly recent memory, whereas memory of an event that happened many years ago may remain intact. Patients repeat themselves in actions and words and may become very emotionally unstable because of their insecurity. As it progresses, dementia may cause patients to become dangers to themselves, e.g. they may turn on the gas but forget to light it. Patients may appear not to recognize close friends or relatives, including spouse.

Action
In the early stages, no action may be required but, where dementia is becoming difficult to live with, the patient and the carer may need counselling and support.

Tests

Investigations for general health, for example, heart and lung disease, are important. Therefore, chest X-ray, ECG, and routine blood tests should be part of the investigation of these patients. An ECG (electrocardiogram) is a test of the electrical impulses in the heart. It detects heart abnormalities that may relate to dementia. Conditions such as brain tumours may appear as dementia and these need to be excluded before definitive diagnosis of dementia or Alzheimer's disease can be made. Rarely brain biopsy may be performed.

Medications and treatment

Some agents are being developed for treating dementia. Treatment should be directed at heart disease and other causes where appropriate.

Further advice

Long-term planning is necessary for patients and for the carers to alleviate the effects of this distressing disease.

Associated conditions

Some conditions, such as Huntington's chorea, may be associated with dementia.

Dental abscess and caries ♥

These are the main dental disorders that are referred to doctors.

Symptoms

The main symptom of dental abscess is severe pain in the mouth adjacent to a tooth. There will be associated temperature and trismus (spasm of the jaw). Dental caries (tooth decay) may lead to a variety of symptoms which are best seen by a dentist.

Action
Where possible, dental diseases should be treated by a dentist. Occasionally, you may need medical advice.

Tests
Dental X-rays will determine the extent of an abscess.

Medications and treatment
Antiseptic mouth washes may help resolve some of the symptoms but antibiotics are required for dental abscess. Draining an abscess is usually definitive in terms of treatment.

Further advice
The best way to prevent dental disease is to avoid eating sweet foods. Regular brushing and the use of dental floss will help prevent tooth and gum disease.

Associated conditions
Gum disease, particularly gingivitis (inflammation of the gums); aphthous ulcers are small ulcers which may appear in the mouth; and fungus infection of the mouth (thrush) may also cause pain and soreness.

Depression

 Depression is probably the most common psychiatric disease. It exists in a range of forms from mild through to very severe. Depression can sometimes be divided into two types, endogenous depression with no outside precipitating factor, or reactive depression. Many patients do not fall simply into either of these two categories, however.

Symptoms
These include a feeling of slowness, sadness, inability to make decisions, poor sleep particularly with early morning waking, lack of self-esteem, lack of self-worth, sometimes excessive sleeping,

slow metabolism, constipation, poor appetite, changes in the sense of taste, sometimes excessive comfort eating with weight gain, loss of libido (impotence), hypochondriasis, addiction to alcohol or prescription drugs, suicide.

Action
Depressed patients are sometimes too depressed to motivate themselves to seek medical advice. A friend or relative, however, should encourage depressed patients to see their depression as an illness rather than as personal failure, and to seek medical advice.

Tests
Clinical examination and psychometric tests may be useful. There are recognized depression rating scales which help to diagnose the condition. Medical examination should try to exclude organic causes for depression such as brain tumour, heart and lung disease, hormonal disturbances such as underactive thyroid, or associated causes such as alcoholism or drug addiction.

Medications and treatment
The treatment consists of attacking the underlying organic cause, dealing with any associated drug addiction or alcoholism, counselling and psychotherapy, antidepressant medication, and ECT (electro-convulsive therapy). Anafranil, Asendis, Aventyl, Bolvidon, Faverin, Fluanxol, Gamanil, Lentizol, Liskonum, Lustral, Marplan, Molipaxin, Motival, Nardil, Norval, Parnate. Parstelin, Priadel, Prothiaden, Prozac, Seroxat, Surmontil, Tofranil, Triptafen

Further advice
Depression often lifts spontaneously even without the use of medication. Depression may be worse in the winter (seasonal affective disorder) or may clearly be associated with a sudden loss or bereavement.

Associated conditions
Bipolar depression (manic depressive psychosis) is where the patient swings from a low mood to a high mood. Agitated depression

is depression mixed with anxiety. Anxiety states probably exist on their own and are usually best treated with anxiolytic drugs for short periods only. Persistently elevated mood such as occurs in mania or hypomania usually responds to treatment with lithium. Anxiety states or mania may appear as phobias or obsessive compulsive disorders. Severe hypochondriasis in depression may result in a hysterical conversion syndrome whereby severe organic symptoms are presented to mask an underlying depression.

Dermatitis and eczema

 Eczema and dermatitis are related conditions where there is itching and scaling of the skin with thickening. The condition is made worse if you scratch the affected area. Dermatitis may be an allergic phenomenon, e.g. contact dermatitis, where allergy to factors, such as soap powder, may bring it on. Eczema may also have an allergic component but, fundamentally, it is a disease associated with an allergic or atopic family, i.e. patients with eczema may suffer from or have relatives with asthma or hay fever.

Symptoms
Itchy or scaly rash which may bleed on contact. The rash may be found in the folds of skin such as behind the knees and in the elbows, and in areas where there is contact with chemicals, such as on the hands.

Action
Avoiding contact by wearing rubber gloves or using barrier creams may often be helpful. Simple remedies may resolve the conditions but severe conditions may require medical intervention.

Tests
The main test for this condition is biopsy of the skin or patch tests to check for skin allergies.

Medications and treatment
Eczema and dermatitis often respond to mild steroids such as Eumovate and hydrocortisone, or stronger steroids such as Betnovate or Dermovate. Strong steroids should be used with extreme caution.

Further advice
Anxiety and stress may provoke these conditions, so you should try to control these as part of your general disease management.

Associated conditions
Seborrhoeic dermatitis, which is similar to dermatitis, may affect the scalp. Blepharitis is an eczema condition affecting the eyes.

Diabetes mellitus ♥♥

 Diabetes mellitus is a condition caused by inter-action of genetic, viral, and possibly dietary components resulting in failure of the pancreas gland to produce enough insulin. Type 1 diabetes occurs usually in young adults who require insulin, whereas type 2 diabetes occurs in the older age group who may be maintained on diet and tablets alone.

Symptoms
These include weight loss, thirst, passing a lot of urine, infections especially of the urine and genitalia and particularly with thrush or other fungi, weakness, tiredness, loss of concentration, poor performance at work or school, loss of libido, impotence, infertility. Diabetes may be symptomless and may be detected on routine blood or urine examination. Progressive deterioration of diabetes, with elevation of blood sugar and ketones in the blood (ketoacidosis), may eventually lead to hyperglycaemic coma and death. Hypoglycaemia (low blood sugar) may occur when the treatment of diabetes with excess insulin or tablets results in a low blood sugar, and this too may appear with unconsciousness or coma.

Action

Where diabetes is suspected, urgent medical attention is required, particularly for diabetic coma states. Appropriate first aid depends on whether the blood sugar is high or low. If in doubt, assume the blood sugar is low and treat patients with glucose tablets or an oral solution of sweet tea to elevate blood sugar. Glucagon injections may be given.

Tests

The tests for diabetes include measurement of blood and urine sugar. Urine tests can also be carried out to look for protein and ketones. Blood tests can look for the presence of acidosis and other factors contributing to a deterioration and state of dehydration. Glycosylated haemoglobin tests can check the control of diabetes.

Medications and treatment

The treatment of hypoglycaemia includes the administration of glucose or glucagon as indicated above. The treatment of diabetes involves the use of diet, tablets such as metformin or glibenclamide, and insulin preparations. Diabenese, Diamicron, Daonil, Glibenese, Glucophage, Glurenorm, Rastinon.

Further advice

The management of diabetes involves specialist advice, particularly from dietitians. The pattern of insulin, food, and exercise needs to be adjusted. Self-monitoring of blood sugar and urine is important in maintaining the condition and making appropriate adjustments in treatment.

Associated conditions

Diabetes insipidus is a rare condition where brain damage destroys the production of vasopressin from the pituitary gland in the brain. The symptoms are thirst and the passing of a great deal of urine, but blood and urine tests do not show elevated sugar. Treatment is by the administration of synthetic vasopressin analogues. Hypercalcaemia may also appear with thirst and passing a lot of urine. This is usually associated with disease of the parathyroid glands. Similarly, diseases of the parathyroid may appear with hypocalcaemia where the patients may develop muscular spasms due to a lack of calcium in the circulation.

Disseminated sclerosis

see **Multiple sclerosis**

Diverticulitis

see **Intestinal obstruction**

Drug addiction

see **Addiction to illegal drugs** *and* **Addiction to prescription drugs**

Duodenal ulcer

see **Peptic ulcer**

Ear wax ♥

Ear wax is a benign condition where the external ear is blocked by production of wax glands in the outer ear.

Main symptoms
Deafness on the affected side, occasionally with pain when the wax presses on the eardrum.

Action
It is not usually possible to remove ear wax using cotton buds and it is best not to poke cotton buds into the ear at all. Self-medication with the appropriate drops may be helpful, but syringing by a medical practitioner or nurse is often curative.

Tests
Routine testing is not appropriate.

Medications and treatment
Ear drops, such as Cerumol or Earex, may dissolve wax without the need for syringing.

Further advice
If you are suffering from ear wax, you should avoid swimming or air travel.

Associated conditions
Otitis externa may give rise to similar symptoms but it requires treatment with antibiotics.

Eating disorders including anorexia nervosa, bulimia, and obesity ♥♥♥

 Eating disorders are commonly known as slimming diseases but their roots are to be found in the patient's disturbed emotional integrity rather than purely in an obsession with food and slimming. Like the phobias and obsessive compulsive disorders described above, these eating disorders may represent some underlying anxiety, trauma (such as sexual abuse in childhood), or depression.

Symptoms
The symptoms of anorexia nervosa are persistent weight

loss, deceptive fiddling with food, laxative abuse, loss of secondary sexual characteristics (i.e. reduction in breast size), and eventually amenorrhoea in females (anorexia nervosa occurs rarely in men). The patients are typically manipulative about food and hide food or vomit food after it has been eaten. Anorexia nervosa may end in the death of the sufferer. Bulimia is a similar condition where starvation may be followed by bouts of bingeing, often associated with the vomiting of food. Patients may be of any weight depending on how much food is retained and how the cycle of bingeing and vomiting varies. Thus, unlike the anorexia patients, the bulimics may be of normal weight or even overweight. Patients with anorexia or bulimia will also show other signs of disturbed personality function including attention-seeking and manipulative behaviour.

Action
Where these conditions are suspected, immediate medical advice should be sought.

Tests
Patients with weight loss should be evaluated for organic causes including cancers, diabetes, and overactive thyroid gland. Similarly, patients suffering from repeated vomiting should be evaluated for gastro-intestinal or liver disorders which may cause vomiting.

Medications and treatment
The treatment of these conditions involves a complex interplay of counselling support with psychotherapy, and the use of appropriate antidepressant and sedative medication.

Further advice
These conditions are chronic and recurrent. It has been said that once you suffer from bulimia you will always suffer from it in some shape or form, and the condition may relapse under moments of stress.

Associated conditions
Compulsive eating and severe obesity may be variants of these conditions which may overlap with the obsessive compulsive disorders described above.

Eczema

see **Dermatitis and eczema**

Emphysema

see **Lower respiratory infections, chronic**

Encephalitis

see **Meningitis and encephalitis**

Endocarditis

 Endocarditis is a condition involving infection, usually by bacteria, of one of the valves inside the heart. This commonly affects the valves on the left side of the heart, particularly where these valves have been previously damaged by rheumatic fever. Valve disease can lead to heart failure and its associated symptoms. Endocarditis may arise after dental treatment in a person who has a damaged heart valve.

Symptoms
Minor debility, which progresses with gradual fatigue, anaemia, and weakness. Certain specific symptoms include painful nodules in the fingers and splinter haemorrhages under the nails. Traces of blood in the urine may also occur due to emboli affecting the kidney.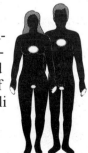

Action
The diagnosis needs to be made by an experienced clinician and treatment initiated.

Tests
These involve blood cultures, cardiac ultrasound, ECG, chest X-ray, kidney investigations, other routine blood tests. Swabs for infection, urine culture.

Medications and treatment
Usually the administration of an antibiotic such as penicillin. This needs to be continued for several weeks. Further treatment may be directed at correcting defects in the heart valve, including surgical treatment. Anticoagulants and other antithrombotic agents may be required.

Further advice
Patients should be advised to take preventative antibiotics before dental treatment.

Associated conditions
Endocarditis may be associated with myocarditis or pericarditis.

Endometriosis

see **Infertility and endometriosis**

Epilepsy and associated conditions ♥♥♥
including narcolepsy, petit mal epilepsy, grand mal epilepsy, and temporal lobe epilepsy

 Epilepsy is a condition caused by abnormal electrical patterns occurring within the brain which may trigger off a major seizure (grand mal) or brief loss of consciousness (petit mal). The cause of epilepsy is usually unknown but, apart from an association with family history, brain tumour, or other increases in brain pressure (e.g. abscess or haematoma) may trigger epilepsy. Epilepsy may be common when the blood sugar is low, such as after excess alcohol or premenstrually.

Main symptoms

Grand mal epilepsy: sudden collapse to the ground followed by spasm and then rhythmic jerking movements often of one side of the body. The seizure may be preceded by an aura or an unusual sensation or taste. Patients may often be incontinent or bite their tongues during a major attack and they may injure themselves in the fall. Petit mal epilepsy: perhaps just brief and repeated moments of loss of concentration and consciousness without collapse or jerky movements. Temporal lobe epilepsy: the symptoms may be similar to grand mal epilepsy but they may also be accompanied by hallucinations, particularly a sensation of smell. Narcolepsy: an irresistible desire and need to sleep.

Action

Where possible, a patient in grand mal epilepsy should be prevented from self-injury. Therefore, if a trained person is available, inserting something between the jaws to prevent biting the tongue may be helpful. It is important to maintain the patient's airway. For grand mal and for other types of epilepsy, you should seek medical assistance or advice as soon as possible.

Tests

These include electro-encephalograph (EEG), brain scan, and routine tests such as blood tests for precipitating factors.

Medications and treatment

There is a wide range of anticonvulsant medications including phenobarbitone, phenytoin, valproate, and carbamazepine. Examples: Ativan; clobazam; Epanutin; Epilim; Lamictal; Mysoline; Sabril; Valium; Zarontin. The practitioner will decide the dose and type of medication. Narcolepsy may respond to amphetamines.

Further advice

If you suffer from epilepsy, you should notify the driving authorities. You should also avoid excess alcohol and take precautions at times of greater risk. You may suffer from epilepsy only premenstrually or at night.

Epilepsy, temporal lobe

see **Epilepsy and associated conditions**

Epistaxis (nose bleed)

 Nose bleeding is a common symptom which usually resolves spontaneously but may sometimes need investigating for underlying causes.

Symptoms
Profuse bleeding from one, or occasionally both, nostrils. It may often occur spontaneously without warning, but typically occurs at moments of high stress and anxiety.

Action
Apply pressure to the appropriate side of the nose, and sit up leaning slightly forward. Putting your head between your knees is not helpful because this will increase the pressure in the nose. You should not lie flat because this will encourage blood to gather in the back of the throat. Persistent heavy epistaxis requires medical attention.

Tests
Nose bleeds may be a symptom of high blood pressure or tumours. Therefore, a brain scan may be required. Investigation of high blood pressure may also be required.

Medications and treatment
The treatment of nose bleeding is essentially surgical, whereby cautery is applied to the bleeding point to arrest bleeding.

Further advice
If you suffer from recurrent nose bleeds, you should avoid persistent nose picking!

Epstein-Barr virus

see **Virus infections, other**

Eye, diseases of the outer

see **Conjunctiva and outer eye, diseases of**

Fibroadenosis

see **Breast, diseases of**

Gallstones

see **Gall bladder disorders**

Gall bladder disorders including ♥♥ gallstones, cholecystitis (inflamed gall bladder)

 The gall bladder is an organ that stores bile which helps to digest fats. The gland itself can become inflamed (cholecystitis) or the bile may gather into various types of stones (gallstones). The stones may cause inflammation or they may block the bile duct causing biliary colic.

Symptoms
Biliary colic is an extremely painful condition usually affecting the

right side of the body under the ribs. It may be associated with jaundice (yellowness of the skin and eyes) and vomiting. Similarly, the presence of gallstones or cholecystitis will be associated with pain on the right side of the upper abdomen with nausea and vomiting, and possibly fever. The pain may radiate through to the back or to the groin. An obstructive jaundice would cause the urine to be dark and the stools to be pale.

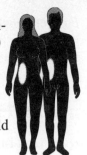

Action
Severe acute obstructive jaundice is an emergency which must be treated urgently. Milder inflammation of the gall bladder may settle down and not require urgent attention.

Tests
Ultrasound of the gall bladder, liver scan, full blood count, sedimentation rate, white count, liver function tests, and tests for hepatitis are all part of the investigation of this condition. Endoscopy, perhaps with the use of special dyes, may be helpful, and laparoscopic investigation of the gall bladder may also be valuable. Cholecystography and cholangiography are investigations which look at the biliary tree, i.e. the tubes taking bile from the gall bladder and liver to the intestines. Cholecystitis may rarely be associated with pancreatitis.

Medications and treatment
These conditions are usually treated surgically, although there are some medications which dissolve gallstones, and antibiotics may be valuable in treating infection of the gall bladder.

Further advice
Where possible, avoid fatty food which usually provokes gall bladder diseases.

Associated conditions
Jaundice due to gall bladder disease may mimic hepatitis so the causes of jaundice should be investigated.

Gall bladder, inflamed

see **Gall bladder disorders**

Gastric ulcer

see **Peptic ulcer**

Gastro-enteritis

see **Bowel infections**

Glandular fever

see **Virus infections, other**

Glaucoma

Glaucoma is a condition caused by increased pressure in the eye which damages the nerve fibres by direct pressure.

Symptoms
There may be no symptoms of glaucoma until vision is substantially impaired in either or both eyes. Acute glaucoma may appear as a painful red eye with some sensitivity to light. Chronic glaucoma may not show symptoms other than gradually impaired vision.

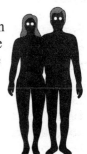

Action
Glaucoma should receive urgent medical attention.

Tests
Pressure in the eye can be measured to detect glaucoma. Precipitating causes such as diabetes should be identified and treated.

Medications and treatment
Eye drops such as Timoptol may be used. Alternatively, glaucoma can be treated by surgery.

Further advice
It is important to diagnose and treat glaucoma properly. Certain eye drops inappropriately given may make the glaucoma worse.

Gout

Gout is a condition caused by excess uric acid level in the blood. It may be genetic or it may be related to alcohol intake.

Symptoms
Classically, the presence of a severely painful joint, particularly in the first joint of the large toe. Gout can affect any joint, and deposits of uric acid may be found in the ear and elsewhere. Uric acid crystals may produce symptoms of renal colic.

Action
If you are suffering from an attack of gout, you should rest, take painkillers if necessary, and drink plenty of non-alcoholic fluids. You should avoid aspirin because, even in low doses, it increases uric acid levels.

Tests
Blood tests to check the uric acid level as well as X-rays of the joint and joint aspiration may help in making a diagnosis. Urine tests will be helpful. Occasionally, uric acid levels can be secondary to other conditions, particularly blood disorders, and these should be checked.

Medications and treatment
The acute pain of gout usually responds to drugs such as colchicine or indomethacin. Long-term prevention is achieved by using allopurinol which lowers serum uric acid levels.

Further advice
It is helpful to avoid alcohol and to drink plenty of non-alcoholic drinks, especially in warm weather. Dietry changes may be helpful and you should reduce your consumption of spinach, strawberries, offal, meat extracts, asparagus, salmon, herrings, anchovies, duck and goose meat.

Associated conditions
Pseudo-gout is a condition which is similar to gout; it usually affects the knees. A number of other conditions may also produce arthritis, including psoriasis and systemic lupus erythematosus.

Grand mal

see **Epilepsy and associated conditions**

Haemophilia and other bleeding disorders

Haemophilia is an inherited condition where lack of a blood-clotting factor (factor 8) causes persistent bleeding. The condition is passed on from mother to son and carried by the daughters of patients with haemophilia. It presents almost exclusively in males, therefore. There are other bleeding disorders, such as von Willebrand's disease and Christmas disease which are similar to haemophilia. Lack of fibrinogen, particularly in severely ill patients in intensive care units, has a similar presentation. Bleeding may also be caused by abnormalities in the platelets, e.g. idiopathic thrombocytopenic purpura.

Symptoms

Persistent bleeding of wounds, bruising, but also internal bleeding, particularly into joints. Therefore, untreated patients or inadequately treated patients may get arthritis in joints such as the elbows and knees. Early symptoms of idiopathic thrombocytopenic pupura may include rash and bruising.

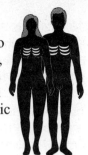

Action

Acute haemophiliac crises need urgent treatment under hospital supervision.

Tests

Blood tests for any bleeding disorder include clotting function and platelet function tests as well as genetic screening and tests for blood-clotting factors such as factor 8 and factor 9.

Medications and treatment

Haemophilia is treated with a concentrated extract of factor 8. In the past, some of these concentrates were contaminated with HIV virus, so haemophiliacs were infected with the virus and some have gone on to develop AIDS.

Further advice

Genetic counselling may be appropriate, and advice on prevention of trauma is invaluable to those suffering from haemophilia. Idiopathic thrombocytopenic purpura may respond to steroids or to removal of the spleen (splenectomy).

Haemorrhoids (piles)

Haemorrhoids are caused by swelling of veins at the end of the digestive passage around the anus. They may be associated with liver failure.

Symptoms
Bleeding on passing motions, feeling of a lump around the back passage, painful itchy sensation, and pain on opening bowels.

Action
Most haemorrhoids respond to self-medication but, if they persist, you should seek medical advice.

Tests
There are no tests for the investigation of haemorrhoids other than tests for liver failure and possibly barium enema. Sigmoidoscopy (telescope into the colon) may be required.

Medications and treatment
Haemorrhoids are usually treated surgically if necessary, but itchiness and soreness can be controlled by ointments including Anacal, Anugesic HC, Anusol, Proctosedyl, Scheriproct, Ultraproct, Uniroid, Xyloproct.

Further advice
Eating a high-roughage diet may prevent or control haemorrhoids.

Associated conditions
Anal fissure may cause pain on opening the bowels. It is caused by a small tear in the anus

Hair loss (alopecia)

Alopecia may be partial or complete. There are many causes of alopecia but, in some cases, the origin may not be known. Pregnancy (hair loss after pregnancy is known as post-partum hair loss), iron or vitamin deficiency, underactive thyroid gland, psoriasis, dermatitis, skin infestation such as lice or scabies, and chemotherapy may all cause hair loss.

Symptoms

Partial or complete hair loss. The hair loss may well be in clumps. There may be associated precipitating factors, such as psoriasis, or symptoms of underactive thyroid gland.

Action

Slight loss of hair, such as might occur after pregnancy, can be ignored because the condition will resolve itself. Severe alopecia needs medical attention.

Tests

Blood tests, such as thyroid function tests, for precipitating causes are appropriate. Skin biopsy may be necessary.

Medications and treatment

Minoxodil lotion has been used to treat alopecia. Thyroid replacement or iron and vitamin replacement should be used to treat precipitating causes.

Further advice

Trying to improve general health, reducing stress, and improving diet may stop alopecia worsening.

Associated conditions

Male pattern baldness may occur early and may result in almost complete alopecia. Minoxodil lotion may be helpful in some cases. Some conditions appear with excessive hair growth; particularly, these are hormonal conditions, such as polycystic ovaries or tumours, that produce excess male hormone. A full hormone investigation is required in such cases.

Hardening of the arteries

see **Cerebral vascular accident**

Head injury

see **Trauma/head injury**

Heart attack

 A heart attack is caused by a reduction in the blood flow to a part of the heart muscle and a subsequent clot in one of the coronary arteries. The factors which may precipitate a heart attack include: family history of heart disease; smoking; obesity; sedentary life style; high blood pressure; high cholesterol; high triglycerides.

Main symptom
Chest pain. The chest pain of a heart attack is typically central in the chest, severe, and vice-like or gripping. The pain may radiate to the left arm and jaw. Any chest pain can, however, indicate a heart attack.

Associated symptoms
Nausea, breathlessness, collapse, loss of consciousness, vomiting, loss of appetite, dizziness, death.

Action
Seek medical assistance immediately. While waiting for medical help, the patient should lie down. Clear patient's airway. Remove dentures. If trained first-aid assistance is available, carry out mouth-to-mouth resuscitation with cardiac massage. Patients should not be given alcoholic drinks or food. Avoid over-warming.

Tests
These include ECG (cardiograph), blood tests for heart enzymes, chest X-ray, blood tests for factors which may cause a heart attack, coronary angiography (X-ray of the coronary arteries using a dye); eventually exercise ECG test.

Emergency medications

The following medicines may be used by a qualified medical practitioner for the treatment of a heart attack: adrenalin, aspirin, bicarbonate drip, calcium chloride, diuretics, eminase, lignocaine, procainamide, streptokinase, TPA.

Other medications

The following medications may be given to a patient following a heart attack: anticoagulants, antihypertensives, anti-obesity drugs, aspirin, lipid-lowering agents.

Further advice

After recovery from a heart attack, you should lose weight, take up light regular exercise, stop smoking, eat a low-fat diet, and treat any other precipitating factors.

Heart failure

 Heart failure is the failure of the heart to pump adequate blood through the body or through the lungs. It may be caused by diseases of the valves such as the mitral valve, aortic valve, or tricuspic valve. These valves function to prevent back-flow of blood within the heart. They may be damaged by rheumatic fever or other infections. Heart failure may also be caused by high blood pressure or heart disease such as that described under angina or heart attack. Heart failure is a complication of having had a heart attack. Some conditions affect the heart muscle (cardiomyopathy) and these can lead to heart failure.

Main symptoms

Shortness of breath, swelling of ankles, fatigue, loss of appetite, poor exercise tolerance, swelling of the abdomen.

Action
Heart failure may be chronic or acute. Acute heart failure needs emergency treatment and patients should be treated in hospital.

Tests
Investigations for heart failure include chest X-ray, ECG, routine blood tests, kidney function tests, lung function tests, tests to identify cause of heart failure such as heart attack or high blood pressure.

Emergency medications
These include diuretics such as adrenalin, frusemide, inotropic drugs, noradrenalin.

Other medications
Medications for the long-term treatment of heart failure include Lanoxin, diuretics, other inotropic drugs, drugs to treat causes of heart failure, anti-arrhythmic drugs.

Further advice
Pay particular attention to fluid intake and output, general health, heart and kidney function. You should take light, regular exercise, stop smoking, reduce alcohol intake, and lose weight.

Heart rhythm disturbances (arrhythmias)

 Arrhythmias are caused by disturbances of the heart's electrical conducting system which can produce irregularities both detectable on ECG and of which the patient is aware. Serious arrhythmias can be fatal. There are various types of cardiac arrhythmias ranging from the simple ectopic beat through to atrial flutter, atrial fibrillation, and ventricular abnormalities, particularly ventricular fibrillation. Ventricular fibrillation is often the fatal end stage of a heart attack. The upper part of the heart is the atrium, while the lower part is the ventricle. Both have muscles which may flutter (mild) or

609

fibrillate (more severe).

Symptoms

The symptoms of arrhythmias depend on the type of rhythm disturbance. The symptoms may range from none at all to a feeling of a missed beat or an extra heartbeat, particularly after stress, fatigue, or high caffeine intake, irregular pulse rate. More severe arrhythmias may produce serious symptoms including collapse and death, the sensation of severe chest pain, breathlessness, or panic. The chest pain produced by arrhythmia may mimic the chest pain of angina or a heart attack and, indeed, may lead to either of these conditions. Some arrhythmias become worse when the patient is in certain situations or positions.

Action

An experienced first-aider may learn to massage the eyeballs or the neck to relieve the arrhythmia. Medical assistance should be sought urgently.

Tests

Tests include investigations for a heart attack and an urgent ECG, blood tests, chest X-ray, and investigation of the coronary circulation by coronary angiography.

Medications and treatment

The treatment of arrhythmias depends on the type of arrhythmia, but includes drugs such as lignocaine, calcium chloride, procainamide, bicarbonate. Milder arrhythmias can be treated with drugs such as Lanoxin, propanolol. Serious arrhythmias require DC shock with a defibrillating machine. A long-term pacemaker may be required.

Further advice

After recovery from arrhythmia, you should follow general advice as for other heart patients including weight loss, reducing nicotine and alcohol intake, and you should take light, regular exercise.

Hepatitis A

see **Liver disorders**

Hepatitis B

see **Liver disorders**

Hepatitis, non-A

see **Liver disorders**

Hepatitis non-B

see **Liver disorders**

Hernia

 A hernia is a swelling of the intestine which protrudes out through abdominal muscle. Hernias may occur in the groin (inguinal or femoral hernia) or where there is a scar (incisional hernia) or around the navel (umbilical hernia). Hiatus hernia is a condition where part of the stomach slides up into the chest and causes indigestion.

Symptoms
The presence of a lump, usually in the groin and occasionally (in men) descending into the scrotum causing an enlarged scrotum. Occasionally these swellings will be painful, particularly where the hernia strangulates or where the blood supply of the hernia is cut off. Strangulated hernia is a surgical emergency.

The hernia most commonly appears after heavy lifting, straining, or coughing, and disappears on lying down. Therefore, the lump usually appears at the end of the day and is not present first thing in the morning.

Action
There is usually no urgency, but a persistent or enlarging hernia needs a medical opinion. The painful hernia may be strangulated and, therefore, could be an emergency.

Tests
Plain abdominal X-ray to check there is no strangulated hernia and thus bowel obstruction. Pre-operative investigations include chest X-ray and full blood count.

Treatment
Hernias are treated by surgery. Wearing a truss is a temporary measure.

HIV infection and AIDS

 The human immuno-deficiency virus is normally a blood-borne virus which, after many years of infection, causes acquired immune deficiency syndrome (AIDS). The virus can be transmitted by unprotected (particularly rectal) intercourse, by blood products, and by infected needles. It is found in all ages and groups of patients (including newborn children who catch it from their infected mothers), but the nature of transmission makes it common in haemophiliacs, needle-sharing drug addicts, and male homosexual patients.

Symptoms
There are almost certainly no symptoms of acquiring HIV infection, although some patients have reported the presence of a rash after accidental needlestick injuries carrying the HIV virus. The period of asymptomatic presentation may persist for many years and varies

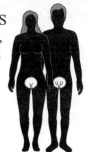

from patient to patient, but the symptoms of AIDS include weakness, fatigue, muscle loss, weight loss, opportunistic infections particularly with fungi such as oral thrush, oesophageal thrush, pneumocystis infections in the lung, septicaemia, endocarditis, and central nervous system effects including dementia, with a gradual progression to death.

Action
Specialist medical advice should be sought where HIV or AIDS is suspected.

Tests
HIV antibody tests on blood can be reported within a few hours. Tests for AIDS would include checking for opportunistic infections and for the presence of activity of T-lymphocytes.

Medications and treatment
Opportunistic infections need to be treated with appropriate antiviral, antifungal, or antibacterial medications. Retrovir is an antiviral drug which has been used in HIV-infected patients to delay progression to AIDS although this is still under research. A number of other interesting antiviral drugs are under development.

Further advice
Prevention of HIV transmission is important, and advice on the use of condoms, safe sex, use of clean needles, and testing of blood products is important.

Associated conditions
There are almost certainly at least two types of HIV virus. Patients presenting with HIV infections may also have other venereal diseases or other blood-borne viruses such as hepatitis.

Hodgkin's disease

see **Lymphomas**

Hypertension

Hypertension or high blood pressure may be related to diseases in other parts of the body such as the kidney or adrenal glands. Hypertension may be an inherited disease, however, or have no known cause (essential hypertension). It is made worse by smoking, obesity, diabetes, high alcohol intake, and may lead to heart disease, stroke, kidney disease, or damage to the eyes.

Symptoms

Hypertension may be symptomless, but symptoms include those caused by stroke or heart disease. Headache may be a symptom of hypertension, as is nose bleeding or heavy bleeding elsewhere such as heavy menstrual bleeding.

Associated symptoms

These include those related to the eyes, kidneys, and other organs which may be affected by hypertension.

Action

Hypertension should be treated by losing weight, stopping smoking, a low-salt diet, and treatment with antihypertensive drugs. If a cause for the hypertension may be identified and treated, investigations should be undertaken immediately.

Tests

These include: chest X-ray, ECG, kidney function tests, tests of the adrenal glands, routine blood tests.

Medications and treatment

Various types of drug lower blood pressure. These include diuretics, ACE inhibitors, and calcium antagonists.

Further advice

You should adopt a healthy lifestyle with light, regular exercise, no smoking, reduced alcohol intake, and weight loss.

Associated conditions
Low blood pressure (hypotension, *see also* shock) may also cause symptoms such as fatigue and headache. In some countries, heart drugs are given to increase blood pressure but this is not standard practice.

Infectious mononucleosis

see **Virus infections, other**

Infertility and endometriosis

Infertility is inability to conceive and may have many causes. Endometriosis may be one of those causes, which is a condition where the lining of the womb may become displaced into other parts of the pelvis and cause disruption of fertility.

Symptoms
Inability to conceive after regular intercourse over a period of 12 months. Infertility may also appear as repeated miscarriage (spontaneous abortion). Endometriosis may appear as infertility or as painful menstruation with pains spreading all over the abdomen and pelvis.

Action
Infertility may require medical advice and intervention if it persists. Endometriosis may settle down but may also require medical intervention.

Tests
Investigation of infertility includes plotting a temperature chart, hormonal tests to check for ovulation, analysis of sperm, post-coital analysis of sperm, immunology tests to check for antibody produc-

tion, pelvic ultrasound to check for ovarian cysts and to prove ovulation. Laparoscopy may involve the removing of ova and preparations for in-vitro fertilization.

Medications and treatment
Endometriosis may respond to hormonal blockers such as bromocriptine. Various hormonal supplements, such as oestrogen, LHRH, or progesterone, may be used to treat infertility depending on where the hormone defect is. LHRH is used to control and stimulate ovulation.

Further advice
Women trying to conceive should take regular exercise, eat a healthy diet, avoid nicotine and alcohol. Endometriosis may resolve on pregnancy.

Associated conditions
The presence of uterine fibroids may cause infertility as may any congenital abnormalities of the womb. Repeated miscarriages may occur with incompetence of the uterine cervix which may respond to suturing. Infertility may also be caused by genetic abnormalities.

Influenza

see **Upper respiratory tract infections, acute**

Intestinal obstruction ♥♥♥
including inflammatory diseases of the bowel, appendicitis, peritonitis, diverticulitis

 Bowel obstruction may be caused by a number of conditions, including appendicitis and diverticulitis, either of which may lead to inflammation of the surrounding sac, i.e. peritonitis. Intestinal obstruction may also occur through cancer, in-

flamed ulcer with stenosis of the pyloris (pyloric stenosis), perforation of the bowel, including perforated duodenal ulcer which leads to peritonitis and intestinal collapse mimicking intestinal obstruction. Diverticulitis and appendicitis are caused by inflammation of material within the gut.

Symptoms

The classic symptoms of intestinal obstruction are vomiting, abdominal pain, and complete constipation, i.e. absence of passing faeces or wind. Bowel perforation, as in perforated ulcer, presents suddenly and dramatically with collapse and abdominal rigidity. The rigidity is caused by peritonitis which can also occur with ruptured appendix or ruptured diverticulum. Appendicitis itself usually presents with central abdominal pain, which shifts down towards the right hip, followed by vomiting and constipation although, occasionally, there may be diarrhoea. Abdominal muscle tension causes guarding (involuntary tension of abdominal muscles) on examination and also complete rigidity of the stomach.

Action

These conditions are surgical emergencies and medical attention should be sought as soon as possible.

Tests

Clinical examination may reveal classical signs, e.g. guarding and rigidity. Plain X-ray of the abdomen may show fluid levels characteristic of bowel obstruction. Ultrasound examination may be useful, and occasionally limited barium studies may help in making the diagnosis. Air in the peritoneum, seen on the abdominal X-ray, signifies perforation with release of air into the peritoneum. Chest X-ray should always be carried out because conditions such as pneumonia may appear with abdominal pain. Blood tests for haemoglobin, urea and electrolytes, liver function, and kidney function should also be performed. White cell count is a good indicator of the presence of infection if it is elevated.

617

Medications and treatment

These conditions are usually treated surgically, although some conditions recover with high doses of antibiotics while awaiting the definitive diagnosis. There is some dispute about the reality of chronic appendicitis because it is usually an acute condition.

Further advice

If you have suffered from diverticulitis, you should eat a high-fibre diet to prevent further pouches developing and becoming infected.

Associated conditions

For gastro-enteritis (bowel infections). Similarly, there may be acute abdominal symptoms with disorders such as cholera, typhoid, or worms.

Iritis and uveitis

 Iritis and uveitis are auto-immune conditions whereby damage is done to the iris or the back of the eye by inflammation.

Symptoms

The symptoms of iritis are a red eye which may be painful and is particularly sensitive to light. The eye may water severely. Uveitis is a similar condition which occurs at the back of the eye. It is also painful and causes difficulty in vision.

Action

If you suspect either of these conditions, you should seek medical attention urgently.

Tests

Examination of the eye will reveal white cells as a sign of inflammation.

Medications and treatment
Steroids, given as drops, tablets, or subconjunctival injection, are used to treat these conditions.

Further advice
It is important to distinguish iritis from conjunctivitis because delay in treatment may result in impaired eyesight.

Associated conditions
Iritis and uveitis may occur as part of a generalized condition such as sarcoid or ulcerative colitis, or ankylosing spondylitis.

Itch

see **Pruritis**

Kidney and bladder, cancer of ♥♥♥♥

The urinary tract may be affected by malignancy, and the organs usually involved are the kidney and the bladder. Some children suffer from a rare type of kidney tumour, but more commonly it occurs in adults.

Symptoms
Passing blood in the urine. This may not be obvious and may only be detectable on routine urine testing (microscopic haematuria). Pain on passing urine or pain in the loins or flank may indicate the presence of a tumour. The symptoms may be similar to those of renal colic.

Associated symptoms
Symptoms of malignancy, such as fever and weight loss, may also be present.

Action
Urgent investigation of any of these symptoms is required.

Tests
Urine analysis, cystoscopy, intravenous pyelogram, biopsy, ultrasound examination of the kidneys, and routine blood tests to look for anaemia.

Medications and treatment
Tumours of the kidney or bladder need to be removed surgically. Radiotherapy may be helpful, and interferon and interleukin may also be used.

Further advice
Tumours of the genito-urinary tract are more common in smokers.

Associated conditions
Warts or papillomas of the bladder may be benign but they may convert to malignant tumours.

Kidney failure

 The kidneys are organs of excretion, and there are several causes of failure. These include acute sudden failure as in glomerulonephritis which may occur after streptococcal infection. Damage to the kidneys through repeated infection, hypertension, or diabetes (diabetic nephropathy) may also cause kidney failure. Congenital abnormalities of the kidneys or polycystic kidneys may also lead to kidney failure.

Symptoms
These include fluid retention, nausea, weight gain, pale skin and anaemia, swelling of the ankles and abdomen, the passing of excess urine or failure to pass urine at all, the passing of blood in the urine (haematu-

ria), breathing problems, heart problems (due to changes in potassium levels), and death.

Action
Suspected kidney failure must be treated as a medical emergency.

Tests
Investigations include routine blood tests to look for causes of kidney failure, concentrating particularly on urea, potassium, creatinine and creatinine clearance. Patients are often anaemic, and this should also be investigated and treated.

Medications and treatment
Treatment of kidney failure includes attention to the cause of the kidney failure, peritoneal dialysis, haemo-dialysis, or kidney transplant. Drugs such as erythropoietin may be useful to treat the anaemia caused by kidney failure.

Further advice
If you are suffereing from chronic kidney failure, you may need to go on special diets which are low in potassium and protein. Special foods are available.

Kidney stones (renal calculus)

 Kidney stones are formed from calcium oxidate or uric acid and they can appear anywhere in the urinary tract from the kidney down to the bladder and urethra. Their appearance may be related to dehydration or conditions where there is an increased calcium level in the blood, hypocalcemia due to overactive parathyroid glands, increased calcium intake with alkalis, or where there is disease of the bones, including malignancy, which releases calcium from bones. Some people have raised calcium in the urine for unknown reasons (idiopathic hypercalciuria).

Symptoms

There may be none. Occasionally, patients may pass bits of gravel, or blood may be detected. Renal colic is a seriously painful condition where a stone becomes trapped in the ureter. Spasm of the ureter, which is trying to expel the stone, results in pain which is continuous and may worsen acutely. The pain may radiate from loin down to the groin and into the genitalia. It may be associated with passing blood or gravel. Late presentation of kidney stones may be with kidney failure. Stones in the bladder may cause irritable bladder and haematuria.

Action

Severe renal colic is a medical emergency. Detection of stones in the urinary tract should always be fully investigated.

Tests

Investigations include cystoscopy, urine measurements for infection, blood, and crystals, intravenous pyelogram (IVP), ultrasound studies, blood tests for calcium and uric acid.

Medications and treatment

The pain of renal colic may resolve with narcotic analgesics. High fluid intake is usually encouraged for the stone to pass naturally. Stones which do not pass naturally may require surgical intervention to remove them.

Further advice

In hot climates, especially, you should drink plenty of non-alcoholic fluids to prevent a high concentration of calcium in the urine.

Associated conditions

Bladder stones may be present without kidney stones. These may form around other bladder abnormalities, e.g. papilloma.

Labyrinthitis

see **Vestibulitis and labyrinthitis**

Laryngitis

see **Upper respiratory tract infections, acute**

Leukaemias

 Leukaemias are conditions where excessive growth in the bone marrow of malignant white cells overwhelms the body's own normal cell production system. Leukaemia may be acute or chronic and may develop from the myeloid or lymphatic blood cell lines. Children usually develop acute lymphoblastic leukamia whereas the elderly may develop chronic myeloid or chronic lymphoblastic leukaemia.

Symptoms
Leukaemia may appear in a variety of ways: excessive bleeding; anaemia; bruising; enlarged glands; enlarged liver; enlarged spleen; persistent infections, particularly shingles. Leukaemia may be detected by routine blood tests.

Action
Where suspected or diagnosed, leukaemia requires urgent specialist attention.

Tests
The tests for leukaemia include blood tests, bone marrow tests, scans of major organs, possible biopsies of lymph glands or spleen.

Medications and treatment
As well as general supportive medications, such as the treatment of anaemia and the use of steroids, specific cytotoxic (powerful cell-killing agents which destroy rapidly growing cells) chemotherapies are used for the treatment of leukaemias.

Further advice
Many types of leukaemia are now treatable and the long-term prognosis is very encouraging.

Associated conditions
There is a range of syndromes, including myelofibrosis (failure of the bone marrow) and polycythemia (excessive red blood cells), which are all related to the leukaemia syndromes.

Lice

see **Skin infestations**

Lipid metabolism, disorders of

 There are rare lipid storage diseases, such as Gaucher's disease, which normally affect children. In adults, the most common problems are elevation of cholesterol and triglycerides, usually as part of an inherited disorder but sometimes due to outside factors, such as alcohol or poor diet.

Symptoms
Usually none, but it may appear with heart disease such as angina or heart attack. Deposits of lipid around the eyes or joints may be noticeable. Furring up of peripheral arteries may appear with intermittent claudication (limping).

Action
A low-fat diet is important but, where a serious lipid disorder is suspected, medical advice should be sought.

Tests
Heart and blood tests for HDL and LDL cholesterol, as well as triglycerides, are important. Other conditions, such as an underactive

thyroid gland, may produce elevation of lipids and these should also be checked.

Medications and treatment

Apart from weight loss and diet, there is a number of medications, particularly the more recently developed drugs, such as Zocor, which lower cholesterol levels. Atromid-S, Bezalip-Mono, Bradilan, Colestid, Lipantil, Lipostat, Lopid, Lurselle, Maxepa, Modalim, Olbetam, Questran-A, Zocor.

Further advice

It is important to drink less alcohol to control elevated lipids. Relatives of patients with elevated lipids should be screened to be checked for familial problems.

Liver, cancer of

see **Liver disorders**

Liver, cirrhosis of

see **Liver disorders**

Liver disorders including hepatitis A, ♥♥♥♥ hepatitis B, non-A non-B hepatitis, cirrhosis of the liver, cancer of the liver

 The liver is the largest organ of the body and is responsible for the removal of toxic substances and the storage of other substances, such as glucose. The liver can be affected by viruses such as glandular fever, hepatitis A or hepatitis B, or a third virus known as non-A non-B hepatitis. There is also a hepatitis C. Hepatitis A is usually contracted by drinking

625

infected water whereas hepatitis B is contracted by receiving infected blood or sexually transmitted disease. Cirrhosis of the liver is a thickening and degeneration of the liver which may occur as a late result of virus infection or due to alcohol. Liver cancers are usually secondary from the bowel, but primary liver cancer may also occur.

Symptoms

The main symptoms of liver disease are jaundice, i.e. yellowness of the skin and eyes caused by an elevated level of bilirubin. Enlargement of the liver may occur such that the liver may be felt below the rib cage. A collection of fluid in the peritoneum (ascites) and the development of haemorrhoids are also signs of liver failure. Blood vessel swelling may also occur around the oesophagus resulting in vomiting of blood. Prolonged liver failure may eventually lead to coma and death. The jaundice that occurs with hepatitis or glandular fever is usually transient, disappearing after a short time. Long-term effects may include depression and sensitivity to alcohol. The spleen may also be enlarged and can be felt under the left rib cage.

Tests

Liver function tests including antibodies for hepatitis viruses and glandular fever viruses are important. Ultrasound or CT scan of the liver will reveal the possibility of cirrhosis or cancer. Endoscopy may be required.

Treatment

Occasionally steroids may be used to treat hepatitis, but the usual treatment is isolation and allowing the virus to settle. Interferon has been used with some success. Rarely, liver cancers may be treated surgically or with chemotherapy. Cirrhosis requires the removal of alcohol from the system and a gradual recovery.

Further advice

Avoiding fatty foods may be helpful for some time after liver infections and cirrhosis. Avoiding alcohol is valuable in all liver diseases because the liver may be particularly sensitive.

Associated conditions

Gilbert's syndrome is a condition which is benign where there is an elevation of bilirubin. Haemachromatosis is a condition where there are deposits of iron in the liver which may cause cirrhosis. There are other types of cirrhosis which are not related to alcohol, e.g. primary biliary cirrhosis.

Lower respiratory infections, acute (pleurisy, pneumonia, tracheitis, acute bronchitis) ♥♥♥

These acute chest infections may be caused by bacteria, viruses, or fungi. They may be secondary to other respiratory infections.

Main symptoms

Cough with production of sputum, chest pain, fever, weakness, and associated debility with vomiting. Conditions such as pleurisy have a chest pain which is noticeably worse on taking a deep breath, and pleurisy may co-exist with pneumonia. The conditions may affect one lobe of the lung or all the lobes of both lungs (double pneumonia).

Action

Severe infections with severe fatigue and prostration require immediate medical treatment. General advice includes resting the patient in bed, avoiding smoking, humidifying the room, and maintaining a sensible room temperature — approximately 20 °C (68 °F). Patients should not be too warm.

Tests

Investigations for suspected pneumonia and other lower respiratory infections include chest X-ray, blood tests including white cell count and sedimentation rate, culture of sputum for bacteria, and fungal swabs from the upper respiratory tract.

Medications and treatment

Antibiotics, including amoxycillin, ampicillin, cephalexin, Ciproxin, erythromycin, penicillin, Septrin, tetracycline, and trimethoprim, can be used for bacterial infections. Antifungal agents are used for fungal infections. Viral infections will not respond to such treatment and need general supportive care, including oxygen, humidifiers, and possibly bronchodilators.

Further advice

You may suffer from repeated lower respiratory tract infections. You should avoid smoking and contact with other irritants such as dust which may provoke chronic lower respiratory infections.

Lower respiratory infections, chronic ♥♥ (including chronic bronchitis, emphysema, and bronchiectasis)

Chronic lower respiratory infections may follow on from lung damage caused by repeated attacks of acute lower respiratory infections. They are more likely where there is poor hygiene and living conditions, cigarette smoking, poor nutrition, and a family history of such infections. Bronchiectasis is a condition where there are lung abscesses, and emphysema where there is breakdown of lung material. The most common is chronic bronchitis, and this is commonly caused by cigarette smoking.

Main symptoms

Chronic cough with overproduction of infected sputum. In addition, shortness of breath, repeated fevers, chest pain, general fatigue, and malaise are also symptoms.

Action

You should seek medical advice to treat the acute exacerbation of chronic bronchitis, bronchiectasis, and emphysema.

Tests
Tests for chronic lower respiratory infections include chest X-ray, sputum culture for bacteria and fungi, ECG, routine blood tests for white count and sedimentation rate.

Medications and treatment
You may need long-term oxygen therapy. In addition, you may require long-term antibiotic treatment, including amoxycillin, ampicillin, cephalexin, Ciproxin, erythromycin, penicillin, Septrin, tetracycline, and trimethoprim, with additional cover during acute exacerbations. Bronchodilators based on aminophylline or salbutamol may be helpful.

Further advice
You should stop smoking, take regular exercise, eat a healthy diet, and improve living conditions where possible to avoid dust, damp, and cold.

Lumbago

see **Backache**

Lung cancer (carcinoma of the bronchus, squamous cell carcinoma, adenocarcinoma, small cell carcinoma, oatcell carcinoma)

Lung cancer, or carcinoma of the bronchus, is the commonest form of cancer. The vast majority of lung cancers occur in cigarette smokers, and passive smoking may be a factor in causing lung diseases. The appearance of mesothelioma (can-

cer of the lung lining) may occur 20-30 years after exposure to asbestos.

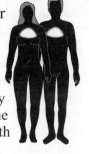

Main symptoms
Persistent cough, weight loss, coughing up blood, repeated chest infections, symptoms of secondary deposits particularly in the brain and bones. Some unusual presentations of lung cancer can occur with fluid retention and joint symptoms.

Action
Diagnosis should be made early. This condition may sometimes be picked up on routine chest X-ray. Examination of sputum for malignant cells can sometimes diagnose this condition.

Tests
Tests involve sputum cytology for malignant cells, chest X-ray, bronchoscopy with biopsy, bone scan, brain scan, routine blood tests.

Medications and treatment
Some lung cancers are amenable to surgery; others respond to chemotherapy and radiotherapy. Infections should be treated with appropriate antibiotics or antifungal medications.

Further advice
Lung cancer is best prevented by avoiding cigarette smoking. If you have suffered from lung cancer and been treated successfully, you should maintain a healthy lifestyle and not smoke.

Lymphomas (including Hodgkin's disease)

Lymphomas are malignant diseases of the lymph glands. There are various types including Hodgkin's disease and the so-called non-Hodgkin's lymphomas.

Symptoms

Lymphomas may appear with swelling of a lymph gland, or the liver or the spleen. Occasionally, the glands may be internal so that an enlarged and malignant gland may not be detectable. The condition may be picked up, therefore, on routine X-ray, e.g. chest X-ray, or other examination. As with other malignant diseases, lymphomas may appear with symptoms of anaemia, weakness, secondary infections such as shingles, or it may invade the bone marrow and be detected by routine blood tests. Hodgkin's disease and other lymphomas are associated with fevers and night sweats, and occasionally with pain in the affected glands when drinking alcohol.

Action

An enlarged lymph gland which is firm, rubbery, and not obviously infected requires investigation.

Tests

These include full blood count, routine liver and kidney tests, chest X-ray, scans of chest and abdomen, biopsy of affected or suspected glands.

Medications and treatment

As with the anaemias, supportive treatment, in the form of treatment of anaemia and use of steroids, is given in addition to cytotoxic chemotherapy and, where appropriate, radiotherapy.

Malaria

Malaria is an infection caused by a protozoan carried by insects, namely the mosquito. Infection is commonly contracted in tropical areas where there is poor sanitation, but the symptoms can appear at any time thereafter.

Symptoms

The symptoms are similar to those of severe influenza, and the diagnosis can often be missed. Fever, shaking, headache, pains in the limbs, abdominal pain, weakness, depression, tiredness, are all symptoms of malaria. Malaria may be mild and recurrent or it may progress to a severe state with haemorrhage, kidney failure, brain haemorrhage, and death.

Action

If you suspect malaria, you should seek immediate medical advice by a specialist in tropical medicine.

Tests

Blood tests to look for malaria parasites can make the diagnosis. Other tests for severe infections might be helpful.

Medications and treatment

Antimalarial drugs, such as pymethamine or chloroquine, are used in the management of the acute case. These and other drugs are also used as preventative measures taken before travelling to potential malaria areas. Avloclor, Daraprim, Fansidar, Halfan, Lariam, Maloprim, Nivaquine, Paludrine.

Further advice

Malaria is normally prevented by taking antimalarial medication prior to, and for four weeks after, a visit to a malaria area. The type of medication taken depends on the area, and updated reports of required medication can be obtained from tropical medicine institutes.

Associated conditions

Tropical diseases include a number of insect-borne infections, such as lyme disease, rocky mountain spotted fever, and a number of other protozoal diseases and infections caused by bathing in or drinking infected water. Any infection in someone who has returned from a tropical country should be investigated for full tropical screen.

ME

see **Myalgic encephalomyelitis**

Ménière's disease (and tinnitus)

 Ménière's disease is a condition whereby the patient suffers from vertigo or dizziness, deafness, and buzzing in the ear (tinnitus). The cause of Ménière's disease is unknown, but it may be related to changes in lymph pressure in the inner ear.

Main symptoms
Tinnitus, deafness, and dizziness or vertigo. These symptoms may occur without warning several times a day and then with remissions for several days or weeks before recurring again without provocation.

Action
If you have a severe attack of Ménière's disease, you should lie down. If the attacks recur, you should seek medical advice.

Tests
Vestibular function tests and brain scan should be carried out to exclude acoustic neuroma, a rare tumour of the eighth cranial nerve which may mimic Ménière's disease.

Medications and treatment
Attacks of Ménière's disease respond to drugs such as Stemetil. Other drugs, such as Serc, may be useful in the long term.

Further advice
You should avoid swimming, diving, and air travel where possible. Cigarette smoking may make the condition worse.

Associated conditions

You may suffer from recurrent attacks of tinnitus without full-blown Ménière's disease. Tinnitus is a distressing symptom which may have no underlying cause and may disappear eventually.

Meningitis and encephalitis

 These serious conditions are caused by bacteria or viruses. Encephalitis is a rare late complication of measles. Meningitis may occasionally follow mumps infection but, often, it is a new infection passed around closed communities.

Symptoms

The symptoms of meningitis include fever, stiff neck, rigidity, rash on the body, deteriorating consciousness, unconsciousness, paralysis, and death. Encephalitis may appear similarly without the stiff neck characteristic of meningitis.

Action

As soon as these conditions are suspected, immediate medical attention is required to maintain the airway, and to begin diagnostic and therapeutic procedures.

Tests

Meningitis is diagnosed by lumbar puncture. Encephalitis may be harder to diagnose. Full blood tests, white count, sedimentation rates, chest X-ray, and skull X-ray are also part of the routine management of this condition. A high white count and raised sedimentation rate (ESR) are signs of infection.

Medications and treatment

Meningococcal meningitis responds to penicillin therapy. Viral meningitis does not respond to antibacterial therapy, and general supportive measures, including ventilation, may be required. Encephalitis is also usually a viral infection and the patient should be treated in hospital with general supportive measures.

Further advice
Meningitis contacts should be swabbed for carrier status. Vaccination is now available for certain types of meningitis.

Menopause, the ♥

The menopause occurs at about the age of 50 years in women and is brought on by a gradual failure of the ovaries to produce hormones. The main hormone involved is oestrogen, and lack of it affects several organs in the body.

Symptoms
Flushing due to excess pituitary hormone, hot sweats, loss of calcium from bone, bone pain and fractures, irritability, unwanted hair growth, dryness of the vagina, and loss of libido. Menstruation becomes irregular and bleeding lighter. Menstruation eventually ceases altogether.

Action
The menopause is a natural process and many women believe that no further action needs to be taken.

Tests
Testing for the menopause, which may begin in the mid- to late thirties, involves hormone tests of oestrogen, progesterone and FSH. Cervical smears may give an indication of the amount of oestrogen present.

Medications and treatment
Hormone replacement therapy using skin patches, vaginal pessaries, hormonal implants, or oral tablets may all be valuable in reversing the menopause. Where a woman has had a hysterectomy, unopposed oestrogen may be used, but otherwise oestrogen and progestogens are given together. These cause re-establishment of

menstruation. Examples include: Cycloprogynova, Duphaston, Estraderm, Estrapak, Harmogen, Hormonin, Ortho Dienoestrol, Ortho-Gynest, Ovestin, Premarin, Prempak, Trisequens, Vagifem.

Further advice
Hormone replacement therapy may slightly increase the risk of breast cancer but probably reduces the risk of heart disease and fractures of the bones, particularly the hip. Worsening premenstrual symptoms may be a sign of the menopause.

Menstrual disorders including ♥♥ heavy bleeding (menorrhagia), intermenstrual bleeding, painful bleeding (dysmenorrhea), dysfunctional uterine bleeding

 Abnormalities of menstruation are very common and, although they may herald diseases of the womb, such as fibroids, they may be related to hormonal fluctuations, and it is often difficult to establish a true causative factor.

Symptoms
Abnormally heavy bleeding, periods which are either too short or too long, cycles which are too short or too long, bleeding between periods (intermenstrual bleeding), bleeding after intercourse (post-coital bleeding), painful menstruation (dysmenorrhea).

Action
Persistent abnormalities in the menstrual cycle should be investigated.

Tests
Clinical examination, ultrasound examination, tests of hormonal function including tests for the menopause should all be carried out.

Medications and treatment

Clinical examination and diagnostic dilatation and curettage (D & C) are part of the management of this condition. The use of hormones may re-establish a normal cycle. Intermenstrual bleeding or post-coital bleeding may be caused by abnormalities of the womb or cervix. Very often the D & C is both investigative and curative, and restarts the normal cycles. The menopause may need to be treated with hormone replacement therapy, including Cycloprogynova, Duphaston, Estraderm, Estrapak, Harmogen, Hormonin, Ortho Dienoestrol, Ortho-Gynest, Ovestin, Premarin, Prempak, Trisequens, Vagifem.

Further advice

The IUCD may cause heavy periods, while taking the oral contraceptive pill may cause particularly light periods.

Middle-ear infection

see **Otitis media**

Migraine (and associated conditions, ♥ migrainous neuralgia and trigeminal neuralgia)

Migraine is a condition where headache is associated with other symptoms described below. The cause of migraine is not known, but it is thought to be precipitated by certain factors such as emotional stress, physical stress, cold, eating certain foods, e.g. cheese and chocolate.

Symptoms

The main symptom of migraine is a severe one-sided headache, but this is not always the typical presentation. The headache is associated with nausea and vomiting, prostration (need to lie down), visual disturbances (teichopsia) and occasionally weakness or numbness of parts of the body. These symptoms are caused by spasm of blood vessels in the brain. Migrainous neuralgia is a condition in which the headache may be associated with pain and watering in one eye (sometimes known as cluster headaches). Trigeminal neuralgia is similar in that there is facial pain on one side.

Action
If you are suffering from migraine, you should lie down in a darkened room and avoid stress or other precipitating factors. The symptoms may resolve spontaneously.

Tests
Nerve conduction studies may be appropriate, as are brain scan and EEG where symptoms are persistent and disabling.

Medications and treatment
Imigran is a relatively new but effective treatment for migraine. Otherwise, there are other ergot medications as well as over-the-counter preparations such as Migraleve. Trigeminal neuralgia and migrainous neuralgia may respond to carbamazepine. Examples: Betaloc; Blocadren; Cafergot; Corgard; Deseril; Dihydergot; Dixarit; Imigran; Inderal; Lingraine; Lopresor; Medihaler-Ergotamine; Midrid; Migraleve; Migravess; Migril; Paramax; Periactin; Sanomigran.

Further advice
Preventing attacks by avoiding precipitating factors may be helpful. Dietary maintenance is often effective.

Motor neurone disease ♥♥♥♥♥
(also called amyotrophic lateral sclerosis)

Motor neurone disease is a progressive neuro-logical condition; its cause is not known. It affects the nerves supplying muscles, and so the symptoms are mainly related to movement rather than to sensation.

Symptoms

Slow, progressive weakness of muscles in certain parts of the body. These muscles may affect speech and swallowing (pseudo-bulbar palsy) or, more commonly, the hands. Weakness and wasting of muscles are characteristic with fibrillation. The condition worsens progressively, and eventually patients will die from the disease.

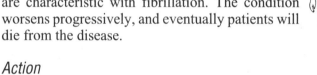

Action

Early diagnosis is important so that support systems can be established to maintain patients who may ultimately become paralysed and need supportive care.

Tests

Biopsy of nerve and muscle may be helpful in making the diagnosis but very often the disease is diagnosed clinically. MRI scan may be helpful.

Medications and treatment

There are no medications which are known to affect the progress of this disease, but treatment of infections, and general support are often required.

Mouth, tumours of the

Tumours of the mouth are quite rare but may occur in people who are heavy smokers or who drink spirits in quantity.

Symptoms
Usually a lump or swelling on the tongue or gum. This may eventually ulcerate or bleed. There may be associated swelling of lymph nodes around the neck.

Action
Seek medical advice urgently for any lump or swelling in the mouth.

Tests
Investigations of these include biopsy to assess the degree of malignancy of the tumour.

Medications and treatment
The treatment of head and neck tumours in general is firstly surgical followed by chemotherapy and radiotherapy.

Further advice
Avoiding smoking and alcohol helps to prevent this condition and you should not smoke or drink alcohol if you are being treated for it.

Multiple sclerosis (disseminated sclerosis)

The cause of multiple sclerosis is not known for certain, although there is a suggestion that it is a degenerative and demyelinating disease triggered by earlier viral infection. The nerve tracts are affected by areas of loss of the fatty sheath (demyelination) which affects nerve conduction. Multiple sclerosis is more common in mild climates and among people with a family history of the condition.

Symptoms

They may vary enormously. Typically, the symptoms are not noticed on both sides of the body at the same time, but they are patchy (i.e. disseminated). Temporary loss of vision may be an early symptom, as may be trigeminal neuralgia. Pain or tingling sensations of heat, or pins and needles anywhere in the body, particularly in the limbs, may also be an early symptom. The symptoms may come and go in bursts with remissions and relapses. The disease progresses at different rates in different people and, while some patients progress inexorably to blindness and paralysis, others remain permanently stable after a brief display of symptoms. Mood changes, from depression to euphoria, may also be associated with the condition. Demyelination affecting the parasympathetic nervous system may cause bowel and bladder problems.

Action

You should seek specialist neurological opinion if your symptoms are alarming and persistent. Self-medication is generally not advisable because there are many unproven treatments available.

Tests

Lumbar puncture and biopsy are the tests which make the diagnosis of this condition. Suspicions may be made on clinical grounds alone. Brain scans, MRI scans, may show a very clear picture of demyelination.

Medications and treatment

While steroids may produce some benefit, and trials of interferon are under way, there are no recognized cures for multiple sclerosis, although general supportive measures are appropriate.

Further advice

Keeping yourself in good health and trying to maintain an optimistic outlook are essential in controlling this condition.

Myalgic encephalomyelitis ♥♥ (ME, yuppie flu, Royal Free disease, post-viral fatigue syndrome)

This condition affects the nerves and the muscles, and usually occurs after a severe virus infection of the glandular fever or Epstein-Barr type.

Symptoms
Classically, fatigue and muscle ache, weakness and depression. True clinical depression may co-exist and make diagnosis difficult. Patients feel permanently exhausted and unable to work or exercise. This sets up a vicious circle from which it may be difficult to escape.

Action
Simple remedies should be tried at first but, if symptoms are persistent, you should seek medical advice.

Tests
There are no diagnostic tests for this condition which adds to the difficulty in treating and managing patients who suffer.

Medications and treatment
High doses of vitamins, sometimes given intravenously, and minerals, such as magnesium, have been tried with some success for this condition. Counselling and psychotherapy may also be of value.

Further advice
Maintaining a healthy diet and regular exercise pattern, as well as a positive attitude may prevent this condition and help recovery from it. You should begin a programme of gentle exercises.

Associated conditions
See infectious mononucleosis, Chapter 15.

Myasthenia gravis

Myasthenia gravis is a disease of the neuromuscular junction. The cause of this condition is not known.

Symptoms

Severe weakness of muscles, particularly affecting the upper limbs, but also the eyes and eyelids. The muscles exhaust very quickly, so that there may be some muscle function after rest but this runs out after a short period of time.

Action

Where this condition is suspected, medical advice should be sought immediately.

Tests

Diagnosis can be made by muscle biopsy and tests using drugs such as edrophonium.

Medications and treatment

Myasthenia gravis is treated with anticholinesterase drugs such as Mestinon or Prostigimin.

Associated conditions

Muscular dystrophies can be similar to myasthenia gravis. These are usually inherited. *See also* motor neurone disease, Chapter 5.

Nails, diseases of

The main conditions affecting the nails are infection (paronychia) and ingrowing toenail. The nails may also be altered by conditions such as psoriasis or calcium and vitamin deficiency. Iron deficiency may cause changes in nail shape.

Trauma to the hands often causes nail disfigurement. Fungus infections may affect the nails.

Main symptoms
Obvious change in the shape, texture, and colour of the nail or an infection next to the nail as in ingrowing toenail or paronychia.

Action
These conditions may respond to self-medication, but, if they persist, you should seek medical attention.

Tests
Biopsy culture of nail scrapings may be required, and investigation of underlying causes (e.g. anaemia or psoriasis) may resolve the cause of nail problems.

Medications and treatment
Nail disorders, such as ingrowing toenail, are usually treated surgically but they may respond to local use of antiseptics and antibiotics. Paronychia should also respond to antibiotics, and fungus infections will respond to local nail paints, such as Trosyl, or antifungal tablets, such as Grisovin. The underlying causes of nail disorders (e.g. anaemia) should receive the appropriate treatment for that condition.

Further advice
Good general health and hygiene will maintain healthy strong nails.

Narcolepsy

see **Epilepsy and associated conditions**

Nasal septum, deviated ♥

Deviated nasal septum is a condition in which the cartilage in the centre of the nose is twisted. This may occur as a result of injury or trauma, but it may also happen spontaneously.

Main symptom
Difficulty in breathing, particularly at night and especially when lying on one side. Symptoms of sinusitis may also occur.

Action
Self-medication may be appropriate, but this condition often needs surgical intervention.

Tests
Examination of the nose is usually enough to make a diagnosis of this condition.

Medications and treatment
Nasal decongestants and antihistamines may improve the symptoms of this condition, but essentially an operation, called a submucous resection, is carried out to correct the twist in the nasal septum.

Further advice
Stop smoking to prevent this and similar conditions from recurring.

Neuralgia, migrainous

see **Migraine**

Neuralgia, trigeminal

see **Migraine**

Neuropathy, including peripheral ♥♥ neuropathy and nerve pressure symptoms, e.g. carpal tunnel syndrome and Bell's palsy

Neuropathy is a condition in which there is interference with, or damage to, the nerves, usually to the hands and feet. Neuropathy may be caused by certain types of vitamin deficiency, diabetes, certain drugs or toxins, and late manifestations of diseases such as syphilis.

Symptoms
The main symptoms of neuropathy are pain, tingling, or loss of sensation in certain areas of the body, usually in the hands and feet. Carpal tunnel syndrome is caused by pressure on a nerve at the wrists and this causes pain in the hands. Bell's palsy is caused by a virus infection of the facial nerve, and this can cause paralysis of the muscles on one side of the face, mimicking a stroke. Patients may have walking difficulties, e.g. foot drop, or difficulty undoing or doing up buttons.

Action
Progressive neuropathy should be investigated and treated but it is not usually an emergency.

Tests
These include excluding vitamin deficiencies, diabetes, and other causes. Therefore, blood tests are carried out to check the blood sugar, anaemia, underactive thyroid gland and other possible causes. Nerve conduction studies are especially useful, e.g. in nerve compression syndrome such as the carpal tunnel syndrome.

Medications and treatment
The underlying causes should be treated specifically, e.g. antidiabetic agents for diabetes, vitamins for vitamin deficiency, and thyroxine for underactive thyroid.

Further advice
Pay particular attention to general health, e.g. alcohol intake and diet. You should exercise regularly.

Neuropathy, peripheral

see **Neuropathy**

Nose bleed

see **Epistaxis**

Oatcell carcinoma

see **Lung cancer**

Obesity

see **Eating disorders**

Osteoarthritis and osteoporosis

 Osteoporosis is loss of calcium from the bones which occurs in older people. Osteoarthritis is loss of cartilage tissue from the joints. It is a degenerative condition and also occurs in the older age groups.

Symptoms
Osteoporosis may appear with fractures, pain, and backache. Osteoarthritis presents with pain, bony swelling in the joints, and stiffness. It can be distinguished from rheumatoid arthritis because

of its occurrence in the older age groups and from the presence of Heberden's nodes (swelling of the last joint) on the fingers. Typically, the hip and the knee are the joints affected, so that difficulty in walking is a main symptom. Osteoarthritis may also affect the hands. There may be an inherited component in the female line of families. Osteoarthritis of the hip may cause pain in the groin. Osteoarthritis of the neck may cause a stiff neck

Action
The symptoms may well respond to rest, improved climate, and to simple painkillers, but persistent symptoms require medical attention.

Tests
X-rays of joints, blood tests to distinguish the condition from rheumatoid arthritis, and measurements of calcium in bone should be carried out to diagnose these conditions.

Medications and treatment
Simple painkillers, such as ibuprofen, or more powerful non-steroidal anti-inflammatory drugs or analgesics may be required. Fractures caused by osteoporosis may need treatment with drugs, such as etidronate, and by hormone replacement to try to improve the calcium retention in bone.

Further advice
A healthy diet, high in vitamins and calcium, and light regular exercise are important in preventing bones and joints deteriorating.

Associated conditions
Backache and its associated conditions are clearly related to conditions such as osteoporosis and osteoarthritis.

Osteoporosis

see **Osteoarthritis and osteoporosis**

Otitis media (middle-ear infection)

Otitis media is an infection of the middle ear which occurs in adults and children. It is usually a bacterial infection.

Main symptoms
Severe pain in the middle ear, deafness particularly in response to changes in air pressure (i.e. while flying), fever, and other symptoms of an infection.

Action
Middle-ear infections usually need treatment, but often they resolve spontaneously when the eardrum ruptures to release the infection. This occurs by the slight tearing of the eardrum, and a sudden decrease in pain. You should seek medical advice, however, to check the integrity of the ear and to prescribe appropriate medications.

Tests
Routine testing is not normally carried out for middle-ear infection. Chronic ear infections with mastoiditis may require more intensive investigation, however, including brain scan.

Medications and treatment
Antibiotics, including amoxycillin, ampicillin, cephalexin, Ciproxin, erythromycin, Flagyl, penicillin, Septrin, tetracycline, and trimethoprim, are best used for middle-ear infections and are usually given by mouth. Antibiotic eardrops are not suitable for this condition.

Further advice
You should avoid air travel during and after middle-ear infection. Avoid swimming, particularly diving deep into swimming pools where bacteria may lurk.

Associated conditions
Otitis externa (external-ear infection) is a similar condition affecting the outer ear. It may respond to antibiotic drops.

Ovary, diseases of the ♥♥♥♥

The ovary may develop cysts and tumours. Polycystic ovaries are a rare cause of amenorrhoea, excess hair, and infertility.

Symptoms
Ovarian disease may be symptomless but, occasionally, there may be abnormal menstrual bleeding, abdominal swelling, and pain. Ovarian cysts may rupture or bleed and this may be an acutely painful condition.

Action
If ovarian disease is suspected, urgent investigation is required.

Tests
Abdominal ultrasound should detect the presence of ovarian disease. Clinical examination and further CT scans may be required.

Medications and treatment
Usually surgery.

Associated conditions
Amenorrhoea may also be a symptom of pregnancy or other uterine disease. It also occurs as part of the anorexia syndrome and may occur at times of emotional stress (e.g. during travel or after moving away from home).

Pancreas, cancer of

see **Pancreas, disorders of**

Pancreas, disorders of, ♥♥♥ including acute and chronic pancreatitis and cancer of the pancreas (for diabetes mellitus see Chapter 16)

 The pancreas gland is a digestive organ which may be involved in acute inflammation (acute pancreatitis) or slower inflammation (chronic pancreatitis). Both these conditions may be related to a high alcohol intake, and pancreatitis may occur as part of a virus disease including the mumps virus. Cancer of the pancreas is an unusual cancer.

Symptoms
Acute pancreatitis: severe upper abdominal pain with associated peritonitis.

Chronic pancreatitis and cancer of the pancreas: possibly low-grade upper abdominal pain and associated jaundice. Any of these conditions may provoke diabetes because of destruction of the islet cells in the pancreas gland. The upper abdominal pain may radiate through to the back and may be indistinguishable from gall bladder disease, indigestion, or even heart disease.

Action
Acute pancreatitis with collapse is a medical emergency. Any patient with low-grade upper abdominal pain and jaundice needs to be considered for chronic pancreatitis or cancer of the pancreas, and investigated accordingly.

Tests
Ultrasound examinations of the pancreas, CT scan, and endoscopy with the use of special dyes all help to diagnose pancreatic disease. Blood tests of amylase are very useful in making the diagnosis of pancreatitis.

Medications and treatment
Aprotinin may be useful in acute pancreatic disorders. Surgical

651

investigation is rarely used although surgery may sometimes be attempted for pancreatic disorders. Acute pancreatitis is normally treated by rehydration and nasogastric tube and by awaiting spontaneous recovery.

Associated conditions

Mumps or gallstones may be associated with pancreatitis. Severe drop in calcium levels can occur with acute pancreatitis as can bruising over the stomach.

Pancreatitis

see **Pancreas, disorders of**

Parkinson's disease

The cause of Parkinson's disease is not known. It results in loss of dopamine-producing nerve fibres in the brain. This causes the symptoms described below. Rarely, Parkinson's-type syndromes can occur after taking certain drugs, particularly phenothiazine types, and after virus infection (post-encephalitic parkinsonism).

Symptoms

These include tremor, usually of the hands, rigidity of the limbs and facial muscles. Patients have difficulty walking, writing, and, on some occasions, talking. For many patients, the rigidity is as serious a problem as the tremor. The disease is usually slowly progressive and affects both sides of the body simultaneously. The tremor occurs at rest and may affect the hands, legs, or head. It usually improves a little with movement (unlike cerebellar disease where the tremor worsens with movement — intension tremor). Rigidity of facial muscles may make the face appear expressionless. Rigidity of the limbs results in a characteristic shuffling gait. The tremor of the hands may be described as a pill-rolling tremor.

Action
There is no urgency to diagnose or to investigate this condition. Many people have benign familial tremors or shaking of the hands for other reasons.

Tests
A diagnosis is usually made clinically, but supported by brain scan and evidence of loss of dopaminergic nerve fibres.

Medications and treament
Dopamine-replacement drugs, such as Sinemet, and other anti-parkinsonian drugs, such as Eldepryl and Artane, are useful in this condition. Also: Akineton; Arpicolin, Celance; Cogentin; Disipal; Eldepryl; Kemadrin; Larodopa; Madopar; Nitoman; Parlodel; Pevaryl; Symmetrel; Tremonil.

Further advice
Maintaining a regular, gentle exercise pattern may reduce the rigidity that this condition causes. You should avoid chest infections which are often very severe because of the difficulty in moving chest muscles.

Associated conditions
Apart from benign tremors, there are other conditions which cause shaking, sometimes wild shaking (chorea). These include Tourette's syndrome and Huntington's chorea.

Parotid gland, swellings of

see **Salivary gland, swellings of**

Peptic ulcer ♥♥
(including gastric ulcer and duodenal ulcer)

 These ulcerous conditions are caused by burning of the lining of the stomach, usually by excess acid. The acid creates a crater or ulcer which is painful. Excess acid may be caused by an inherited overproduction of acid, an overproduction of acid caused by an excess production of hormones such as gastrin, excess alcohol and nicotine. Stress also causes increased acid production. Precursors of ulcers include gastritis and hiatus hernia, where acid is released from the stomach into the oesophagus (reflux), particularly on bending or when lying flat.

Symptoms
The symptoms of ulcers, gastritis, and hiatus hernia include abdominal pain. Typically, duodenal ulcer pain is worse after a meal and the pain is to the right side of the abdomen. Gastric ulcer pain is often relieved by food, as is gastritis. Hiatus hernia usually causes symptoms when increased abdominal pressure — during pregnancy or when bending, for example — pushes acid up into the stomach (reflux). In general, these symptoms can be bracketed under the heading of indigestion. Nausea, vomiting, vomiting of blood, loss of weight, diarrhoea and constipation, chest pain, back pain, pain radiating through from the stomach to the back, may all be symptoms of indigestion, gastritis, and ulcer disease.

Action
Self-medication is usually appropriate in the early stages of this treatment but, where serious symptoms occur, e.g. vomiting blood, suggestions of obstruction, passing blood or altered blood out of the back passage (melaena or black stools) the patient should be investigated.

Tests
Routine blood and liver-function tests are needed as well as investigations of the stomach, including barium meal and endoscopy. Biopsies should normally be taken during an endoscopy where the ulcer is looked at directly.

Medications and treatment
Antacid remedies may relieve symptoms of gastritis or hiatus hernia, but more severe symptoms need more potent drugs, such as cimetidine, ranitidine, or omeprazole. Algicon; Algitec; Alumix; Asilone; Axid; Caved S; Colofac; Colpermin; Cytotec; Gastrocote; Gastrozepin; Gaviscon; Kolanticon; Maalox; Mucaine; Nacton; Pepcid; Piptal; Prepulsid; Pyrogastrone; Roter; Topal are all used to treat and relieve gastric disorders.

Further advice
If you suffer from indigestion, acid symptoms, or ulcers, you should eat a healthy diet low in spicy foods, reduce alcohol intake, reduce smoking, and, where possible, reduce stress.

Associated conditions
Rarely, a tear of the oesophagus can cause pain and vomiting of blood. Oesophagitis is inflammation of the oesophagus and may occur as part of hiatus hernia. Ulcers may progress to become stomach cancer.

Pericarditis

 Pericarditis is inflammation of the pericardium or sac which surrounds the heart muscle. It is usually caused by a virus infection but sometimes occurs after bacterial infection, in association with endocarditis, or after a heart attack. It may also be associated with conditions such as pleurisy.

Main symptom
Chest pain which may mimic the chest pain of a heart attack. Often

this pain is related to posture, and, in this sense, the condition may be discriminated from a heart attack. The pain may radiate to the left arm and the jaw like the pain of a heart attack and may be associated with nausea, breathlessness, collapse, and fever.

Action
Patients should be treated as if they have had a heart attack until the definitive diagnosis of pericarditis has been made.

Tests
An ECG would show signs characteristic of pericarditis, and further investigations would include cardiac ultrasound, chest X-ray, blood tests.

Medications and treatment
These depend on the precipitating cause of pericarditis, and, if a bacterial infection has been found, antibiotics may be appropriate.

Further advice
If you have suffered an attack of pericarditis, you may be unfit and you should build up your exercise training gradually.

Peripheral arterial disease (intermittent claudication) ♥♥♥

Peripheral arterial disease is caused by a narrowing or blocking of the blood vessels in the lower limbs. This appears as intermittent claudication, a condition where there is pain in the legs on walking which is relieved by rest. It may also appear as sudden blockage of one of the arteries to the leg. Factors which precipitate peripheral arterial disease include smoking, obesity, high blood pressure and diabetes. Buerger's disease is a rare form of peripheral arterial disease, which is particularly sensitive to nicotine.

Symptoms

These include pain in the legs, particularly pain that is worse on walking and that is relieved by rest. Pain in the legs at night (rest pain) is also a symptom of this condition. Sudden blockage of an artery will result in a severely painful and white foot which needs emergency treatment. Progressive peripheral arterial disease may eventually lead to ulceration, infection, and gangrene.

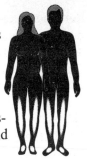

Action

Peripheral arterial disease needs investigation. Sudden onset of blockage of the main artery to the leg should be treated as an emergency. Patients should be rested and attempts made to warm the leg without overheating it.

Tests

Investigation of peripheral arterial disease include: arteriography to look at the state of the vessels, as well as general routine tests including chest X-ray, ECG, blood tests for clotting disorders or possible embolus. Doppler ultrasound methods can be used to assess blood flow in peripheral vessels.

Medications and treatment

Heparin or warfarin may be useful, and emergency surgical procedures may be necessary. In the longer term, several drugs are said to function as peripheral vasodilators to improve the blood supply. Examples: Hexopal, Opilon, Trental.

Further advice

Treatment of underlying conditions e.g. anaemia or diabetes is also part of the management of this condition. You should give up smoking, lose weight, take light, regular exercise, and reduce alcohol intake.

Associated conditions

Apart from Buerger's disease, some people have poor circulation. This may be associated with conditions such as SLE or scleroderma, but other people, particularly young women, have Raynaud's phenomenon where the small arteries in the hand are particularly sensitive to cold.

Peritonitis

see **Intestinal obstruction**

Petit mal

see **Epilepsy and associated conditions**

Phobias and obsessive compulsive disorders ♥♥

Phobias, such as claustrophobia (fear of closed spaces) or agoraphobia (fear of open spaces or of going out), are irrational fears. Obsessive compulsive disorders may be similar in that they are irrational, and very often the patient is compelled to undertake repetitive actions for fear that something bad will happen to them.

Symptoms

Specific phobias, such as fear of spiders or fear of birds, usually do not trouble the sufferer unless they are placed in the particular situation of stress. Claustrophobia will mean that patients will avoid travelling by air or by underground, and fear of flying may be a specific phobia in itself. Agoraphobia usually presents as a gradual withdrawal from social life and going out. In general terms, the phobias may represent some underlying trauma, anxiety, or depressive state. Obsessive compulsive disorders usually appear as a need to carry out repetitive actions such as hand washing (which may be more than 100 times a day), or checking that lights are switched off, or the gas switched off, or that doors are locked. Some patients have a series of set rituals which they must follow before they can go out. The eventual climax is that they are unable to go out, i.e. they are agoraphobic, because the ritual takes them all day. Some people need to dress and wash in exactly the same pattern each day and become disturbed if they cannot follow this procedure. Like the phobias, the obsessive compulsive disorders mask an underlying anxiety, trauma, or depression. The possibility of sexual abuse at some stage of the patient's life might also be considered.

Action
Where these conditions are disturbing the patient's normal life in terms of working or socializing, then professional help is required.

Tests
Psychometric testing and evaluation by a clinical psychologist and psychiatrist are necessary to evaluate these conditions. As in all psychiatric conditions, clinical examination should exclude the possibility of some underlying organic condition, such as a brain tumour which may appear with psychological features.

Medications and treatment
Psychotherapy combined with certain antidepressant drugs, such as clomipramine, may be helpful in the management of these conditions.

Further advice
These conditions may be chronic and patients may relapse under stress.

Associated conditions
Certain types of manic disorder such as kleptomania or nymphomania may be a variant of an obsessive compulsive disorder rather than part of true mania.

Piles

see **Haemorrhoids**

Pituitary gland, disorders of the ♥♥♥

 The pituitary gland is situated just below the brain. It controls many hormonal functions in the body including the thyroid growth hormones, sex hormones, and the hormones of the posterior pituitary gland. The pituitary gland can be damaged or destroyed by trauma or by tumour. Tumours of the pituitary gland may produce excess hormone or may destroy the controls of the other hormonal systems.

Symptoms

The symptoms of pituitary disease include a lack of pituitary function where the tumour has destroyed the pituitary gland. Thus, patients will develop symptoms of underactive thyroid gland, failure of ovulation with infertility, amenorrhoea, and impotence (due to lack of sex hormones), and collapse and wasting similar to Addison's disease due to lack of cortisone in the blood. Occasionally, excess hormone is produced by the pituitary gland, the most common of which is excess growth hormone resulting in a condition known as gigantism or acromegaly with overgrowth of the bones and jaw. Destruction of the posterior pituitary gland not only causes diabetes insipidus but also failure of lactation.

Action

Where pituitary failure or hyperactivity is suspected medical advice should be sought as soon as possible.

Tests

Pituitary function tests include routine blood tests for levels of hormones such as thyroid, oestrogen, testosterone, growth hormone, and insulin stress test for the ability of the pituitary gland to produce growth hormone in response to stress.

Medications and treatment

Excess growth hormone or prolactin production may respond to drugs such as bromocriptine, but often surgery is needed to remove tumours of the pituitary gland, thereby treating gigantism or acromegaly. Underactive pituitary glands necessitate treatment of the cause as well as replacement of hormones, particularly cortisone and thyroxine. Children will also need growth hormone supplements. Additional hormones will be required for the treatment of impotence and infertility.

Further advice
Insulin stress tests need to be carried out with caution. Overactive pituitary glands may also cause diabetes.

Pleurisy

see **Lower respiratory infections, acute**

Pneumonia

see **Lower respiratory infections, acute**

Pneumothorax

 Pneumothorax is a condition in which air enters the space between the lung and the chest wall. Pneumothorax may be a spontaneous event arising from rupture of the lung or it may occur as a result of trauma. In the latter case, a dangerous type of pneumothorax may occur with increasing pressure and compression on the lung.

Symptoms
The classic symptom of pneumothorax is a sudden onset of severe chest pain and breathlessness. This can occur in otherwise fit and healthy individuals with no predisposing factors, although it may be exacerbated by changes in air pressure, such as during air travel or

deep-sea diving. The patient may collapse through the shortness of breath and the pain. Pneumothorax caused by trauma will clearly also appear with symptoms of trauma itself, e.g. puncturing wound of the chest, gunshot wound, and so on.

Action

Immediate medical attention is required. Trained paramedics may wish to attempt to relieve the pressure caused by pneumothorax in an emergency situation by application of a needle which releases air from the chest and relieves lung compression.

Tests

Investigations for pneumothorax include chest X-ray, bronchoscopy, pleural biopsy.

Medications and treatment

The treatment of pneumothorax is surgical, but short-term oxygen and antibiotics may be required. Trauma needs to be attended to in its own right.

Further advice

If you are prone to recurrent spontaneous pneumothorax, you should avoid changes of barometric pressure or consider having preventative operations to obliterate the space between the lung and the chest wall.

Associated conditions

Haemothorax or haemopneumothorax is an additional complication of this condition where blood enters the space between the lung and the chest wall.

Polymyalgia rheumatica, and temporal arteritis ♥♥

These conditions are related but their cause is not known.

Symptoms

The symptoms of polymyalgia rheumatica are pain and weakness in the muscles, particularly the shoulders and around the pelvis. Temporal arteritis presents with pain and swelling in an artery on the head and may cause severe headache. The conditions often exist together, or one may lead to the other. A classic symptom of polymyalgia is inability to comb the hair because of weakness in the arm muscles. The muscles may be extremely painful.

Action

Where this condition is suspected, medical advice should be sought immediately.

Tests

A raised sedimentation rate occurs in these conditions, so that blood tests to check for this, for anaemia, and for other possible causes, including muscle enzymes, should be carried out. X-rays may be required. A biopsy of the temporal artery may be needed to make the diagnosis for temporal arteritis.

Medications and treatment

This condition usually responds to steroids. You may need to take the steroids for a prolonged period, occasionally in quite high doses.

Further advice

You should undergo gentle physiotherapy to encourage the use of your muscles.

Post-viral fatigue syndrome

see **Myalgic encephalomyelitis**

Pregnancy and its complications ♥♥♥

 The main complications of early to mid-pregnancy are ectopic pregnancy and antepartum haemorrhage. In addition, threatened miscarriage (threatened abortion) is also a symptom of pregnancy.

Symptoms

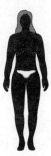 Ectopic pregnancy usually presents with abdominal pain and some vaginal bleeding. Threatened abortion will also appear with pain and bleeding. Later in pregnancy antepartum, haemorrhage may appear with catastrophic abdominal pain and bleeding. All of these conditions may mimic other acute surgical abdominal emergencies.

Action

Patients should lie down, and medical attention should be sought immediately.

Tests

Abdominal ultrasound, vaginal examination, tests for haemoglobin, and other routine blood tests may be included in the investigation of these conditions.

Medications and treatment

Ectopic pregnancy is treated by surgery. Threatened abortion may settle but may progress such that a dilatation and curettage is required. Antepartum haemorrhage may also settle but may be catastrophic or require surgical intervention.

Further advice

Some of these conditions may be prevented by reducing activity, e.g. by avoiding driving or air travel during pregnancy. The use of the IUCD may lead to ectopic pregnancies.

Associated conditions

Chorio-carcinoma and hydatidiform mole are conditions where pregnancy may be mimicked and may appear with bleeding and abdominal pain.

Premenstrual tension

 PMT is a hormonal condition which is found in women of all age groups. PMT symptoms may merge into, and overlap with, menopausal symptoms in the older age groups. Symptoms of premenstrual tension include fluid retention, breast tenderness, mental irritability, insomnia, hypersomnia, hyperphagia (excessive eating), and frank depression.

Action
Persistent premenstrual tension should be investigated.

Tests
Hormonal tests may reveal imbalances between oestrogen and progesterone that may be responsive to medication.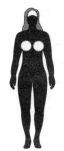

Medications and treatment
Diuretics, vitamin B$_6$, evening primrose oil, and hormones such as oestrogen and progesterone. The contraceptive pill may improve the symptoms of PMT.

Further advice
Avoiding alcohol and improving diet is said by some to reduce the symptoms of PMT.

Presenile dementia

see **Dementia**

Prostate, diseases of the ♥♥♥♥

 The prostate gland is found at the neck of the bladder in men. It is likely to become enlarged (benign prostatic hypotrophy) or to develop tumours (carcinoma of the prostate). Both of these occur more frequently as men get older.

Symptoms

The symptoms of prostate disease are difficulty passing urine, poor stream of urine, difficulty starting urination, difficulty stopping urination, dribbling after urination, and incontinence. Retention of urine, with total inability to pass urine may occur. Cancer of the prostate may additionally appear with other symptoms of malignant disease such as secondary metastases to the bones causing bone pain.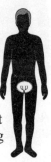

Action

Symptoms may come and go in the early stages, and may be made worse when there is urine infection. If the symptoms persist for more than a month, you should seek medical advice.

Tests

Tests include routine blood tests, tests for evidence of tumours in the bone (alkaline phosphatase), tests for prostatic cancer (acid phosphatase), and also prostate-specific antigen. Physical examination, as well as cystoscopy, intravenous pyelography, and studies of bladder function may also be included.

Medications and treatment

Benign prostatic hypotrophy is usually treated by surgery, although recently Proscar tablets have been made available, and these can reduce the size of the prostate gland. Prostatic cancer may respond to hormonal treatment, and rarely castration is advised to slow down the progress of the disease because the cancer grows in the presence of androgens (male hormones).

Further advice
After prostate surgery, you may suffer from impotence and incontinence.

Pruritis (itch) ♥
and skin allergy (including urticaria)

Pruritis or itch may be a symptom of other conditions but it may be a condition in its own right without any known underlying cause, or associated with generalized allergy. Severe allergy may result in urticaria, a condition where there is generalized swelling of skin and underlying tissues. Very commonly, drugs may cause allergies, skin rashes, and skin eruptions. These may be itchy.

Main symptom
Itching.

Actions
If possible, do not scratch, and seek medical advice.

Tests
Allergy tests and skin biopsies are very important.

Medications and treatment
Antihistamines and steroid creams, including Betnovate, Calmurid, Clarityn, Epogam, Eumovate, Eurax, Hismanal, Phenergan, Piriton, Sudafed, Triludan, Zaditen, and Zirtek, may provide symptomatic improvement in cases of pruritis, but a full investigation is necessary if symptoms persist for more than a few days.

Further advice

Hot showers may make symptoms worse and, generally, sunlight is bad for itchy skin. Take extra care about medications, such as penicillin, where allergy is suspected.

Psoriasis

 Psoriasis is a skin disorder distinct from, but in many ways similar to, eczema. Its cause is not known. Psoriasis is not contagious.

Main symptoms

An itchy, scaly rash, predominantly on the outside of the elbows, knees, in the hair, and on the hands. It is associated with changes to the hair and nails. Psoriasis can appear on any part of the body and may be quite extensive. The rash is quite red in appearance and may have a violet hue.

Action

Simple remedies may help psoriasis, and self-medication may be appropriate.

Tests

The main tests for psoriasis are skin biopsy in which a microscopic examination of the skin will confirm a diagnosis.

Medications and treatment

Self-medication with coal tar may be appropriate but prescription drugs, such as Dovonex, may be needed for the more severe cases. Cytotoxic drugs may also be useful. Ultraviolet A light is often used in association with psoriasis treatments. Steroids may result in some improvement.

Further advice

Stress and exposure to sunlight may worsen psoriasis. Diet may also affect the condition.

Associated conditions
Psoriasis may cause changes to nails as well as hair loss.

Pulmonary embolus

 Pulmonary embolus is caused by a blood clot which travels to the lung and may block the lung or one of the blood vessels in the heart. Factors which may precipitate pulmonary embolus include deep-vein thrombosis and any blood-clotting disorder, previous or recent surgery, injury or damage to the veins in the leg or pelvis. Pulmonary embolus is a common complication of prolonged bed rest and hospitalization, particularly post-operative.

Main symptoms
These include onset of chest pain which may appear in a similar way to a heart attack. There is severe shortness of breath, and there may be collapse and sudden death. Pleuritic chest pain (that is, chest pain which is worse on taking a deep breath) may be a symptom of pulmonary embolus. Patients may cough up blood.

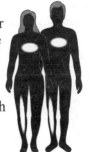

Action
Pulmonary embolus is a medical emergency. Patients should be rested and medical attention sought immediately. It is important to distinguish pulmonary embolus from a heart attack because different resuscitating methods will be required.

Tests
Investigations for suspected pulmonary embolus include: chest X-ray, lung perfusion scans (to test how much lung tissue is working), ECG, arteriography, blood tests for causes.

Medications and treatment

The treatment of pulmonary embolus includes urgent resuscitation and lung ventilation if required. Dissolving the clot and preventing further clots may require anticoagulant therapy which should be continued for several months. Prevention of pulmonary embolus is achieved by using heparin pre-operatively in surgical patients.

Associated conditions

Small multiple pulmonary emboli may appear without any symptoms. Eventually they may cause shortness of breath and possibly late presentation with full pulmonary embolus or pulmonary hypertension.

Pyelonephritis

see **Renal tract, infections of**

Rectum, cancer of the

see **Bowel cancer**

Renal calculus

see **Kidney Stones**

Renal tract, infections of the (pyelonephritis and cystitis)

Cystitis (infection of the bladder) has been dealt with in Chapter 8 above.

Serious infection of the kidney (pyelonephritis) can occur when cystitis remains untreated and the infection ascends, or due to metastatic spread of bacteria.

Symptoms
Fever, pains in the loin or bladder, passing of infected urine or bloody urine.

Action
Minor urinary tract infections may respond to a high fluid intake, urine alkalinizers, and bedrest and hot-water bottle. More serious infections require medical intervention.

Tests
Tests include examination of the urine and culture for infection, routine blood tests for infection, intravenous pyelography, ultrasound studies particularly where kidney abscess is suspected.

Medications and treatment
Infections will normally respond to antibiotics. Severe, recurrent kidney infections may require surgical intervention to remove the damaged kidney or to correct a urinary tract abnormality which may be congenital.

Further advice
You should drink plenty of non-alcoholic fluids to prevent and treat urinary tract infections.

Associated conditions
Kidney cysts or abscesses may be present, and these may need to be treated separately.

Retina, detached

see **Retina, diseases of**

Retina, diseases of the, ♥♥♥ including detached retina, retinal artery thrombosis, retinal vein thrombosis, hypertensive and diabetic retinopathy

 The retina is a delicate membrane at the back of the eye, and is subject to a number of diseases. Detachment may occur after trauma or in someone who is very short-sighted. Hypertension and diabetes cause haemorrhages and exudates in the retina. Blockage of blood vessels to the retina can also cause damage. Rarely, tumours of the retina (retinoblastoma) may occur. These may have an hereditary factor.

Symptoms
There may be no symptoms of retinal disease until it is picked up on routine medical examination. Detachment of the retina may appear with sudden loss of vision in one eye and a film moving upwards across the field of vision. Thrombosis of the retinal artery and retinal vein may cause sudden blindness in all or part of the field of vision. Severe hypertensive diabetic retinopathy will eventually appear as loss of vision and blindness in the affected eye.

Action
Urgent specialist medical advice is required for any of these conditions.

Tests
Examination of the eye, tests for predisposing factors such as hypertension, diabetes, routine blood tests, clotting screen and search for cause of thrombosis or embolus, angiogram of the retinal vessels.

Medications and treatment
Detached retina is usually treated by bed rest and laser therapy to re-attach the damaged retina. Hypertensive or diabetic retinopathy is

treated by attention to the primary disease and by laser therapy to prevent new vessel formation and more extensive damage. Thrombosis of the retinal artery or vein may resolve spontaneously but bed rest and attention to clotting factors may be required.

Further advice
Good management of hypertension and diabetes will prevent damage to the eyes. Detached retina may indicate that you should avoid contact sports in the future.

Associated conditions
Retinoblastoma is treated by removal of the eye and treatment with drugs or radiotherapy.

Retinal artery thrombosis

see **Retina, diseases of**

Retinal vein thrombosis

see **Retina, diseases of**

Retinopathy, hypertensive and diabetic

see **Retina, diseases of**

Rheumatoid arthritis

 Rheumatoid arthritis is an inflammatory joint condition which is more common in women than men, particularly young women. Its cause is unknown.

Symptoms

Pain, stiffness, and swelling of joints, particularly the small joints of the hands and feet. In the morning after rest, the stiffness in the joints may be particularly noticeable. Other joints may also become involved, including the neck, shoulders, elbows, wrists, knees, and ankles. Rheumatoid arthritis may even affect the jaw joint. In some cases, the disease progresses to a severe condition with involvement of other organs such as the heart, lungs, and eyes. In others, it burns itself out but leaves some disability, particularly in the hands.

Action

If you suffer from persistent pain and stiffness in the hands or feet, you should seek medical advice.

Tests

Blood tests including rheumatoid factors, full blood counts, sedimentation rate, and tests of heart and lung function are included in the investigation of rheumatoid arthritis. X-rays will show characteristic erosion of bone and joint.

Medications and treatment

Steroids probably have little place in the management of this condition. Non-steroidal anti-inflammatory drugs, including aspirin, Distamine, Myocrisin, and Nivaquine, are often helpful, and severe cases may need more radical treatment such as gold or penicillamine. Occasionally cytotoxic chemotherapy may be used to treat rheumatoid arthritis.

Further advice

Many patients claim that they benefit from a vegetarian diet, and a diet high in essential fatty acids and oils. You should try to exercise and maintain a good standard of general health.

Associated conditions

Bornholm disease is an arthritis caused by a virus that affects the ribs. It may appear as chest pain.

Rhinitis

see **Upper respiratory tract infections, acute**

Royal free disease

see **Myalgic encephalomyelitis**

Salivary gland, particularly the parotid gland, swellings of

The parotid gland is a large salivary gland on each side of the jaw. There is a number of causes of swelling of the parotid gland including chronic infection, benign tumour, malignant tumour, and mumps (acute parotitis).

Symptoms
Swelling of the gland or glands and pain. Mumps and chronic parotitis may be associated with fever. The gland is often exquisitely painful.

Action
Seek medical advice to make the diagnosis.

Tests
Chronic infections of the parotid gland or suspected tumours may be investigated by arteriography or a sialogram.

Medications and treatment
Mumps and parotitis should be treated with painkillers and antibiotics, including amoxycillin, ampicillin, cephalexin, Ciproxin, erythromycin, Flagyl, penicillin, Septrin, tetracycline, and trimethoprim, where necessary. Benign or malignant tumours of the parotid gland

require surgical intervention.

Further advice
Chronic parotitis may be associated with a high alcohol and nicotine intake, so you should drink less alcohol and stop smoking.

Associated conditions
Stone in the salivary duct may also cause swelling of the salivary gland and this needs to be investigated surgically. Mumps may be associated with other conditions such as swelling of the testicles (orchitis), inflammation of the pancreas gland (pancreatitis), and inflammation of the eyes (uveitis).

Sarcoidosis

Sarcoidosis is a granulomatous disease whereby granulomata appear in various organs, including the lymph nodes, lungs, liver, spleen, eyes, bones. Granulomata are internal 'abscesses' sometimes of unknown cause. The cause of sarcoidosis not known.

Symptoms
There may be no symptoms with sarcoidosis but, occasionally, it appears with chest symptoms due to enlargement of lymph nodes in the chest. There may also be fever, arthritis, eye symptoms such as uveitis, skin rash, liver failure, enlargement of the spleen, or changes in the heart. Sarcoidosis may cause elevation of calcium in the blood or urine and so it may appear with thirst and frequency of urination or kidney stones.

Action
Sarcoidosis needs to be investigated and managed in a specialist centre.

Tests
These include chest X-ray, Kveim test, blood test measuring sedi-

mentation rate, calcium levels, liver function, lung function tests, eye tests and examination, cardiac investigation.

Medications and treatment

The main drugs used for treatment of sarcoidosis are steroids. Patients may not require any steroids but, occasionally, maintenance doses of Prednisolone of about 5 to 20 mg a day are required.

Further advice

If you are suffering from sarcoidosis, you may be vulnerable to infections, particularly if you are taking steroids. Therefore, you should try to maintain a good standard of general health and look out for any long-term side effects of the steroids.

Scabies

see **Skin infestations**

Scarlet fever

see **Upper respiratory tract infections, acute**

Schizophrenia

 Schizophrenia is disturbed mental function and is not the split personality that many believe it to be. The disturbance of mental function may be severe enough to cause a schizophrenic psychosis or it may be mild. Schizophrenia may have a genetic or biochemical basis for its origin.

Symptoms

These range from a mild delusion with paranoia which may include hallucinations, particularly auditory hallucinations. Patients may hear voices which may be critical voices. These voices may be

677

scolding the patient or instructing the patient to carry out certain activities or functions. The voices are often described as coming from an electrical source such as a radio or television; schizophrenic patients may become obsessed with electricity and the thought that they are somehow wired up and are being listened to. The paranoia may increase or the patient may develop a frozen or catatonic state. Holding conversations with these unheard voices may be part of the deterioration into full schizophrenic psychosis which may appear to the layman as frank madness. Milder forms of schizophrenia may be difficult to detect and may appear as a depressive disorder. Here the patient simply cannot carry out normal working tasks and withdraws.

Action
Professional medical help is necessary as soon as this condition is suspected.

Tests
Full evaluation by psychiatrists and clinical psychologists are necessary to help detect this condition. As with all psychiatric disorders, organic conditions, such as brain tumour, should be excluded as a cause for bizarre presenting symptoms.

Medications and treatment
Neuroleptic drugs, such as Largactil, are valuable in the management of this condition. Medication should be accompanied by supportive psychotherapy. Surgical and electrical treatments are rarely used for the management of this condition nowadays. Anquil, Clopixol, Clozaril, Depixol, Dolmatil, Dozic, Fentazin, Heminevrin, Largactil, Melleril, Moditen, Nozinan, Orap, Serenace, Stelazine, Sulpitil.

Sciatica

see **Backache**

Septicaemia ♥♥♥♥♥

 Septicaemia is a condition of generalized infection. Theoretically, any bacterium or fungus can affect the blood stream, usually in unwell or immuno-compromised patients. Toxic shock can occur in patients who have infection with certain types of gram-negative bacteria. These can occasionally be caused by infected tampons.

Symptoms
The symptoms for septicaemia are similar to those of influenza with fever, headache, shaking, chills, weakness, collapse, and death.

Action
Where septicaemia is suspected, urgent medical attention is required.

Tests
Blood cultures can help to diagnose the infecting agent and help with instituting appropriate treatment.

Medications and treatment
Antibacterial, antifungal medication should be given, usually by intravenous infusion. Monoclonal antibodies are available for treatment of gram-negative toxic shock.

Further advice
Septicaemia can be prevented in hospitals by adequate aseptic techniques and by awareness of the likelihood of diagnosis so that early treatment can be instituted.

Associated conditions
Bacterial endocarditis may be associated with septicaemia.

Shock ♥♥♥♥♥
(collapse, hypotension, anaphylactic shock)

 Shock is caused by a sudden drop of blood pressure which may result from a severe allergy (anaphylactic shock), severe trauma as in a road traffic accident, loss of blood, or anything which precipitates a sudden decrease in blood pressure.

Main symptoms
Collapse, weakness, headache, inability to walk, inability to move limbs. Shock may result in death.

Action
Patients should be laid flat to improve the blood supply to the brain. Medical attention should be sought immediately. Patients should not be overwarmed with blankets because this will worsen shock. Obvious bleeding should be stopped where possible.

Tests
Investigations into the cause of shock should proceed immediately. These include ECG, chest X-ray, search for bleeding points, search for causes of allergy.

Medications and treatment
The main treatment for shock is to increase blood volume by giving plasma, blood, or fluids. Adrenalin, noradrenalin, isoprenaline, and other inotropic drugs will also bring up blood pressure.

Other medications
These can be used to treat the cause of shock, e.g. steroids, adrenalin, antihistamines for allergic shock, and specific treatments for heart attack if this is the cause.

Sinusitis

see **Upper respiratory tract infections, acute**

Skin allergy

see **Pruritis**

Skin infections

 Bacteria, fungi, and viruses can cause skin infections. Bacterial infections usually give rise to acne, cellulitis, or impetigo. Fungus infections are quite common in the form of ringworm, athlete's foot, dhobi itch, and simple fungal plaques. The most common viral infections of the skin are herpes simplex, or cold sore, as well as herpes zoster or shingles. Occasionally, bacterial infections may cause a granuloma or swelling. All these conditions are contagious.

Main symptoms

Spots and a possible itchy rash. Dhobi itch affects the groin and athlete's foot affects the spaces between the toes. Acne is most common on the face, chest, and back whereas impetigo can often affect the face. Cellulitis is a spreading skin infection which can occur anywhere. Cold sores are usually found on the upper lip and are made worse at times of stress or menstruation.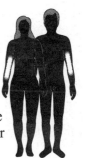

Action

Self-medication with a local cleansing agent may resolve a bacterial infection and over-the-counter antifungal preparations can also be used. Cold sores often disappear spontaneously but may require prescription medication.

Tests

In difficult cases, scrapings may be taken for microscopic examination.

Medications and treatment

Antibiotics, particularly tetracycline and clindamycin, are useful for skin infections such as acne. Erythromycin is useful for treating acne as well as cellulitis and impetigo. Antifungal agents, such as Canesten, are useful for fungal infections, and Zovirax Cream valuable in the treatment of cold sores.

Further advice

Pay particular attention to hygiene, including washing clothes regularly, and avoid poor diet high in chocolate.

Associated conditions

Acne rosacea is a condition similar to acne which also responds to tetracycline therapy. It is not thought to be due to a bacterial infection and its cause is unknown.

Skin infestations (lice and scabies)

 These conditions are caused by skin infestation with small insects. They occur in areas of poor hygiene or when people live in very close communities such as in boarding schools.

Main symptoms

An itchy rash, and small eggs or insects can often be seen on the skin.

Action

Improve general hygiene, including washing sheets and blankets, but persistent infestation requires medical attention.

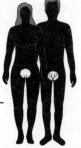

Tests
Skin biopsies are often used; examination of insects and eggs under the microscope will fix the diagnosis.

Medications and treatment
Ascabiol, Clinicide, Lyclear, Quellada.

Further advice
Attention to general hygiene, avoiding overcrowding, and regularly washing hair and linen should prevent this condition.

Associated conditions
Pubic lice are a venereally contracted condition where insects may be seen on the pubic hair.

Skin rash associated with fever ♥

Skin rash associated with fever is most commonly caused by a virus infection. Notably these include measles, German measles, chickenpox, and shingles. In all cases the rash is generally contagious on the body or torso.

Main symptoms
Rash and fever. The rash of measles is slightly redder than the rather pink rash of German measles. Chickenpox consists of small fluid-filled blisters whereas shingles, which is caused by the same virus as chickenpox, affects one side of the body only and in one limited area. There is often considerable pain associated with shingles. Chickenpox may affect the lungs; German measles can cause glandular swelling, particularly at the back of the neck; while measles can cause reddening of the eyes and infection of the brain (encephalitis).

Action
Most of these virus infections are self-limiting, and, apart from

medical attention to make the diagnosis, will respond to bedrest.

Tests
Occasionally blood tests may be required to confirm the diagnosis. Chest X-ray or lumbar puncture may be considered if complications occur.

Medications and treatment
Shingles responds to Zovirax and, recently, doctors have started to use Zovirax for chickenpox. Measles and German measles do not respond to current antiviral therapy. German measles is severely damaging to the unborn child, and so pregnant women should avoid contact with German measles. Shingles pain may continue for a very long time but it can be alleviated by painkillers. Encephalitis is a rare but late complication of measles. Glandular fever treated with ampicillin may result in a rash, and scarlet fever may cause a rash with fever.

Skin tumours, warts, and swellings

Any swelling or tumour of the skin can be alarming. In this category we include skin tumours, such as malignant melanoma, basal cell carcinoma, squamous cell carcinoma, haemangiomas, lipomas, warts, and naevi. Of these, only malignant melanoma is particularly serious although, occasionally, lipomas may turn out to be liposarcomas which are malignant.

Many skin conditions, including melanoma and basal cell carcinoma, are made worse by exposure to sunlight and therefore occur in fair-skinned people living in tropical areas. Many warts are caused by viruses but, in general terms, the remainder of the skin lesions in this category have no known cause.

Main symptoms
A lump or bump in the skin which may bleed or ulcerate. Particularly serious signs to look for are the failure of a cut to heal, bleeding of

a skin lesion, itching, change in size, shape, or colour, and the presence of associated or satellite lesions. These may indicate malignancy. Lipomas are usually painless lumps; warts have a crusty appearance; haemangiomas are collections of blood while naevi are often like large moles.

Action
You should seek medical attention if the lump or ulcer changes in any way.

Tests
The main test of any skin lesion is a biopsy. An incision is carried out and the fragments are examined under a microscope.

Medications and treatment
Most of these conditions require surgical excision. Occasionally warts may respond to local wart remedies. Malignant conditions may need chemotherapy and/or radiotherapy.

Further advice
In general, you should avoid overexposure to sunlight and wear sunblocks.

Slipped disc

see **Backache**

Small cell carcinoma

see **Lung cancer**

Spondylitis

see **Backache**

Sports injuries and trauma

 There is a wide range of sports injuries, from tennis elbow to torn cartilage conditions. Repetitive strain injury falls into this category and may affect the fingers in typists and keyboard operatives, for example. Bone fractures may also be caused by sports injuries, and fracture is usually easily diagnosed. Tendon and cartilage injuries, particularly in the knee, are very common in sports. Inflammation of the bursa, or sac of fluid, causes conditions such as tennis elbow or golfer's elbow where there is pain particularly on gripping or movement. A similar condition is the carpal tunnel syndrome where there is pressure on the nerve in the wrist.

Symptoms

Symptoms of a fracture include severe pain, swelling, inability to move, and occasionally cracking or crepitus. When bone breaks through the skin surface, it is known as a compound fracture. Cartilage injuries, particularly in the knee, appear with locking of the knee, pain and swelling, and discomfort on exercise. Tennis elbow and other conditions, such as bursitis, appear with pain on gripping or moving the affected joint. Carpal tunnel syndrome presents with pins and needles in the hand (usually excluding the little finger) particularly at night and in women during pregnancy and at the time of the menopause. Repetitive strain injury presents with pain and stiffness in the fingers. Any joint may be affected by a sports injury, and others commonly affected are the shoulder and ankle. Neck ache and stiff neck may result from certain types of injury.

Action

Most sports injuries respond to rest and treatment with ice. Failure to respond after a short time will require medical intervention.

Tests

X-rays are required if fracture is suspected. Clinical examination is usually sufficient to diagnose cartilage injury. Arthroscopy (looking into a joint) would be very helpful.

Medications and treatment

Torn cartilages can be removed through an arthroscope, or extensive open surgery will be required. Minor conditions, such as tennis elbow, may respond to injections of local anaesthetic and corticosteroids. Less serious injuries will respond to analgesics, analgesic creams and sprays, and non-steroidal anti-inflammatory drugs including: Algesal, Brufen, Feldene, Feldene Gel, Froben, Indocid, Intralgin, Mobiflex, Naprosyn, Nurofen, Orudis, Ponstan, Proflex, Relifex, Rheumox, Stugam, Traxam, Voltarol. Carpal tunnel syndrome may require surgical intervention but occasionally responds to diuretic treatment to reduce pressure on the joint.

Further advice

Make certain that you warm up and train properly to help prevent sports injuries. Trying to exercise through an injury to improve it rarely works, and rest, physiotherapy, and treatment with ice are invaluable in the treatment of all sports injuries. Occasionally steroid injections are helpful but they should not be overused.

Squamous cell carcinoma

see **Lung cancer**

Stomach cancer

Stomach cancer is decreasing in frequency but it remains a common cause of death, particularly among men. It may develop from previous ulcer disease although this is uncertain. Certainly high spirit intake and nicotine may provoke stomach cancer.

Symptoms
There may be no symptoms of stomach cancer. Alternatively, it may proceed insidiously with slight indigestion, loss of weight, anaemia, and symptoms of peptic ulcer. Vomiting blood, or passing blood, or altered blood (melaena) in the stools may be a symptom of this condition. Symptoms may also appear from secondary spread to the lungs, bone, or liver.

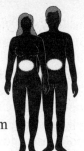

Action
Persistent indigestion should be investigated if it does not respond to self-medication.

Tests
The best test to exclude stomach cancer is endoscopy (telescope into the stomach) and biopsy. It is important, therefore, that this is done before treating ulcers because anti-ulcer treatment may take away the symptoms of stomach cancer. Blood tests, liver-function tests, and chest X-ray are all used to investigate this condition.

Medications and treatment
Stomach cancer is treated surgically with the addition of chemotherapy and radiotherapy where appropriate. Supportive treatment is required.

Further advice
Prevention of stomach cancer is best achieved by attention to diet, alcohol, and nicotine intake.

Associated conditions
Cancer of the oesophagus is similar and will appear with dysphagia (difficulty in swallowing). Cancer of the small intestine is unusual. For cancer of the colon or rectum.

Stroke

---

see **Cerebral vascular accident** *and* **Cerebrovascular acident**

Testes, diseases of the, ♥♥♥♥♥
including cancer of the testes (seminoma or teratoma), epididymitis, torsion of the testicle, orchitis, and varicocoele

 Scrotal lumps may be due to lumps in the testis itself which may be benign or malignant; or enlargement of the epididymis, either an epididymal cyst or an inflamed epididymis (epididymitis). Enlarged veins in the scrotum may appear as a varicocoele which is rather like varicose veins. Inflammation of the testes may occur, for example after mumps infection, resulting in orchitis.

Symptoms
The presence of a painful or painless lump in the scrotum may be alarming. Pain usually indicates infection, e.g. orchitis, epididymitis, or torsion of the testicle. A painless lump is more likely to be a cyst of the epididymis or possibly a malignancy, e.g. seminoma or teratoma. Infections may also appear with urinary symptoms such as pain on passing urine. Blood in the semen may also be a symptom of these conditions.

Action
Torsion of the testicle, where the blood supply may be cut off, is an emergency, and, if this is suspected, medical advice should be sought urgently.

Tests
Clinical examination, ultrasound of the testicles, routine X-ray, bone scan, analysis of semen and urine may be included in the investigation of these conditions.

Medications and treatment
Infections are treated with antibiotics. Suspicion of malignancy requires biopsy. Epididymal cysts may be drained, and torsion of the

689

testis requires immediate interventionist surgery. Varicocoele requires surgical operation to correct the presence of veins.

Further advice
Men should examine themselves to detect and prevent these conditions.

Associated conditions
Undescended testicle may occur where the testis is on a short cord and fails to descend directly into the scrotum. Surgery is required in these conditions. Inguinal hernias may enter the scrotum and produce a scrotal lump.

Thyroid gland, diseases of the

 The thyroid gland controls the rate of metabolism of the body, and an underactive thyroid gland (myxoedema or hypothyroidism) produces a slow, sluggish metabolism whereas an overactive thyroid gland (thyrotoxicosis or hyperthyroidism) will produce a fast metabolism.

Symptoms
The symptoms of an underactive thyroid gland are coldness, tiredness, weight gain, depression, sleepiness, loss of hair particularly from the eyebrows, dry skin, elevated cholesterol, heart disease, carpal tunnel syndrome, anaemia, and infertility. The symptoms of an overactive thyroid gland are anxiety, hypertension, weight loss, excessive appetite, sweating, rapid pulse, and insomnia.

Action
Either of these conditions may come on insidiously without being noticed by the patient's friends or relatives. Where suspected, medical attention should be sought as soon as possible.

Tests
Thyroid function tests and other routine blood tests including full

blood count will make the diagnosis. Examination of
the thyroid gland itself to look for goitres, cysts, or
tumours, is important, using clinical examination and
other means such as ultrasound. Pituitary function
might also need to be investigated.

Medications and treatment

Myxoedema is easily treated with thyroid replacement
Tertroxin or Eltroxin. An overactive thyroid may respond to a single dose of radioactive thyroxine, or surgery may be
necessary, particularly where a cyst or tumour needs to be removed.
Carbimazole may also be used to treat an overactive thyroid.

Further advice

Continuous assessment may be required to establish the correct dose
of treatment. An overactive thyroid gland may often swing to be
underactive during or after treatment.

Tinnitus

see **Ménière's Disease (and tinnitus)**

Tonsillitis

see **Upper respiratory tract infections, acute**

Tracheitis

see **Lower respiratory infections, acute**

Trauma/head injury ♥♥♥♥

Head injury is common, particularly in road-traffic accidents, among motorcyclists, cyclists, and pedestrians. Some of the symptoms of head injury may be delayed.

Symptoms

Obvious trauma may be associated with bleeding from the ear or nose. Loss of consciousness may occur, and this is usually associated with more serious disease. Signs of raised brain pressure, e.g. headache, vomiting, deteriorating consciousness, require urgent attention. Blood clots in the brain, e.g. extradural or subdural haematomas, may cause delayed or very late symptoms which may appear with a slowly progressive dementia or epilepsy. Head injury may damage certain brain functions causing, for example, loss of smell, diabetes insipidus, loss of taste, loss of memory (anterograde or retrograde amnesia).

Action

Patients with obvious head injuries should be moved by skilled medical or paramedical personnel only to prevent further damage, particularly to the spinal cord. Ventilation may be required.

Tests

Investigations include CT brain scan, MRI scans, skull X-rays, X-rays looking for injuries elsewhere, arteriography of brain blood vessels.

Medications and treatment

General supportive treatment, including the use of dexamethasone to reduce brain pressure, and antibiotics for infection, are included as part of the medical support for these patients.

Further advice

After a head injury, you may develop late symptoms, such as depression or epilepsy.

Tuberculosis

Tuberculosis is an infection by the tubercle bacillus and it usually causes diseases of the lungs although it may affect other parts of the body including the brain, the gut, and adrenal glands. It is associated with poor general nutrition and hygiene.

Symptoms
These include weight loss, fever, cough, production of sputum and blood.

Action
If it is suspected, tuberculosis must be fully investigated and treated under medical supervision.

Investigations
These include chest X-ray, sputum tests for tubercle bacilli, biopsy of suspected glands, stool tests for possible bacilli, blood tests particularly for changes in white cells and sedimentation rate. Investigations of tuberculous meningitis or cerebral tubercle would include lumbar puncture and brain scan.

Medications and treatment
There is a number of antituberculous drugs available, including Myambutol, Mynah, Rifadin, Rifater, Rifinah, Rimactane, Rimactazid, Zinamide, and streptomycin which is given by injection. Patients should be encouraged to rest, stop smoking, and, where possible, be isolated from susceptible contacts.

Further advice
If you are suffering from conditions that lower the immunity, such HIV infection or AIDS, you may also contract tuberculosis. You should be given appropriate supportive and immunological treatment. Tuberculosis can be prevented by a suitable programme of screening and vaccination as well as by pasteurization of milk and improved social and housing conditions. Alcohol and diabetes may lower the immunity and predispose to tuberculosis. Occasionally

tuberculous pleurisy, tuberculous laryngitis, or tuberculous infections of the gynaecological tract may occur.

Ulcerative colitis

see **Bowel disorders, inflammatory**

Upper respiratory tract infections, ♥ acute (including rhinitis, coryza, influenza, laryngitis, tonsillitis, sinusitis, scarlet fever)

These upper respiratory tract infections are very common causes of minor illness. Most of them are caused by viruses (especially coryza and influenza) and some are caused by a bacterial infection (particularly sinusitis and tonsillitis). They may often co-exist or, indeed, one of these infections may lead on to one of the others. It is appropriate, therefore, to consider them together because treating one will treat all.

Main symptoms
Sore throat, blocked and runny nose, nasal discharge, hoarseness, cough, fever, shivering, shaking, aches and pains, malaise.

Action
Many of these conditions will respond to self-medication for a few days at least, and a number of preparations are listed at the end of this chapter for self-treatment of these conditions. Symptoms which persist for more than seven days may require medical treatment, however.

Tests
Minor infections which do not respond to self-medication may require medical attention. Tests where necessary would include

sinus X-ray, chest X-ray, analysis of sputum or discharge for bacteria.

Medications and treatment

Bacterial infections are treated with antibiotics including amoxycillin, ampicillin, cephalexin, Ciproxin, erythromycin, Flagyl, penicillin, Septrin, tetracycline, and trimethoprim. Viral infections will respond to supportive treatment. Paracetamol and aspirin are useful to control fever and aches and pains in the limbs, and you should drink plenty of non-alcoholic fluids.

Further advice

Bed rest in the acute stage of an upper respiratory infection is useful. You should not get too warm even though you may feel shivery.

Associated conditions

Allergic rhinitis may appear like an acute rhinitis (nose infection), but it is caused by allergy. It will respond to antihistamine treatment, and patients should avoid allergic precipitating factors.

Urticaria

see **Pruritis**

Uterine prolapse

Prolapse of the womb occurs through loss of ligamentous support of the womb, and occurs after childbirth, particularly after multiple childbirth or difficult childbirth.

Symptoms

A feeling of having a swelling in the genital area, frequent urinary infections, stress incontinence (release of urine on coughing, sneezing, or laughing), heavy menstrual bleeding, and a dragging sensation.

Action
Symptoms may resolve, particularly if they have been there for a short time after pregnancy. Pelvic floor exercises may improve the symptoms.

Tests
Tests for bladder function including urine tests for infection (cystometry), investigations using dyes, and flow rates of urine may be helpful.

Medications and treatment
Prolapse may respond to the insertion of a vaginal ring to support the womb. Greater degrees of prolapse may require surgery.

Further advice
Continuing pelvic floor exercises can prevent and treat prolapse, particularly after pregnancy.

Uterus and cervix, diseases of

Diseases of the uterus and cervix include cancer of the womb, cancer of the cervix, fibroids, cervical erosions, and pelvic inflammatory disease.

Symptoms
These conditions may be symptomless. Inflammatory disease may appear with chronic pelvic pain and vaginal discharge. Fibroids may appear with heavy periods and abdominal pain. Cancer of the cervix may be picked up on routine cervical smear but it may also appear as post-coital bleeding. Cervical erosions, warts of the cervix, and other disorders of the cervix may also appear with post-coital bleeding.

Action
Investigation of pelvic pain, abnormal bleeding, or abnormal dis-

charge should be carried out under medical supervision.

Tests
Vaginal swabs, low and high, abdominal ultrasound, pelvic examination, and routine blood tests may be included in the investigation of these conditions.

Medications and treatment
Pelvic inflammatory disease should be treated with antibiotics. Disorders of the cervix may require cautery or surgical treatments such as cone biopsy. Malignancies will require biopsy and further surgery including hysterectomy on occasions. Further treatment with chemo- and radiotherapy may also be required. Fibroids may respond to hormonal treatment but often hysterectomy is required. Fibroids may be removed leaving the womb intact (myomectomy).

Further advice
Women should have regular cervical smears and any problems should be investigated immediately.

Associated conditions
Womb infections are likely to occur after childbirth, particularly if there are retained products of conception.

Uveitis

see **Iritis and uveitis**

Vaginal diseases and infections

 This class of diseases includes cystitis, fungus infections (thrush), discharges from the vagina, trichomonal vaginitis, vaginismus, and overlaps with pelvic infections. Bartholin cysts are present as a lump in the vagina.

Symptoms

Usually vaginal discharge. Vaginismus presents as a spasm of the vagina on examination or during or after intercourse. Cystitis presents as pain on passing urine, sometimes with blood and cloudy, infected urine.

Action

These conditions should be investigated as soon as possible.

Tests

Low vaginal and high vaginal swab for microbiology are useful, as is a midstream urine specimen for diagnosis of cystitis. Abdominal ultrasound may be required to look for deeper pelvic infections.

Medications and treatment

Trichomonas infections respond to metronidazole. Thrush usually responds to an antifungal cream. Cystitis will require antibiotics, and deeper pelvic infections may require prolonged courses of antibiotics. Vaginismus or muscular spasm may require both physical and psychological intervention.

Further advice

Trichomonas may be a venereal disease, and the partner may also need treatment. Thrush is more common in those on the contraceptive pill and after taking broad-spectrum antibiotics. Thrush and cystitis may also be more common in people with diabetes.

Varicose veins

 Varicose veins are caused by failure and incompetence of the veins in the legs which result in swelling of the veins and a collection of blood in those veins. Varicose veins may be precipitated by a family history, pregnancy, constipation, and a sedentary lifestyle.

Symptoms

Swelling of the veins in one or both legs which may sometimes be painful or bleed. Occasionally, varicose ulceration may be seen together with pigmentation on the inside of the ankle. Occasionally, varicose veins may bleed profusely.

Action

Bleeding varicose veins should be treated by local pressure. Avoid using a tourniquet because this may make the matter worse. Less urgent varicose vein treatment includes support stockings, injections, and surgery which is the main treatment for the condition.

Tests

Investigations include venograms and Doppler ultrasound.

Medications and treatment

Paroven, for example, may relieve the pain from aching legs.

Further advice

After surgery, you should exercise regularly.

Associated conditions

Varicose veins are not usually associated with deep-vein thrombosis but there may be a superficial inflammation of the veins in the form of thrombophlebitis. Varicose veins in the scrotum can appear as a varicocoele.

Venereal diseases

The range of venereal diseases includes non-specific urethritis, trichomonas vaginitis, gonorrhoea, syphilis, hepatitis B, and HIV infection. All of these may be sexually transmitted.

Symptoms

The symptoms of gonorrhoea or urethritis include discharge from the urethra in men or vagina in women. Syphilis may appear as a hard lump (chancre) on the penis or in the vagina. Genital warts appear with the presence of painless warts around the vagina, anus, or on the penis. Herpes presents with sores inside or outside the genitalia. Hepatitis B infection usually presents with jaundice while HIV infection presents after many years with immune deficiency - AIDS. Minor conditions, such as trichomonas vaginitis, appear with a white vaginal discharge. These conditions may all be asymptomatic, i.e. they may be carried by a person who does not have symptoms but can still infect others.

Action

If any of these symptoms appear, you should seek medical advice immediately.

Tests

Blood tests to check for infectious agents, swabs of vagina or urethra and cervix to check for bacteria; smears may see changes due to warts or viruses.

Medications and treatment

Trichomonas infections usually respond to metronidazole. Urethritis, gonorrhoea, and syphilis respond to antibiotics. Virus infections such as HIV, herpes, and warts may require specific antiviral therapy, such as acyclovir; e.g. Zovirax. Warts may respond to interferon.

Associated conditions

HIV infections may be transmitted nonsexually, e.g. by blood transfusion or accidentally by contamination among health-workers. Similarly, hepatitis B can be transmitted accidentally.

Vestibulitis and labyrinthitis ♥

 These conditions are caused by infection or inflammation of the balance mechanism of the inner ear (labyrinth). The infection is often a viral infection, but attacks of labyrinthitis or vestibulitis may occur without obvious infective cause.

Main symptoms
Vertigo, dizziness, and nausea, which may be associated with deafness and buzzing in the ears.

Action
Acute attacks may respond simply to bedrest. A viral infection should be treated in the same way as acute upper respiratory tract infections such as sinusitis. Severe symptoms or symptoms that persist for more than seven days require medical attention.

Tests
If medical attention is required, labyrinthine function tests may be performed as well as hearing tests and brain scan.

Medications and treatment
Drugs such as Serc, Stemetil, or Stugeron may be useful for controlling the severe symptoms of labyrinthitis or vestibulitis.

Further advice
If you are prone to recurrent attacks, you should avoid smoking and drinking alcohol, and any other factors, such as air travel, which may bring on the attacks.

Associated conditions
See tinnitus, Ménière's disease.

Virus infections, other, including Epstein-Barr virus and infectious mononucleosis (glandular fever)

Virus infections, such as measles and chicken-pox, have been covered in the section on skin disorders. Glandular fever and Epstein-Barr viruses are common causes of minor virus infections. But they are most commonly associated with a severe post-viral syndrome, sometimes known as myalgic encephalomyelitis (ME) or yuppie flu.

Symptoms

The symptoms of glandular fever include swollen glands, sore throat, vomiting, severe headache, general debility, occasionally skin rash particularly where an ampicillin has been used, and occasionally swelling of the liver and spleen with jaundice and intolerance of alcohol. Epstein-Barr virus is similar but the symptoms are often not as severe. The symptoms of ME include profound lethargy, weakness, depression, with aches in the muscles.

Tests

There are specific blood tests to look for Epstein-Barr and glandular fever (infectious mononucleosis) viruses. A Paul Burnell test is specific for glandular fever. Clinical examination will reveal enlargement of glands and occasionally liver and spleen. Liver function tests may be carried out. A similar picture can be obtained with the Epstein-Barr virus. ME is difficult to diagnose on specific testing, and the diagnosis is often made by clinical history.

Action

These conditions will often resolve without specific medication, and supportive therapy can include non-alcoholic fluids and analgesics, such as aspirin and paracetamol. If symptoms persist or are severe, you should seek medical advice.

Medications and treatment

Apart from general supportive treatment, antidepressant medication may be helpful in ME. High doses of vitamins and minerals such as magnesium may be helpful in the treatment of prolonged post-viral symptoms.

Further advice
These viruses may be transmitted by oral contact, such as kissing and probably through infected saliva transmitted by sneezing. There are no vaccines available to prevent their spread.

Associated conditions
There is a number of other virus conditions which may appear with similar symptoms but, in general, these conditions are self-limiting and improve after seven to ten days.

Vocal cords (larynx), swellings of

Swellings of the vocal cords can be malignant (carcinoma of the larynx) or benign, (particularly laryngeal warts and singers' nodules). All are more common in smokers, and singers' nodules are common among public speakers and in people who use their voices for professional purposes. Some people have multiple laryngeal papillomata (warts on the larynx) which may be viral in origin.

Main symptoms
Hoarseness and loss of voice. Some singers find that they are unable to reach notes that are usually achievable.

Action
You should be referred to an ear, nose, and throat specialist if one of these symptoms persists for longer than would be expected from just a simple upper respiratory infection such as laryngitis. Laryngitis would normally resolve after one to two weeks.

Tests
Direct laryngoscopy, i.e. examination of the vocal cords, should be carried out by an experienced ear, nose, and throat specialist.

Medications and treatment
After biopsy of the lesion, surgical removal or laser treatment may be appropriate. Some patients with multiple papillomata respond to interferon therapy.

Further advice
You should rest your voice, stop smoking, and reduce alcohol intake.

Associated conditions
Other conditions, such as laryngeal pouches or laryngitis, may give rise to similar symptoms.

Warts

see **Skin tumours, warts, and swellings**

Yuppie flu

see **Myalgic encephalomyelitis**

A